Essentials of
VETERINARY BACTERIOLOGY AND MYCOLOGY

Sixth Edition

Essentials of
VETERINARY
BACTERIOLOGY
AND MYCOLOGY

Sixth Edition

G. R. Carter • Darla J. Wise

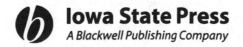

Iowa State Press
A Blackwell Publishing Company

Gordon R. Carter, D.V.M., M.S., D.V.Sc., is Professor Emeritus, Virginia-Maryland Regional College of Veterinary Medicine, Virginia Polytechnic Institute and State University, Blacksburg, Virginia. His area of expertise is pathogenic microbiology. He has published many scientific papers and is the senior author on more than a dozen textbooks. He has served on the faculties of the University of Toronto and Michigan State University and has served as a consultant of infectious diseases of animals for several international agencies.

Darla J. Wise, Ph.D., is Assistant Professor, Department of Biology, Concord College, Athens, West Virginia. Dr. Wise has published articles in the areas of immune responses, characterization of enzymes associated with host–pathogen relationships, and DNA-based methods of disease diagnosis. She is associate editor of *Proceedings of the West Virginia Academy of Science*. She has a patent in the area of molecular biology.

Iowa State Press
2121 State Avenue, Ames, Iowa 50014

Orders: 1-800-862-6657
Office: 1-515-292-0140
Fax: 1-515-292-3348
Web site: www.iowastatepress.com

First edition, 1976 (Michigan State University)
Second edition, 1982 (Michigan State University)
Third edition, 1986 (Lea and Febiger)
Fourth edition, 1991 (Lea and Febiger)
Fifth edition, 1995 (Williams and Wilkins)
Sixth edition, 2004

Library of Congress Cataloging-in-Publication Data

Carter, G. R. (Gordon R.)
  Essentials of veterinary bacteriology and mycology / G. R. Carter, Darla J. Wise.—6th ed.
    p. cm.
  Rev. ed. of: Essentials of veterinary microbiology. 5th ed. 1995. Includes bibliographical references and index.
    ISBN 0-8138-1179-1 (alk. paper)
    1. Veterinary bacteriology. 2. Veterinary mycology. 3. Veterinary virology. I. Wise, Darla J. II. Carter, G. R. (Gordon R.). Essentials of veterinary microbiology. III. Title.
    SF780.3.C37 2003
    636.089'6014—dc22
                                              2003015555

The last digit is the print number: 9 8 7 6 5 4 3 2 1

Contents

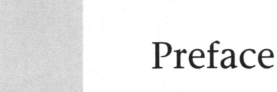

Preface

In this edition, we have somewhat simplified some chapters in the Introductory section. However, because of the theoretical and practical importance of genetics and genetic engineering for future veterinary microbiology, the pertinent chapters have been expanded.

A taxonomic approach has been used in the presentation of the major pathogenic bacteria. Although the emphasis on taxonomy may seem at times burdensome, it helps show the correlation between genetic relatedness and the kind of disease produced.

We have attempted to provide the latest information on all facets of the principal bacterial and fungal pathogens of veterinary interest. As in earlier editions, a special effort has been made to emphasize practical applications. The book is primarily directed to undergraduate veterinary students.

Veterinary microbiology is traditionally taught by means of lectures and laboratory exercises. This text provides the more important facts of introductory and pathogenic microbiology for the didactic portion. In the interest of economy, the number of illustrations has been kept to a minimum. If laboratory exercises are adequate, students will have an opportunity to observe and study the microscopic and cultural characteristics of important microorganisms.

We have found that the teaching of the pathogenic portion of the course can be made more interesting and relevant to veterinary practice by the use of case reports and scientific papers describing outbreaks of infectious disease. These can be used Socratically as the principal way for conveying the lecture material, or employed on occasion to stimulate interest.

We decided, as have other authors, to forgo the listing of references at the end of chapters. This was done because of the easy availability of a plethora of references both old and current via the Internet. This also contributes to a less expensive book.

A glossary has been added at the end of many chapters to explain terms with which many readers may not be familiar. The individual glossaries have been placed in a Cumulative Glossary at the back of the book.

We would like to express our appreciation to the Virginia-Maryland Regional College of Veterinary Medicine and Concord College for the use of various facilities including office space and communications.

Dr. Yasuko Rikahisa had prepared a chapter for the previous edition and Dr. G. William Klaus two chapters. We substantially revised these chapters. Some of their material from the previous edition was retained and is gratefully acknowledged.

We acknowledge the valuable help of Ms. Linda Cox and Dr. M. M. Chengappa of the College of Veterinary Medicine, Kansas State University, on many practical aspects of veterinary bacteriology and mycology.

The help of the staff of Iowa State Press in the many aspects of preparing the final manuscript is gratefully acknowledged.

G. R. Carter
Darla J. Wise

PART I

Introductory Bacteriology

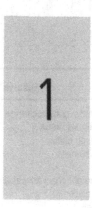

1

Morphology and Classification of Bacteria and Archaea

Microbes or microorganisms comprise a large, diverse group of unicellular organisms that are placed together because they are microscopic in size (i.e., they cannot be seen without the aid of a microscope). Included in this group are bacteria, Archaea, fungi, protozoa, viruses, and some algae. The world's oldest fossils, which are more than 3.5 billion years old, are those of unicellular organisms resembling today's blue-green bacteria or cyanobacteria.

PROKARYOTES AND EUKARYOTES

With regard to intracellular organization, the cells of all living things are either eukaryotic or prokaryotic. Eukaryotic cells have a membrane-bound nucleus (a "true" nucleus), whereas prokaryotic cells contain a nucleiod region in which the chromosome is physically located within the cell. Bacteria and Archaea are prokaryotes, and all of the other groups are eukaryotes (Eukarya, protists). Important features comparing prokaryotes and eukaryotes are listed in Table 1.1.

Recent studies employing ribosomal ribonucleic acid (RNA) gene sequences have shown that there are three phylogentically distinct lineages of cells, two that are prokaryotic and one that is eukaryotic. Thus, two cate-

gories of prokaryotes are recognized, the Eubacteria and the Archaea. The group containing the eukaryotes is Eukarya. Some of the features that distinguish bacteria, Archaea, and eukarya are given in Table 1.2.

The vast majority of bacteria are single-celled, although some filamentous forms are considered multicellular. They occur in several different morphologic forms and typically possess a cell wall containing peptidoglycan but lack a defined cell nucleus and membrane-bounded organelles. A variety of means for obtaining nutrients is observed in the bacteria, the majority of which obtain their nutrients from their environment. However, others are able to make their own food through photosynthesis or chemosynthesis. Bacteria are widely distributed in nature, and a relatively small number are pathogenic.

The Archaea comprise a group of organisms that was once thought to be older than the bacteria. Further analysis of this group revealed that, in fact, this was not the case; however, the name Archaea was already accepted for the group. The Archaea are more closely related to eukaryotes than are the bacteria. These microorganisms lack a cell nucleus and membrane-bounded organelles, possess cell walls comprising materials other than peptidoglycan, and thrive in "extreme environments." From this last characterization, the Archaea are often referred to as extremophiles. Archeae

Table 1.1   Differences between Prokaryotic and Eukaryotic Cells

Characteristics	Prokaryotic Cells	Eukaryotic Cells
Nucleoplasm bounded by a membrane	−	+
Nucleolus	−	+
Mode of reproduction (method of chromosomal division)	Asexual (binary fission)	Asexual and sexual (mitosis and meiosis)
D-amino acids, diaminopimelic acid, and muramic acid	+*	−
Cytoplasmic ribosomes (small and large subunits)	70S (30S & 50S)	80S (40S & 60S)
Endoplasmic reticulum	−	+
Mitochondria	−	+
Chloroplasts	−	+†
Golgi apparatus	−	+
Cytoplasmic streaming	−	+
Cytoplasmic membrane lipids	Typically, sterols absent	Sterols present
Organelles with nonunit membrane	+	−

*Except for mycoplasmas and chlamydiae.
†Plants and algae.

3

Table 1.2   Comparison of Bacteria, Archaea, and Eukarya

Characteristics[a]	Bacteria	Archaea	Eukarya
Cell wall	Peptidoglycan	Peptidoglycan or protein, only	Plants: polysaccharide Animals: none Fungi: chitin
Cell wall: Amino acids	D-isomers	L-isomers	L-isomers
Cell wall: Muramic acid	+	−	+
Cell membrane	Straight-chain fatty acids ester linked to glycerol	Branched hydrocarbons ester linked to glycerol	Straight chain fatty acids ester linked to glycerol
Protein content	High	Low	High
Lipids	Phospholipids	Glycolipids, nonpolar isoprenoid lipids, phospholipids, and sulfolipids	Phospholipids
Sterols	−[b]	−	+
Ribosome sensitivity to diphtheria toxin	−	+	+
Methanogenesis	−	+	−
Nitrification	+	−	−
Chlorophyll-based photosynthesis	+	−	+
Fatty acids	+	−	+
Plasmids	+	+	−
Histone proteins	−	+	+
Ribonucleic acid polymerases	One type; simple; four subunits	Several; complex; eight to 12 subunits	Several; complex; eight to 12 subunits
Transcription factors required	−	+	+
Sensitivity to chloramphenicol, streptomycin	Yes	No	No

[a]Not all representatives within a domain will demonstrate a given property.
[b]*Mycoplasma*, *Ureaplasma*, *Spiroplasma*, and *Anaeroplasma* have sterols.

have been isolated from environments such as extreme salt, boiling sulfur springs, and methane-producing bacteria. To date, no pathogenic Archaea have been identified.

The fungi are a very diverse group that can be single-celled (yeast and some molds) or can take macroscopic multicellular forms (such as mushrooms). The cell wall of fungi is composed of chitin or cellulose. Unlike the bacteria and Archaea, the fungi possess a cell nucleus and membrane-bounded organelles. Like some of the bacteria and Archaea, fungi absorb their nutrients from the environment. Fungi are also found widely distributed in nature. A relatively small number of members of this group are pathogenic. Some have been found to produce beneficial antibiotics. Introductory aspects of the fungi are discussed in Chapter 35.

Protozoa are single-celled organisms that have a cell nucleus and membrane-bounded organelles. Protozoa do not typically have cell walls. Like the fungi, they obtain nutrients from their environment; however, some are capable of making their own; for example, by photosynthesis. Protozoans are widely distributed in nature, and a small number are pathogenic.

Viruses are acellular microbes that, on their own, are not capable of any of the activities of the other microbes, such as metabolism. They are composed of nucleic acid surrounded by a protein coat. Viruses are capable of replication only when they have infected particular cell types. Those viruses capable of invading cells may become pathogenic.

Algae are a very diverse group containing single-celled and multicellular varieties. They possess a cell nucleus, a membrane-bounded organelles, and a cell wall composed of cellulose. All algae are capable of making their own food by photosynthesis. They are widely distributed in fresh water and oceans. Although some algae produce toxins, they rarely cause disease.

BACTERIAL TAXONOMY AND CLASSIFICATION

Taxonomy is defined as the science of classification (orderly arrangement of organisms). Biological classification, in general, is based on natural, evolutionary relationships between organisms. Traditionally, in higher organisms, taxonomy has been based on readily observable structures and other features. This approach is not sufficient for the classification of the prokaryotes. Instead, prokaryotes traditionally have been classified on the basis of phenotypic characteristics observed in the laboratory, such as morphology, cultural and staining characteristics, biochemical activity, oxygen requirements, and so forth. The modern phylogenetic classification of microorganisms is based on molecular criteria.

GENETIC BASIS FOR CLASSIFICATION

Genetic information of bacteria is coded in deoxyribonucleic acid (DNA) base sequence. The genetic nature of bacteria undergoes frequent variation by mutation, conjugation, transduction, and selection in different environments leading often to relatively rapid evolution.

DNA Base Compositions

The proportions of the four DNA bases in the total DNA of an organism can be determined. By convention, the base composition of a DNA preparation is expressed as the mole percentage of guanine–cytosine (GC) to the total amount of DNA. Because GC + AT (adenine–thymine) = 100% of the DNA, if the GC content is 40%, the AT content is 60%. Determination of GC percentage is relatively simple and is of some value in taxonomy: All the Enterobacteriaceae, including *Escherichia coli* and *Salmonella*, have GC percentages ranging from 50% to 54%. Similarity of base composition, however, does not necessarily signify DNA homology. The genomes of all vertebrates have a GC percentage of 44%, which is the same as some microorganisms.

DNA Hybridization

DNA sequence homology between two organisms can be quantified by procedures that determine the extent of formation of molecular hybrids from two DNA strands of different origin. This approach has been useful in demonstrating the relative order and degree of DNA similarity of closely related groups of bacteria. However, this technique is too specific to be used to study the relationships of dissimilar bacterial groups. Hybridization between DNA molecules of two *E. coli* strains would be close to 100%, but hybridization of *E. coli* with a *Salmonella* strain would be about 45%. The phylogenetic definition of a species generally includes strains with approximately 70% or greater DNA–DNA relatedness.

DNA Fingerprinting

DNA fingerprinting is used for identifying microorganisms at the species and strain levels. **Restriction enzymes** are used to cut a molecule of DNA at locations where a specific base sequence occurs. The resulting restriction fragments are separated by gel electrophoresis. Comparison of the number and size of fragments from different organisms indicate the extent of their genetic similarity.

Sequence Comparison: 16S rRNA

16S rRNA is a large nucleotide (~1500 bases) of the ribosomes of prokaryotes. It contains highly conserved (stable) sequences of nucleotides and, also, more variable sequences. The former, more stable sequences are useful for comparisons at the higher taxonomic ranks. Comparisons of the variable regions are useful to determine divergence at the strain or species level. Alternative phylogenetic markers have been provided, such as 23S rRNA, but 16S rRNA continues to be the standard for elucidating bacterial phylogeny. The eukaryotic counterpart of 16S rRNA is 18S rRNA.

A practical application employing 16S rRNA is ribotyping. In this procedure, microorganisms are identified by analysis of DNA fragments generated from restriction enzyme digestion of genes encoding their 16S rRNA.

The polymerase chain reaction (PCR), described in Chapter 4, is particularly useful for increasing the amount of microbial DNA for the nucleic acid analyses referred to above.

BACTERIA

Bacteria are single-celled organisms that are mainly distinguished from the eukaryotic organisms by the characteristics listed in Table 1.1. They constitute an enormous and varied group and are considered to share a distant common ancestor. By far, the majority occur as free-living organisms in nature, with only a few species having medical or veterinary significance. Some idea of the size and diversity of the group can be gathered from the several volumes of *Bergey's Manual of Systematic Bacteriology*, the latest edition of which is referred to later in the chapter. This compendium of microbial taxonomy lists and describes all recognized bacteria. It currently divides the prokaryotes into two domains (the Archaea and the bacteria) and a number of phyla, referred to later. The principal kinds of bacteria are described briefly below.

Rickettsia and Chlamydia

Although rickettsia and chlamydia differ from each other phylogenetically, they have a number of features in common:

- They are coccoid to rods in shape, with a diameter of 0.3–0.7 μm.
- With the exception of one rickettsia (*Rochalimaea*), they are obligate intracellular parasites and, thus, require living cells for cultivation.
- They contain both DNA and RNA.
- Both have gram-negative-type cell walls (peptidoglycan).
- Both cause a number of important diseases in animals and humans.

They differ as follows:

- Rickettsia multiply by binary fission; chlamydia have a distinct life cycle (see Chapter 31).
- Rickettsia are mainly transmitted by arthropods; chlamydia are mainly airborne.
- Both groups are susceptible to a number of antibiotics, but chlamydia are not susceptible to penicillin.
- Chlamydia are more limited biosynthetically than rickettsia.
- Rickettsia can oxidize glutamate; chlamydia cannot.
- Rickettsia are closely related to human mitochondria and thus are thought to have an

ancestor that originally participated in an **endosymbiotic** relationship with eukaryotic cells.

Mycoplasmas

These highly **pleomorphic** organisms lack cell walls (resistant to penicillin) and are the smallest of the Eubacteria. They are of particular evolutionary interest because of their small genomes and simple cell structure. Some important features are:

- They consist of five genera that require sterols and three that do not.
- They grow in culture media, although supplementation with other factors, such as serum, may be required.
- Although they do not stain gram-positive because of the absence of a cell wall, they are considered to be phylogenetically related to low mol % GC (guanine plus cytosine content) gram-positive bacteria.
- They include facultative anaerobes and obligate anaerobes.
- They contain **lipoglycans** that resemble the lipopolysaccharides of gram-negative bacteria.
- There are more than 100 species, and many are parasitic on plants and animals.

Cyanobacteria (Blue-Green Algae)

Although once considered algae, their typically prokaryotic cell structure identifies them as bacteria. They perform oxygenic photosynthesis and possess plant-like chlorophylls in **thylakoid membranes**. They are different from photosynthetic bacteria, which perform **anoxygenic** photosynthesis and possess bacteriochlorophyll, but not from thylakoid membranes. On occasion, livestock, pets, and wild animals may ingest toxic cyanobacteria and be fatally poisoned.

Other Free-Living Bacteria

The rest of the free-living bacteria include the phototrophic, gliding, sheathed, and appendaged bacteria; rod, coccal, and spiral-shaped bacteria; and both gram-positive and gram-negative bacteria. The phototrophic bacteria (purple bacteria and green bacteria) perform anoxygenic photosynthesis and possess a unique pigment system containing bacteriochlorophyll.

METHODS EMPLOYED FOR OBSERVING BACTERIA

The microscope is an essential investigative tool of microbiology. The units of measurement employed in microbiology are the micrometer ($\mu m = 10^{-6}$ m), the nanometer (nm $= 10^{-9}$ m), and the angstrom ($\text{Å} = 10^{-10}$ m). A variety of different microscopes, each with different features, allow microbiologists to examine microbes. These are described below.

Bright-Field Microscope

The conventional microscope has three objectives: low power, high power (high dry), and oil immersion. A total magnification of 1000× can be obtained using the oil-immersion lens on a typical bright-field microscope. This scope is used for the routine examination of stained bacterial smears and **wet mounts**. The resolution of the light microscope is limited by the wavelength of visible light, which is about 0.5 μm; images less than 0.2 μm cannot be clearly resolved.

Dark-Field Microscope

Dark-field illumination can be used in the conventional microscope by substituting a dark-field condenser for the conventional condenser. This special condenser obliquely reflects a powerful source of light onto a wet preparation. Very small objects, including microorganisms, scatter the light and can be seen as brilliant images against a dark background. Extremely small and slender organisms such as spirochetes, which cannot be seen with the conventional microscope, can be readily visualized using this method. Living organisms and their movement can be seen.

Fluorescence Microscope

Various fluorescent dyes are used to stain microorganisms. The technique, known as immunofluorescence (fluorescent antibody, or FA, procedure), is widely used in clinical microbiology for the identification of microorganisms. Fluorescent antibody reagents are prepared by coupling a fluorescent dye to a specific antibody. This conjugate will unite with its corresponding **antigen**. The union of antigen bound with antibody is observed by the presence of fluorescence detected with the ultraviolet light of a fluorescence microscope.

PHASE-CONTRAST MICROSCOPE. When light waves pass through transparent objects, such as cells, they emerge in different phases, depending on the properties of the materials through which they pass. In phase-contrast microscopy, a phase condenser and phase objective lens convert differences in phase into differences in intensity of light. Thus some structures appear darker than others. This method is useful in studying the fine detail of unstained living microorganisms.

Electron Microscopy

TRANSMISSION ELECTRON MICROSCOPE. The principle of this instrument is analogous to that of the light microscope. Instead of visible light, the electron microscope employs a beam of electrons that is focused by an electromagnetic field instead of by glass lenses. Because of the short wavelength, it can resolve objects as small as 0.0004 μm.

Because biologic materials are mainly composed of the elements carbon, hydrogen, nitrogen, and oxygen, which have low electron–scatter-deflecting ability, special techniques are necessary to make specimens stand out against background.

HIGH-VOLTAGE ELECTRON MICROSCOPY. This method allows thicker specimens to be examined by obtaining a stereo image. The higher-accelerating voltage of 1000 kV (1 MV) or higher results in improved resolution and penetration power. In comparison, the conventional electron microscope operates at 60–80 kV.

SCANNING ELECTRON MICROSCOPY (SEM). The object is scanned with a flying spot of electrons, and the emergent secondary electrons are collected and shown on a screen of the cathode-ray tube. Three-dimensional images are obtained, but internal detail is not provided by SEM.

X-Ray Microanalysis

When an electron hits a specimen, characteristic x-rays are released from each element. In x-ray spectroscopy, an x-ray detector is used to monitor the distinct x-ray pattern produced by the interaction between the electron beam of the microscope and the chemical elements in specific areas of the specimen. This method is especially suitable for localizing specific elements in the microorganism.

Staining Procedures

Staining methods are used to determine the morphologic form of bacteria and their affinity for certain dyes. Bacteria are divided into two major groups on the basis of Gram stain. Briefly, the procedure for Gram stain is as follows: cells are first fixed to a glass slide by heat, stained with a basic dye (crystal or methyl violet) that is washed off with an iodine–potassium iodide solution (**mordant**), and then rinsed with water and cautiously decolorized with acetone or ethyl alcohol. The smear is then counterstained with safranin. The results:

- Gram-positive organisms retain the basic dye following decolorization with acetone or alcohol and appear deep violet.
- Gram-negative organisms, however, do not retain the violet stain but take up the counterstain (safranin) and stain red to pink. As a general rule, organisms that give a doubtful reaction are gram-positive.
- The gram-positive cell wall presents a permeability barrier to elution of the dye–iodine complex by the decolorizing agent. Aging gram-positive cells appear gram-negative after a Gram stain because autolytic enzymes attack the cell wall.

Gram stain differentiates between gram-positive and gram-negative organisms on the basis of differences in the structure of their cell wall. Gram-negative organisms have more lipid in their cell walls. Gram-positive bacteria have a thicker peptidoglycan layer, which renders them more resistant to mechanical damage. Because of these structural differences, the two groups vary in their reaction to the Gram stain and in their susceptibility to enzymes, disinfectants, and antimicrobial drugs.

Not all bacteria can be satisfactorily stained by the Gram method. The cell walls of mycobacteria contain lipids and waxy substances (mycolic acid) that make them difficult to stain. However, when they are stained by a special procedure, the acid-fast stain, they retain the carbolfuchsin even after exposure to a strong acid–alcohol (HCl and ethanol) solution.

The leptospira and treponemes are very slender and cannot be satisfactorily resolved following Gram staining, but they can be demonstrated by silver staining. Negative staining, employing nigrosin or india ink, is used for demonstrating capsules. Capsules appear clear and unstained, surrounded by dark inert particles. For demonstrating flagella (around 0.02–0.03 μm in diameter), a mordant is used before staining; this precipitates onto flagella and thus thickens them. Because the Gram stain may not disclose spores produced by such organisms as *Bacillus anthracis*, special spores stains may be required.

BACTERIAL STRUCTURE

Shape and Structure of Bacteria

The five basic morphologic forms of bacteria are the coccus, which is spherical or ovoid; the rod, which is straight and cylindrical; the spiral, which includes vibrios (comma-shaped), spirillum (curved, spiral-shaped rod), and spirochete (elongated, tightly coiled); the filamentous bacteria, which form long, thin cells or chains of cells; and the appendaged bacteria. There is considerable variation in these basic forms. The morphology of all but the free-living appendaged bacteria is depicted in Fig. 1.1.

The cocci are found in different arrangements, depending on the plane of cell division. The staphylococci occur in bunches or clusters, the streptococci form chains, and the pneumococci are predominantly paired. Some of the micrococci occur in groups of four, or tetrads (*Aerococcus viridans*); others are grouped in packets of eight (*Sarcina*).

The various species of the Enterobacteriaceae occur as rather regular rods, but some of the smaller organisms such as *Pasteurella*, *Brucella*, and *Haemophilus* are both bacillary and coccobacillary. Some members of the genera *Bacillus* and *Clostridium* have rods in chain formation. The corynebacteria are remarkably pleomorphic and produce club-shaped forms. The actinomycetes (*Actinomyces* and *Nocardia*) have both bacillary and filamentous branching forms. The anaerobic *Fusobacterium* has a characteristic elongated spindle shape. The curved bacteria (vibrio) have a single turn, with some comma and S-shaped forms. The spiral forms have a series of twists or turns and are tightly or loosely coiled (*Treponema* and *Leptospira*).

The size of bacteria also varies considerably. Most rod forms range from 2 to 5 μm in length by 0.5 to 1 μm in

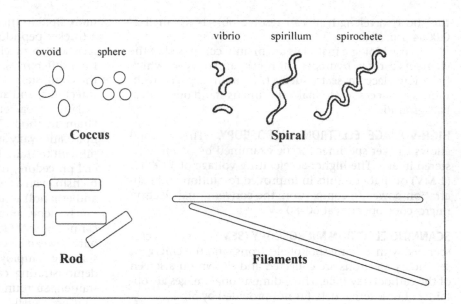

FIGURE 1.1 Basic morphologic forms of bacteria.

width; spirochetes may be longer (up to 20 μm) and narrower (0.1–0.2 μm). Cocci are approximately 1 μm in diameter. The size of a single type of bacteria can vary somewhat, depending on the medium and the growth phase. They are usually smallest in the logarithmic phase of growth. It is of interest that an *Escherichia coli* bacterium has a volume of approximately 1 μm^3 and a weight of approximately 10^{-12} g, whereas a liver cell has a volume of approximately 1000 μm^3 and a weight of approximately 10^{-9} g. For convenience, bacteria can be roughly grouped according to size. For example: large: Spirochetes, *Bacillus*, *Clostridium*; medium: Enterobacteriaceae (e.g., *Escherichia coli*, *Proteus*), pseudomonads; small: *Brucella*, *Pasteurella*, *Haemophilus*; very small: *Rickettsia*, *Chlamydia*, and some elements of mycoplasmas.

With regard to size, it is of interest that a remarkably large bacterium, *Thiomargarita namibiensis*, has been discovered recently. Single, spherical cells are 100–300 μm in diameter but may be as large as 700 μm. The organism inhabits Namibian shelf deposits.

BACTERIAL ULTRASTRUCTURE

Except for the mycoplasmas, bacteria are enclosed by the cell envelope, which is made up of the capsule (if present), the cell wall, and the cytoplasmic membrane. The cell envelope surrounds the cytoplasm of the prokaryotic cell. The cytoplasm contains various granules, ribosomes, the nucleiod, and in some, bacterial **mesosomes**. Many bacteria have flagella, and some gram-negative varieties have pili or fimbriae (Fig. 1.2).

The cytoplasmic membrane is a thin, elastic, trilaminar structure consisting mostly of lipoprotein and proteins imbedded in a phospholipid bilayer. Mesosomes are saclike invaginations of the cytoplasmic membranes. Their tubu-

FIGURE 1.2 Principal structures of bacteria.

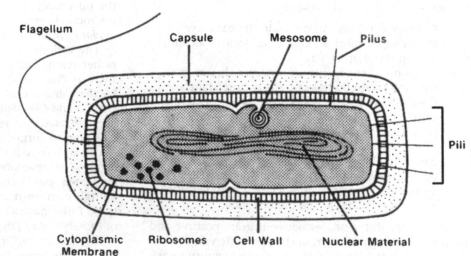

lar and circular structures, which are attached to DNA chromatin, are thought to have a role in cell division. The principal structural features of bacteria are shown in Figs. 1.2 and 1.3.

Cell Envelope

This includes the cytoplasmic membrane, the cell wall, and the capsule.

Capsules

These are amorphous, polymeric, often-gelatinous materials lying outside the cell wall. Most bacterial capsules are polysaccharides, but those of several species consist of polypeptide; some bacteria, such as *Bacillus megaterium*, have both compounds in their capsule. Special staining procedures, including negative stains, are used to demonstrate capsules. The capsules of mucoid strains of *Pasteurella multocida* and *Streptococcus equi* consist almost wholly of hyaluronic acid. Virulence may depend to some extent on the antiphagocytic properties of the capsule, as with *Bacillus anthracis*, *Pasteurella multocida*, and *Streptococcus pneumoniae*. Capsules vary chemically, and thus are antigenically diverse. This is important, as will be shown later, in vaccine production and in laboratory diagnosis.

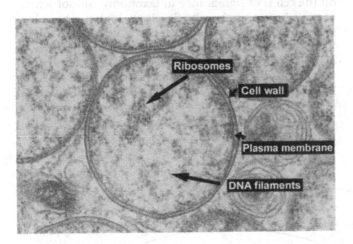

FIGURE 1.3 Transmission electron micrograph of *Rickettsia.*

Cell Wall

There are basic differences between the cell walls of gram-positive and gram-negative bacteria. The cell wall makes up approximately 20% of the total dry weight of the bacterium. It gives the organism its shape and a rigid structure that protects the cell's internal structures from severe chemical and physical actions.

The cell wall is permeable, and the cytoplasmic membrane is selectively semipermeable, determining which molecules will be excreted from the cell and what concentration of the different solutes will be maintained. Movement of substances across the membrane takes place by simple diffusion and by more complex transport systems.

The supporting role of the cell wall can be demonstrated if its formation is prevented by penicillin or if it is destroyed by **lysozyme**. The structures that remain are bound by the cytoplasmic membrane only and are called protoplasts (gram-positive) or spheroplasts (gram-negative). Unless placed in a hypertonic milieu, protoplasts and spheroplasts swell and burst.

The cell wall confers shape and rigidity to the bacterial cell. This rigid structure is provided by peptidoglycans. These very large polymers are composed of two kinds of building blocks: N-acetylglucosamine and N-acetylmuramic acid disaccharide polymers, and peptides consisting of four or five amino acids; namely, L-alanine, D-alanine, D-glutamic acid, and either lysine or diaminopimelic acid (Fig. 1.4). The latter is unique to bacteria.

GRAM-POSITIVE BACTERIA. Cell walls range from 150 to 800 Å in thickness. In addition to the peptidoglycan, some gram-positive organisms possess polysaccharides and teichoic acids. Teichoic acids are polymers of glycerol phosphate or ribitol, and in many bacteria, they are linked to peptidoglycan. They are major surface antigens that may serve as virulence factors. All gram-positive bacteria have lipoteichoic acid linked to the cytoplasmic membrane. Table 1.3 compares some major envelope structures of gram-positive and gram-negative bacterial cells. A diagram of the cell walls of both types of organisms is shown in Fig. 1.5.

GRAM-NEGATIVE BACTERIA. The cell wall is approximately 100 Å in thickness, high in lipid content (11%–22%), and appears as a unit membrane; thus, it is called the outer membrane. A major protein of the outer membrane,

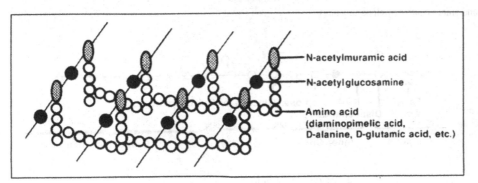

- N-acetylmuramic acid
- N-acetylglucosamine
- Amino acid (diaminopimelic acid, D-alanine, D-glutamic acid, etc.)

FIGURE 1.4 Schematic peptidoglycan structure.

Table 1.3   Principal Components of the Cell Walls of Gram-Positive and Gram-Negative Bacteria

Characteristic	Gram-Positive	Gram-Negative
Peptidoglycan	Thick	Thin
Tetrapeptide	Most have lysine	All have diaminopimelate
Cross-linkage	Generally through pentapeptide	Direct bond
Teichoic acid and/or teichuric acid	+	−
Lipoproteins	−	+
Lipopolysaccharide (LPS)	−	+
Outer membrane	−	+
Periplasmic space	−	+
Polysaccharide	+	+
Protein	+ or −	+

called porin, forms transmembrane pores or diffusion channels allowing passage of small hydrophilic molecules through the outer membrane. A relatively small amount of peptidoglycan is present in the inner rigid layer, but a large amount of a lipopolysaccharide (LPS), often referred to as endotoxin, occurs external to the outer membrane. Endotoxin is important in the pathogenesis of some diseases. The serologic specificity of the O-antigens of gram-negative bacteria resides in the terminal repeating units or O side chains (major surface antigens with diverse **epitopes**) of the polysaccharide. The lipid moiety of the LPS, called lipid A, is the toxic component. The basic structure of LPS is shown in Fig. 1.6.

PERIPLASM.   The periplasm is the space between the plasma membrane and the cell wall, and it is visible in gram-negative organisms but difficult to see in gram-positive bacteria. The periplasm contains various hydrolytic enzymes and binding proteins that specifically bind sugars, amino acids, and inorganic ions. These enzymes and proteins aid transport of various compounds into and out of the bacterial cytoplasm, and they are released by osmotic shock.

S-LAYERS.   S-layers, also called the bacterial surface layers, are one of the most abundant cell envelope surface components. S-layers are present in the Eubacteria, as well as the Archaea. S-layers are composed of either a single protein or glycoprotein, depending upon the species. Some researchers believe that because of their simplicity, S-layers represent the simplest biological membranes evolutionarily. As a result, they are the subject of intense investigation with regard to their genetics, structure, synthesis, and function. Furthermore, they are being examined for potential uses in areas such as biotechnology, molecular nanotechnology, and nanoelectronics.

Appendages

FLAGELLA.   These are long, whiplike structures of locomotion. They are composed of three parts: filament, hook, and basal body. The basal body is embedded in the plasma membrane and gives the flagella its rotary motion, which propels the organism. The distribution of flagella on the cell is of significance in taxonomy. Monotrichous bacteria have a single polar flagellum, lophotrichous bacteria have tufts of several flagella at one pole, amphitrichous bacteria have flagella at both poles, and peritrichous organisms have a number of flagella distributed all around the cell surface. The diameter of a flagellum is 10–20 nm, and special staining procedures are used to

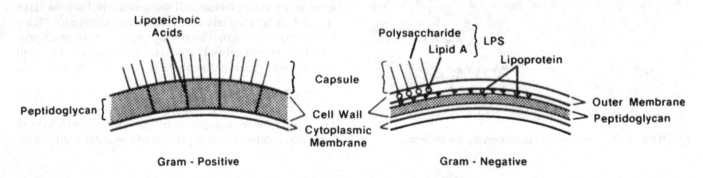

FIGURE 1.5   Diagram of gram-positive and gram-negative envelope structures.

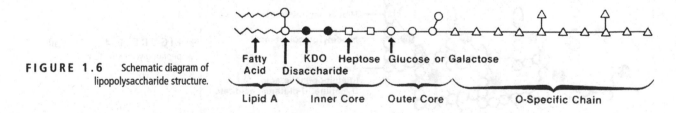

FIGURE 1.6   Schematic diagram of lipopolysaccharide structure.

KDO: 2-keto-3-deoxyoctonic acid

demonstrate them. They are composed entirely of a protein subunit called flagellin, which differs in primary structure from one species to another. The surface of flagella has protein antigens with diverse epitopes. For example, H-antigens are used in the serologic classification of some bacterial species.

Most of the organisms that produce capsules (species of *Klebsiella, Haemophilus, Pasteurella,* and *Bacillus)* are nonmotile. None of the cocci of medical importance is motile. Motility is determined in the laboratory by the examination of wet preparations from cultures under the microscope (hanging-drop method) and by observing the kind of growth obtained when a semisolid agar medium is stabbed with an inoculum of the organism being examined. Diffuse growth into the agar indicates motility.

AXIAL FILAMENT.   This is a flagellum-like filament located in the periplasmic space between the inner and outer membranes of spirochetes. The spiral organisms move by a traveling helical wave along axial filaments.

PILI (FIMBRIAE).   These are shorter, thinner, and straighter than flagella and are attached to the plasma membrane of mostly gram-negative bacteria. They are composed of a protein monomer called pilin, which is 4–20 nm in diameter and can only be seen by electron microscopy. The pili enable some bacteria to adhere to epithelial cells, thus leading to colonization of mucous membranes.

The sex pili (see Chapter 4) occur in fertility (F) factor (+) cells found in the Enterobacteriaceae and a few other bacteria. They adhere to F (−) cell surfaces and make possible the transfer of genetic material from F (+) to F (−) cells during bacterial conjugation.

Endospores   Members of the genera *Clostridium* and *Bacillus* have the capacity to produce highly resistant, thick-walled spores (Fig. 1.7). They occur when vegetative cells are deprived of some factor or nutrient necessary for growth. In anthrax, spores are produced by *Bacillus anthracis* when the organisms are exposed to oxygen.

Spore formation begins with realignment of DNA material into filaments and invagination of plasma membrane, forming a structure called the forespore. The forespore is further surrounded by the plasma membrane. At this point, the forming endospore is surrounded by a double membrane. The facing side of these two plasma membranes is the peptidoglycan synthesizing side, and spore cortex, a poorly polymerized peptidoglycan that is synthesized in the space between the two layers of plasma membranes. Spore coat, a keratin-like protein rich in cysteine, is formed outside the spore cortex. In some microorganisms, an exosporium is formed outside the spore coat. When spore formation is completed, the mature spore is released by the disintegration of the envelope of the mother cell, or sporangium. Each spore germinates into a single vegetative cell when conditions for growth are favorable. In gram-stained preparations, spores appear as ovoid, refractile, nonstaining objects either within the cell or free of it.

The location of the mature spore in the cell may be central, terminal, or subterminal, depending upon the organism, and is useful for identification of the microorganism. The remarkable heat resistance of spores is thought to be the result of the dehydration of the spore protoplast. The irradiation resistance may be related to a high level of cysteine disulfide bonds in the spore coat protein, and dehydration resistance is caused by keratin-like spore coat protein.

Relatively large amounts of calcium and dipicolinic acid, a compound unique to spores and a derivative of diaminopimelic acid (a component of peptidoglycan), occur in the spore.

Bergey's Manual of Systematic Bacteriology

Bergey's Manual of Systematic Bacteriology, a standard reference work for microbiologists, contains detailed descriptions of most known bacteria. Many different features, including morphologic, staining, cultural, and biochemical characteristics as well as oxygen requirements, DNA base compositions, and DNA homology were used to key and identify bacteria. Volumes of the first edition of *Bergey's Manual of Systematic Bacteriology* were published in 1984 and 1986. This reference is currently undergoing revision, and five new volumes should all be published within several years. Volume 1 became available in June 2001. This second edition will incorporate, along with the conventional information referred to earlier, the results of ribosomal RNA analysis.

The proposed content of the new volumes is, briefly, as follows:

Volume 1: *The Archaea and Deeply Branching and Phototrophic Bacteria;* none of these are of veterinary or medical significance.
Volume 2: *The Proteobacteria;* many gram-negative pathogenic bacteria are in this category, which begins with *Rickettsia.*
Volume 3: *The Low G + C Gram Positives;* this volume begins with the *Clostridia.*
Volume 4: *The High G + C Gram Positives;* this volume begins with the Actinimycetes.
Volume 5: *The Plantomycetes, Spirochaetales, Fibrobacteres, Bacteroides and Fusobacteria;* this volume begins with the *Chlamydia.*

With regard to nomenclature, the classic binomial (Linnaean) system by which organisms are given a genus

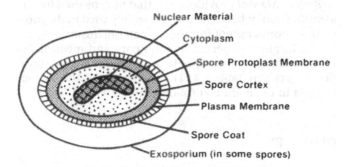

FIGURE 1.7   Basic structure of a bacterial endospore.

Table 1.4   Location of Bacterial Genera in Phyla in Proposed Taxonomic Outline

Domain	Phyla	Genra
Archaea	Phyla AI and AII	None of veterinary or medical significance.
Bacteria	Phylum BI to BBXI	None of veterinary or medical significance.
	Phylum BXII *Proteobacteria*	*Rickettsia, Ehrlichia, Aegyptianella, Anaplasma, Cowdria, Ehrlichia, Neorickettsia*
		Bartonella, Brucella, Afipia
		Burkholdera, Alcaligenes, Bordetella, Taylorella
		Neisseria, Chromobacterium, Eikonella, Kingella, Simonsiella
		Spirillum
		Fancisella
		Legionella, Coxiella, Rickettsiella
		Pseudomonas, Acinetobacter, Morazella
		Enterobacteriaceae (14 genera)
		Actinobacillus, Haemophilus, Pasteurella, Mannheimia
		Lawsonia
		Arcobacter, Campylobacter, Helicobacter, Wolinella
	Phylum BXIII *Firmicutes*	*Clostridia*
		Mycoplasma, Eperythrozoan, Haemobartonella, Ureaplasma
		Spiroplasma
		Acholeplasma
		Erysipelothrix (Genera incertae sedis)
		Bacillus, Listeria, Staphylococcus
		Lactobacillus, Enterococcus, Streptococcus
	Phylum BXIV *Actinobacteria*	*Actinomyces, Actinobaculum, Arcanobacterium*
		Micrococcus
		Dermatophilus
		Corynebacterium, Mycobacterium, Nocardia, Rhodococcus
		Streptomyces
	Phylum BXV *Planctomycetes*	None of veterinary or medical significance.
	Phylum BXVI *Chlamydiae*	*Chlamydia, Chlamydophila*
	Phylum BXVII *Spirochaetes*	*Spirochaeta, Borrelia, Treponema, Brachyspira, Serpulina, Leptospira*
	Phylum BXVIII *Fibrobacteres*	None of veterinary or medical significance.
	Phylum BXIX *Acidobacteria*	None of veterinary or medical significance.
	Phylum BXX *Bacteroides*	*Bacteroides, Prevotella*
		Flavobacterium, Capnocytophaga, Riemerella, Weeksella
	Phylum BXXI *Fusobacteria*	*Fusobacterium*
		Streptobacillus

*Adapted from Boone DR and Castenholz RW, editors: *Bergey's Manual of Systematic Bacteriology*, Vol. 1, 2nd ed. Springer, New York, 2001.

and species name is used. The taxonomic levels or ranks used in the current *Bergey's Manual* are hierarchical ones. The hierarchy of taxonomic categories generally employed in the upcoming new edition are as follows:

Domain: There are two domains, Archaea and Bacteria.

Phylum: A major category within a domain.

Class: Consists of related orders.

Order: Contains a group of related families.

Family: Contains closely related genera.

Genus: Contains closely related species.

Species: Contains strains of bacteria that have many characteristics in common.

Subspecies: Some species may be further subdivided into subspecies on the basis of small but consistent differences.

Strain: A strain consists of the descendants (clone) of a single isolate in pure culture. For each species, there is a type strain, which usually is the particular culture from which the species description was originally made. Type strains are available in various culture collections.

Biovar: A strain with special biochemical or physiologic properties.

Serovar: A strain with distinctive antigenic properties.

In addition to generic (genus) and species names, well-known trivial names, such as tubercle bacillus (*Mycobacterium tuberculosis*), often appear in medical literature.

Since 1980, valid names of all bacterial species have been published in the *International Journal of Systemic Bacteriology*.

Bergey's Manual provides a key that may be used for the identification of bacteria. It is not widely used in diagnostic laboratories except for uncommon organisms.

The location of genera of veterinary and medical significance in the various phyla in the proposed classification is given in Table 1.4. The discussion of the various bacteria in the main text follows this generic order.

GLOSSARY

anoxygenic Does not form oxygen as a product of photosynthesis.

antigen Molecule or substance that is recognized by an animal as foreign (nonself) and elicits an immune or specific antibody response.

endosymbiotic Relationship of an organism that lives in a symbiotic relationship within another organism or cell.

epitope Local chemical configuration on the antigen molecule (antigenic determinant) that elicits a specific antibody.

lipoglycans Long-chain heteropolysaccharides linked to membrane lipids and imbedded in the cytoplasmic membranes of many mycoplasmas.

lysozyme Enzyme, also known as muramidase, present in many body fluids, that breaks down murein, a component of the cell walls of gram-positive bacteria.

mesosome Bacterial structure associated with an invagination of the plasma membrane. It is the site of respiratory enzymes.

mordant Chemical (in the Gram stain iodine) that fixes a dye (crystal violet in the Gram stain) by combining with it to form an insoluble compound.

pleomorphic Assuming various forms.

restriction enzymes Bacterial enzymes that recognize and cleave specific DNA sequences.

thylakoid membrane Flattened membrane discs in which chlorophyll and other components for photosynthesis are located.

wet mounts Suspension of clinical material in saline or other solutions to facilitate microscopic examination.

2 | Bacterial Nutrition and Growth

CHEMICAL AND PHYSICAL REQUIREMENTS FOR GROWTH

Of the vast number of bacteria, a relative few are **pathogenic**. Many microorganisms never cause an infection simply because the host tissue does not provide the physical or chemical conditions necessary to support growth. However, some tissues provide an acceptable environment for the growth of opportunistic and frankly pathogenic microorganisms. An understanding of the chemical and physical requirements for growth of a microorganism better enables one to grow it in the laboratory, identify it, and advise regarding treatment.

Nutritional Categories

Microorganisms may be divided into two major categories according to their ability to use various forms of energy and carbon for biosynthesis. The two major categories are autotrophs and heterotrophs. Sometimes the autotrophs are subdivided into those that use light energy (photosynthetic) and those that use the energy associated with chemical reactions (chemolithotrophic).

PHOTOTOSYNTHETIC MICROORGANISMS. These organisms are capable of using light as a sole energy source and either carbon dioxide or more reduced organic molecules as a carbon source for growth.

AUTOTROPHS. Autotrophs are divided into two major categories, based on the source of energy for their metabolism. Photoautotrophs are capable of using light as a sole energy source and either carbon dioxide or more reduced organic molecules as a carbon source for growth. Autotrophic (chemolithotrophic) microorganisms are those that cannot use light as an energy source but that can use inorganic molecules as the sole source of energy, and they may use either carbon dioxide or more reduced organic molecules as a carbon source for synthesis and growth.

There are no known strict autotrophic microorganisms that are animal pathogens.

HETEROTROPHS. In contrast to autotrophs, heterotrophs cannot use light or inorganic compounds for energy, and their carbon source for growth needs to be obtained directly from their environment in the form of biomolecules. Specifically, the heterotrophs use reduced organic molecules (such as sugars, amino acids, fatty acids, and nucleic acids) both as a source of energy and as a source of carbon for synthesis and growth. Only a few heterotrophs cannot be cultivated in artificial (synthetic) media in the laboratory. All pathogenic microorganisms, both **opportunistic** and strict pathogens, are heterotrophs, and the large majority of these are saprophytes (they feed on dead organic matter).

Nutrient Requirements

Nutrients for microbial growth may be divided into two classes: essential nutrients, without which a cell cannot grow, and nonessential nutrients, which are used if present. All essential nutrients must be provided in an artificial medium for cultivation of a microorganism.

All cells must have a source of carbon and a source of energy to grow. In addition, all cells must have a nutritional source of nitrogen, phosphorus, sulfur, sodium, potassium, iron, magnesium, and manganese and trace quantities of many other minerals. These nutrients are essential for the growth of all microorganisms. Some microorganisms are able to grow on media that contain only those nutrients just listed. These organisms are known as prototrophs. For example, some enterobacteria will grow in a medium containing only glucose (as a carbon and energy source), ammonium ion (as the sole nitrogen source), phosphate ion (as a phosphorus source), sulfate ion (as a sulfur source), and trace amounts of other minerals. These cells form all the polysaccharides, fats, proteins, and nucleic acids necessary for growth solely from the carbon and energy available in the glucose molecule. These cells have a very complex metabolism with powerful biosynthetic capabilities.

Other microorganisms require complex organic compounds to grow. These organisms are known as auxotrophs. For example, they may need certain amino acids, fatty acids, nucleotides, or vitamins. These microbes are not able to make these compounds from a simple carbon and energy source (like glucose); therefore, these compounds must be supplied in the growth medium. These organic compounds are called preformed nutrients because they must be offered to the cells in a preformed state. If a microbe requires many preformed nutrients for growth, it is said to be fastidious. Fastidious microbes lack powerful synthetic capabilities. An example of an auxotroph (fastidious bacteria) is *Haemophilus parasuis*, which requires the coenzyme NAD^+ for growth.

Even though a microorganism is capable of making everything it needs from a simple sugar such as glucose, it will usually grow more rapidly in the presence of many preformed nutrients. For example, *Salmonella* species are capable of growth on a glucose plus mineral salts medium, but they will grow many times faster if provided with the preformed nutrients found in yeast and beef extracts. In general, microorganisms preferentially take in preformed nutrients rather than making them on their own because this saves energy.

Both pathogenic and nonpathogenic microorganisms associated with animals can range from nutritionally prototrophic to those that are extremely fastidious.

Hydrogen Ion Concentration

Some bacteria of veterinary significance are acidoduric; that is, they have the ability to survive (but not grow) for short periods of time in very acidic environments. For example, gastric fluids may have a pH value of 1.0, and gastrointestinal (GI) pathogens must first survive these stomach fluids before growing and exerting their adverse effects in the intestines. Although some microbes are acidoduric, very few are able to grow at these extremes in pH. An exception is *Helicobacter*, which lives in the stomach and can cause gastroenteritis.

Each microorganism has a pH range within which growth is possible, and each usually has a well-defined optimum pH at which the cells grow at their maximum rate. Most bacteria of medical or veterinary significance grow best at a neutral or slightly alkaline pH (pH 7.0–7.5), the pH of most mammalian fluids and tissue.

When one prepares a medium for laboratory growth of a microbe, its initial pH (hydrogen ion concentration) is often above or below the pH that will support optimum growth of that microorganism. It is then customary to adjust the pH with an inorganic acid or base before the medium is sterilized. Autoclaving sometimes alters the medium pH; therefore, it is best to check the pH after the autoclaved medium has cooled.

It is desirable to maintain a relatively constant medium pH during microbial growth. However, some growing microbes excrete organic acids that increase the acidity (decrease the pH) of the growth medium, and some microbes excrete ammonium ions that increase the alkalinity (increase the pH) of the growth medium. Buffers are salts of weak acids or bases. If buffers are present in the growth medium, they respond to the microbial addition of acids or bases by taking up or giving off hydrogen ions, helping to keep the pH constant. Amino acids are good buffers, and they are naturally present in many complex laboratory media.

Carbon Dioxide Concentration

All microorganisms require carbon dioxide (CO_2) for both survival and growth. This is supplied either exogenously (from the environment outside the cell; the earth's atmosphere normally contains about 0.03% CO_2) or endogenously (from within the cell; produced by decarboxylation reactions during catabolism).

Some microorganisms initiate growth in the laboratory and reproduce at a more rapid rate when the CO_2 concentration is increased above that normally found in the atmosphere. This phenomenon is characteristic of many pathogens of veterinary significance. These microbes may be grown in a CO_2 incubator by using compressed CO_2 to replace about 10% of the atmosphere inside the incubator. Alternatively, one may seal the inoculated cultures inside a jar with a lighted candle (candle jar) and allow the candle to burn to extinction; this method decreases the amount of O_2 available and raises the CO_2 levels from 0.03% to about 3% (see Microaerophiles below).

Oxygen Concentration

When oxygen is dissolved in fluids, it forms a variety of ions, such as the toxic superoxide radical. As a consequence of metabolism in the presence of O_2, toxic hydrogen peroxide is also formed. Therefore, cells capable of growth in the presence of O_2 must have a way to detoxify these harmful forms of oxygen. Microorganisms accomplish this by producing enzymes that break down the toxic molecules or change them into a form that is less toxic. Superoxide dismutase, catalase, and peroxidase are examples of such enzymes.

Cells that grow in the presence of air usually use O_2 to support a respiratory type of metabolism. Other types of microbes normally live where there is only a small amount of O_2; consequently, they have only a limited ability to detoxify oxygen radicals, and their cultivation in the laboratory must be under conditions in which the O_2 concentration is artificially lowered. Still other microbes live only in environments that exclude O_2; these microbes usually lack this detoxification ability, and their laboratory cultivation must be in the complete absence of O_2.

The terms that follow reflect an organism's ability to grow in the presence of O_2 and, in some cases, even to use O_2 to its metabolic advantage.

STRICT (OBLIGATE) AEROBES. These are microorganisms that can only grow in the presence of air (O_2). Strictly aerobic pathogens are not common; some occur on the mucosa of the upper respiratory tract. They have an unusually high capacity to detoxify the toxic forms of O_2; that is, they produce large amounts of extremely active catalase and superoxide dismutase. In the laboratory, strict aerobes are usually cultivated on the surface of solid media or in well-aerated liquid media. These microbes are incapable of supporting growth from the energy supplied by fermentation. All accomplish a respiratory type of metabolism and use only O_2 as a terminal electron acceptor.

FACULTATIVE ANAEROBES. These are able to grow in either the presence or the absence of air (O_2), but they grow better when oxygen is present. Many bacteria, including most pathogens, are facultative anaerobes. They may begin to grow in well-oxygenated tissue (or laboratory media) and rapidly use the dissolved oxygen. However, they then continue to grow in the absence of O_2, but at a slower rate. Because facultative anaerobes are able to grow in the presence of air, they must have the ability to detoxify the toxic forms of O_2. In the laboratory, facultative anaerobes are usually cultivated under aerobic conditions, but they may grow in the absence of O_2 and at all intermediate oxygen concentrations. These microbes are able to support growth from the energy supplied by either fermentation or a respiratory catabolism.

There are many facultative bacteria associated with the animal body. For example, bacteria normally found on an animal's skin or within its intestines are often facultative. These bacteria are common opportunistic pathogens that cause tissue infections when the skin or gut wall is broken or abraded.

MICROAEROPHILES.   These microbes require oxygen, but they will not grow in air that normally contains 20% oxygen. Only a few bacteria are microaerophiles, but some of these are important animal pathogens, such as some *Brucella*, *Actinomyces*, and *Campylobacter* species. Cultivation in the laboratory is often achieved in liquid or on solid media held in an atmosphere containing about 6% oxygen. Laboratory cultivation is also possible in semisolid media (0.1%–0.4% agar). The agar prevents oxygen from freely mixing through the tube. Oxygen can only diffuse from the surface; thus, the medium is stratified, with an oxygen gradient having the most oxygen-rich layer at the surface. After inoculating the medium by stabbing deeply with a loop or needle, microaerophiles begin to grow in a discrete band located from a few millimeters to several centimeters below the surface, where the oxygen concentration is the most favorable (Fig. 2.1). Microaerophiles use a strictly respiratory catabolism, with O_2 being the only terminal electron acceptor used.

STRICT (OBLIGATE) ANAEROBES.   These anaerobes lack the ability to grow in the presence of air, and often even small amounts of O_2 are toxic. In healthy animals, anaer-obic environments are commonly found in the oral cavity (especially between the teeth and gums) and in the intestines (where the facultative microbes scavenge all available O_2). Strict anaerobes are among the normal microflora of these environments. Most infections initially contain a mixture of facultative anaerobes and anaerobes, and the facultative bacteria quickly use up the available O_2. This leaves an anaerobic environment that favors the growth of strict anaerobes. Only a relatively few species are strict anaerobes. The best known anaerobes of veterinary significance are in three genera: *Bacteroides*, *Clostridium*, and *Fusobacterium*.

The reasons why strict anaerobes are intolerant of O_2 are not completely clear, but it may be that they lack the ability to remove toxic forms of oxygen (most strict anaerobes lack superoxide dismutase). For this reason, anaerobes are cultivated in an artificially reduced medium in an atmosphere that contains little or no oxygen. Reducing agents are commonly added to the medium to depress the oxidation reduction (redox) potential of the medium and to hold it at the correct state of reduction. Anaerobic jars and cabinets with controlled atmospheres are used in the laboratory for the isolation and growth of anaerobes.

Although some strict anaerobes are capable of anaerobic respiration (using inorganic terminal electron acceptors other than oxygen), those of veterinary significance appear to support growth only from energy supplied by fermentation.

Temperature

Temperature is one of the most important environmental factors affecting the growth and survival of microorganisms. At cold temperatures, metabolic rates are very slow, and cells will survive for long periods of time. As the temperature rises, enzymatic reactions inside the cell proceed at faster rates, and growth also becomes more rapid, until the optimum growth rate is achieved. Just above that optimum temperature, however, proteins, deoxyribonucleic acid (DNA), and ribonucleic acid (RNA) become irreversibly denatured, and the growth rate falls rapidly to zero. Continued increases in temperature will kill the microbe.

The optimum growth temperature of most microbes associated with mammals is from 35° to 37°C, but some (such as *Yersinia* species) still grow well at room temperature (25°C). These are called mesophiles (optimum growth from 28° to 38°C); this category contains most known microorganisms.

Pathogens that have an optimum growth rate at the body temperature of one animal may not grow or may be killed when transferred to another animal that has a body temperature just a few degrees higher. This may help to explain the species specificity of some microbial pathogens. The higher temperature at an inflammatory site may be less favorable for microbial growth.

If the temperature is elevated above the maximum at which growth is possible, then vegetative cells (but not **endospores**) die. Our knowledge of these lethal temperatures is used in **pasteurization** and in the sterilization

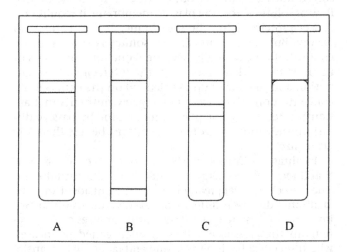

F I G U R E   2 . 1   Growth of aerobes **(A)**, anaerobes **(B)**, microaerophiles **(C)**, and facultative anaerobes **(D)** in semisolid agar.

of instruments and other articles by autoclaving (steam heat under pressure).

The effect of cold temperatures on microorganisms is also of considerable significance. As the incubation temperature is lowered, enzymatic reactions inside the cell proceed at slower rates, and growth rates are decreased until cells reach the minimum temperature at which growth is possible. Unlike elevated temperatures, however, temperatures below the minimum growth temperature cause no damage. On the contrary, cold temperatures preserve microorganisms. Storing cultures in a refrigerator (about 4°C), in a freezer (about −10°C), or in a liquid nitrogen container (about −196°C) are common methods for the long-term preservation of microbial cultures.

MOVEMENT OF NUTRIENTS INTO CELLS

Movement through the Capsule and Cell Wall

The capsule surrounding many microorganisms is a loose matrix that permits the diffusion of all soluble molecules but does not allow transfer of colloid-sized particles. Thus, the capsule does not prevent entry of most available nutrients into the cell.

The gram-positive cell wall is also a permeable but rigid matrix that allows for diffusion of soluble nutrients.

The outer membrane of gram-negative cell walls, however, is thought to be a barrier to large molecules. Interspersed throughout this outer membrane are a large number of only a few types of proteins (Fig. 2.2). The concentration of each protein in the outer membrane varies considerably, depending on the types of nutrients in the environment. One type of protein, which is almost always present in large numbers, is called a porin. The porin molecules appear to form water-filled channels that span the outer membrane, and these channels are of sufficient diameter to allow passage of molecules having a molecular weight up to 800–900 **daltons** (Da). Therefore, small hydrophilic nutrients (like inorganic ions, mono- and disaccharide sugars, amino acids, and di- and tripeptides), as well as small non-nutrient molecules, can easily diffuse through these channels (pores). Thus, it is believed that the outer membrane of the gram-negative cell wall acts as a molecular sieve.

Other proteins present in the outer membrane of the gram-negative cell wall occur in smaller numbers than the porins. A number of these minor proteins seem to be receptor proteins (Fig. 2.2) that facilitate entry of molecules too large to pass through the pores (such as iron chelates, vitamin B_{12}, and degradation products of nucleic acids). These membrane-bound receptor proteins occur in larger amounts when their substrate is present in the medium. Still other minor outer membrane proteins appear to have a structural function.

Neither the outer membrane of the gram-negative cell wall nor the cytoplasmic (plasma) membrane should be thought of as static structures. There is evidence that optimal cell growth occurs only when the outer membrane of the gram-negative cell wall and the plasma membrane are in a partially fluid state.

In the region between the outer membrane and the plasma membrane of the gram-negative cell, there is a rigid, girder-like polymer called peptidoglycan (Fig. 2.2). This region is referred to as the periplasm. Within the periplasm are three types of proteins. First, there are hydrolytic enzymes, such as proteases, RNA and DNA nucleases, phosphatases, phosphodiesterases, and lactamases (which destroy the β-lactam antibiotics such as penicillin). The function of the hydrolytic enzymes is to cleave intermediate-sized nutrients so that they are small enough to pass through the plasma membrane. Second, there are binding proteins that specifically bind sulfate, some sugars, and amino acids and that act in concert with the plasma membrane to help translocate these nutrients into the cell. Third, there are the chemoreceptor proteins that allow motile gram-negative cells to detect certain nutrients in the environment, so that they may direct their movement toward the nutrient source. Thus, periplasmic proteins play a predominant role in both detecting nutrients and transferring them into the cell.

Translocation (Movement) across the Plasma Membrane

Most microorganisms function best when surrounded by water containing dissolved inorganic ions. Most microbes also require reduced organic molecules that are used as a carbon and energy source. For the cell to use these nutrients, they must first be moved across the plasma membrane. The term translocation is used here to indicate the general movement of nutrients across the plasma membrane, regardless of whether energy is required to accomplish that movement. Translocations accomplished without the expenditure of energy are called diffusion, whereas those requiring energy are called transport.

PASSIVE AND FACILITATED DIFFUSION.   Passive diffusion is probably the simplest method of moving solutes (dissolved nutrients) into or out of the cell. It allows the free flow of solutes across the plasma membrane, it requires no carrier protein within the membrane, and it requires no energy. But passive diffusion of solutes is slow, and the concentration eventually becomes equal on both sides of the membrane. Therefore, both the intercellular concentration and the rate of uptake depend on the extracellular concentration. There are relatively few nutrients that are translocated across the plasma membrane by passive diffusion; they must, with few exceptions, be less than 100 Da in size.

Facilitated diffusion is similar to passive diffusion in that it requires no energy and the solute concentration inside the cell is never greater than on the outside. However, facilitated diffusion differs from passive diffusion in two important ways: first, facilitated diffusion uses carrier proteins in the plasma membrane, often called permeases, which specifically bind the solute and facilitate its translocation, and second, facilitated diffusion is more rapid than passive diffusion. Facilitated diffusion of soluble nutrients appears to be rare in bacteria.

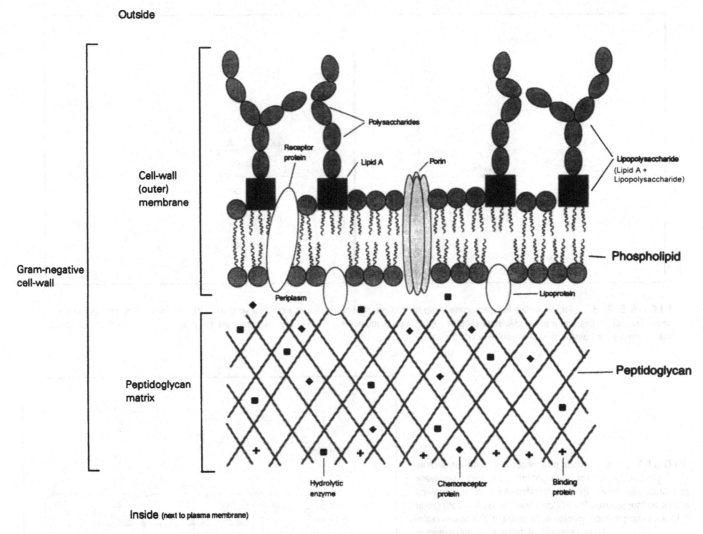

Outside

Inside (next to plasma membrane)

FIGURE 2.2   Representation, as viewed in cross section, of the gram-negative cell wall (not drawn to scale). The wall has two main layers: an outer membrane, composed of a phospholipid bilayer containing embedded proteins and lipopolysaccharides, and a rigid peptidoglycan matrix containing various types of functional proteins.

Glycerol is the only nutrient known to enter *Escherichia coli* by facilitated diffusion, and it appears that the same mechanism is also used for glycerol translocation in *Salmonella typhimurium* and species of *Klebsiella, Shigella, Pseudomonas, Bacillus, Nocardia,* and every other bacterium studied to date.

Both passive and facilitated diffusion probably play minor roles in nutrient translocations.

Energy-requiring translocations are only accomplished by actively metabolizing cells, and these types of translocations are called active transport mechanisms. There are two types of active (energy-requiring) transport mechanisms: one is called coupled transport and the other group translocation.

Coupled Transport.   The cell uses energy in the form of adenosine triphophate (ATP) to move compounds across the plasma membrane, usually from outside to inside. Similar to facilitated diffusion, coupled transport requires membrane-bound carrier proteins (also called permeases)

that specifically bind one type of nutrient and assist in its translocation across the membrane. Also like facilitated diffusion, the nutrient translocated by coupled transport enters the cell in an unaltered state. However, unlike facilitated diffusion, coupled transport requires energy that is provided by the proton motive force. The processes involved are shown schematically in Fig. 2.3.

Group Translocation.   There are three main features of group translocation: first, similar to facilitated diffusion and coupled transport, group translocation requires a membrane-bound carrier protein to specifically bind one type of nutrient and assist in its translocation across the membrane; second, like coupled transport, group translocation requires energy, but this energy comes from a high-energy metabolic intermediate, such as the hydrolysis of ATP; and third, unlike coupled transport, the nutrient enters the cell in a chemically altered (usually phosphorylated) state (Fig. 2.4). The cell does accumulate a useful nutrient in much greater concentration than its precursor

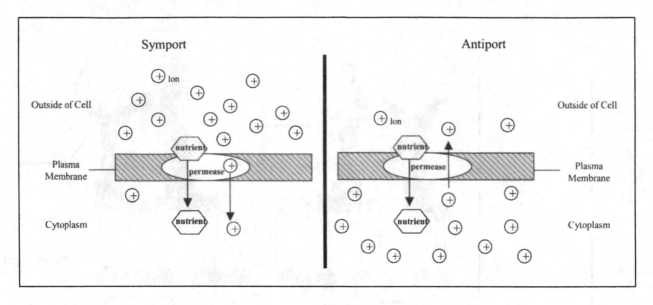

FIGURE 2.3 Proton motive force associated with the movement of nutrients into a cell. In a symport *(left)*, the ion and nutrient move in the same direction, in this case into the cell. In an antiport *(right)*, the ion and nutrient move in opposite directions. The proton gradient in either case provides the energy for the translocation of the nutrient into the cell.

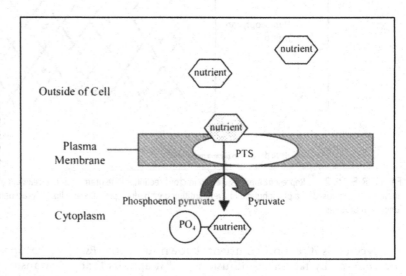

FIGURE 2.4 Group translocation of a nutrient, such as glucose. The nutrient is brought into the cell via a permease associated with the PTS (phosphotransferase system) that consists of at least four proteins. The PTS then transfers a phosphate group (PO_4) from phosphoenol pyruvate to the nutrient. This results in the formation of a phosphorylated nutrient and pyruvate.

on the outside, so the overall effect appears similar to that accomplished by active transport.

The best studied examples of group translocations involve certain sugars, such as β-glucosides, fructose, glucose, N-acetylglucosamine, and mannose. Each of these molecules appears to be phosphorylated during transport by the phosphotransferase system (PTS). The mechanism, illustrated in Fig. 2.4, involves at least four separate proteins that carry the high-energy phosphate group from phosphoenolpyruvate (a common catabolic intermediate) to the incoming sugar.

Because group translocation does not require intermediates that are produced in great quantities except during cellular respiration (such as ATP and high-energy electrons), this transport mechanism is thought to occur predominantly in fermenting organisms. *Micrococcus, My-*

cobacterium, and *Nocardia* appear to lack a PTS. Facultative anaerobes of veterinary significance known to contain a PTS include *Escherichia, Salmonella, Staphylococcus,* and *Vibrio.* In addition, a PTS is found in the strict anaerobes *Clostridium* and *Fusobacterium.* Group translocation is confined to prokaryotes.

ESTABLISHMENT AND GROWTH OF PURE CULTURES

Pure Culture Isolation

The establishment and maintenance of pure cultures are absolute requirements for the study of bacteriology. The microbiologist may spend considerable time and energy in obtaining pure cultures from environmental, clinical, and other sources to study the microbial characteristics. Sometimes a pure culture can be obtained by physically separating (streaking or spreading) the culture on the surface of a general-purpose medium (Fig. 2.5). Sometimes, however, other bacteria will outgrow the sought-after microbe on such a plate medium, or the sought-after bacterium may be present in such small numbers that it would be unlikely to appear as an isolated colony on a streak or spread plate. This common situation requires the use of either a selective medium or an enrichment culture to isolate the suspected bacterium or pathogen.

SELECTIVE AND DIFFERENTIAL MEDIA. An ideal selective medium is one that will preferentially grow only one type of microorganism. One must first determine the type of microbe that is suspected, then choose a medium that will both encourage the growth of the suspected pathogen and inhibit the growth of all other organisms common to that environment. In order to choose a satisfactory selective medium for that microbe's growth, one must make sure that all the cell's nutritional requirements are supplied by that medium. Then one can select the inhibitory agent that will prevent the growth of the other microbial competitors.

There are many kinds of selective media, but most employ some chemical agent that is added to the growth medium. To be selective, the organism you wish to isolate (the suspected pathogen) must be resistant to that chemical agent, and the organisms whose growth you wish to inhibit (e.g., the normal flora) must be susceptible to that chemical agent. Antibiotics, dyes, detergents, and sodium chloride are commonly used for selective growth inhibition.

A differential medium is one that allows the growth of several different organisms, which for growth or metabolic reasons, appear differently on or in the medium. Therefore, based on a metabolic activity of one, it can be observably distinguished from the others that may be present. Differential media contain substances such as blood or an acid–base indicator that only certain types of microbes will respond to in a characteristic way. For example, blood agar is the most commonly used differential medium. On this medium, bacteria can be differentiated on the basis of whether or not they lyse red cells (produce hemolysins) and on their characteristic colony morphology.

Sometimes a medium may be both differential and selective. For example, a medium may contain blood (to differentially detect α- and β-hemolysis produced by streptococcal colonies) as well as an antibiotic (that will selectively inhibit growth of other gram-positive cocci). Another widely used differential and selective medium is MacConkey agar, which contains lactose and growth inhibitors. It distinguishes between lactose fermenters (e.g., *E. coli*) and nonfermenters (*Salmonella*).

When microbiologists use the term selective medium, they generally are referring to a solid medium contained in a Petri dish or test tube. These are usually inoculated with a loop or a small volume of liquid. When organisms are few, larger volumes must be examined for the suspected microorganism, and this requires enrichment culture.

ENRICHMENT CULTURE. This culturing technique is used for the growth of microbes that are present in very small numbers and that may represent only a very small proportion of all types of microorganisms present in a mixed culture. Usually, a relatively large volume (from 1 to 10 mL) is inoculated into a type of broth that provides a selective environment favoring the growth of one kind of microorganism; for example, selenite broths favors the growth of *Salmonella* spp.

DETERMINATION OF CULTURE PURITY. A pure culture is defined as one that contains cells of only one type of bacteria. One can attain this purity by microscopic separation and subsequent cultivation of a single cell, but this method is extremely time-consuming and usually impractical. The most practical method for obtaining a pure culture is the streak plate. Using this method, one can start with a mixed culture and physically separate one from all others (see Fig. 2.5). During incubation, individual cells will grow and each form a colony. The colony resulting from the growth of a single cell is a pure culture. A pure culture obtained by the streak-plate method is considered adequate in the clinical microbiology laboratory.

Bacterial Growth Characteristics

When referring to growth, the bacteriologist means an increase in cell numbers. For bacterial numbers to increase, the medium must have the minimum essential nutrients, and the atmosphere surrounding the medium must provide the minimum physical conditions for growth of that cell type. Both the rate of growth and the numbers achieved at the end of growth will increase when any one of the following conditions is raised above minimum levels: the concentration of any one essential nutrient, the temperature, and the concentration of oxygen (unless the bacterium is microaerophilic or strictly anaerobic). Also, growth rate and final numbers will often increase with the

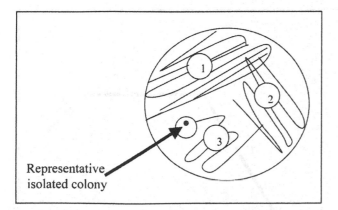

FIGURE 2.5 Streak-plate method for obtaining pure cultures. A loop full of sample is used to inoculate an agar plate, as indicated at **(1)**. The loop is sterilized, and a streak is made as indicated in **(2)**. The loop is sterilized, and a streak is made as indicated in **(3)**. It is in region **(3)** where isolated colonies are obtained; in this region where isolated colonies are obtained, one can be certain that one is working with a pure culture.

addition of preformed nutrients, because cells prefer to use environmentally supplied nutrients instead of making their own.

However, the rate of growth will either decrease or stop when nonessential or essential nutrients are depleted; when waste products accumulate to toxic levels; or when the concentration of heat, hydrogen ions, or oxygen (for some) is lowered below optimal levels. The same conditions that slow or stop microbial growth may also cause cell death.

GROWTH IN LIQUID MEDIA.   When a small number of cells from a pure culture are inoculated into a liquid medium (broth), the cells exhibit a characteristic growth curve that can be thought of in four phases (Fig. 2.6). Note that Fig. 2.6 shows the change in the logarithm of viable cell numbers versus time.

During the lag phase, cells are shifting their metabolism to grow on the new medium. There are two important characteristics of the lag phase: (1) cells are rapidly making new DNA and RNA and inducing the synthesis of new enzymes needed for cell division, and thus, there is a great deal of metabolic activity (including synthesis) taking place; but (2) as shown in Fig. 2.5, there is no increase in cell numbers. The initiation of cell division marks the transition between the lag phase and the exponential growth phase.

During the exponential growth phase, cell division occurs at a maximum rate for the growth conditions provided by that medium and those environmental conditions. This is called the exponential phase (log phase), because cell numbers are increasing (doubling) at an exponential rate. In other words, the logarithm of the cell numbers increases linearly with time.

The rate of cell division during exponential growth is often called the doubling time. This is the time that it takes for one doubling in cell numbers. The doubling time of any culture is affected greatly by the environmental (nutritional and physical) conditions provided. The doubling time is also affected by the cell's genetic ability to carry out efficient catabolic and anabolic pathways; therefore, growth rates are often characteristic of microbial cultures. For example, *Escherichia coli* has a doubling time of about 20 minutes in nonsynthetic media under optimal conditions, whereas the doubling time of *Mycobacterium tuberculosis* may be as long as 24 hours in nonsynthetic media under optimal conditions. Its cousin, *M. leprae*, has a doubling time of 2 weeks.

This rate of cell division does not continue indefinitely, however. A test tube, flask, or plate is a closed system; that is, each contains a limited amount of medium. Eventually, the cells may run out of nutrients, or cellular waste products may build up to toxic levels, or the population density may become so great that the rate of diffusion of nutrients between cells becomes limiting. When the rate of cell division slows below exponential levels, the cells make a transition from exponential growth to the stationary phase.

In the stationary phase, there is no net increase or decrease in cell numbers. What happens depends on the bacterial type. Some just stop growing but fully maintain their viability. Others reach a state in which the rate of new cell formation is equal to the rate of cell death. Regardless of the cause, the effect is always a lack of change in viable numbers.

Eventually, cells begin to die, initiating the death phase. During this phase, the rate of cell death in the population is exponential. Cell death is defined as the loss of a cell's ability to form a colony when transferred to a plate. However, the rate of death is not always equal to the rate of growth of the same population.

GROWTH ON SOLID MEDIA.   Growth of microorganisms on the surface of a solid medium follows the same growth characteristics shown in Fig. 2.5. However, cells usually cannot become as widely dispersed as in a liquid medium, so they remain tightly packed together in a colony after many divisions. Under these conditions, nutrient diffusion rapidly becomes limiting, especially at the center of

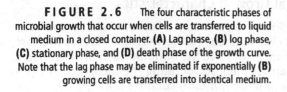

FIGURE 2.6   The four characteristic phases of microbial growth that occur when cells are transferred to liquid medium in a closed container. **(A)** Lag phase, **(B)** log phase, **(C)** stationary phase, and **(D)** death phase of the growth curve. Note that the lag phase may be eliminated if exponentially **(B)** growing cells are transferred into identical medium.

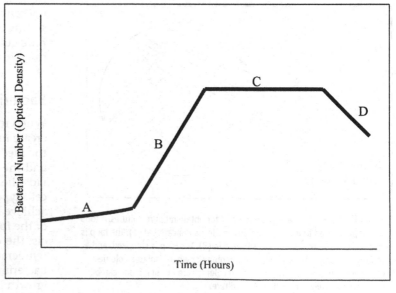

the developing colony, and those cells rapidly reach the stationary phase. However, at the colony's edge, cells continue to grow exponentially even while those at the center are in the death phase. For reasons that are not clearly understood, bacterial colonies usually do not continue to expand indefinitely across the surface of a plate.

GLOSSARY

dalton Unit of mass used to express masses of atoms, molecules, and nuclear particles. It is equal to one-twelfth of the weight of the carbon 12 atom; it is also called atomic mass unit.

endospore Structure formed within certain gram-positive bacteria, such as *Bacillus anthracis*, that is extremely resistant to heat, drying, and other harmful influences.

opportunistic Microorganisms that do not normally cause disease, for example, many bacteria of the normal flora of animals, but that can be pathogenic under certain circumstances such as trauma and impairment of the immune system.

pasteurization Heating of milk or other liquids to the point that potential pathogens are killed. It has been particularly effective in the prevention of tuberculosis and brucellosis in humans (see Chapter 9 for more detail).

pathogenic Having the capacity to cause disease in a susceptible host.

3 Bacterial Metabolism

Metabolism refers to all of the chemical reactions occurring within the living cell. Metabolism starts with nutrients brought in from the environment, and the ultimate product is a new cell. Basically, metabolism can be divided into two parts: catabolism and anabolism. Catabolism refers to those metabolic reactions that break down the nutrient, serving as the cell's chemical energy source. Anabolism denotes those metabolic reactions that use the energy provided by catabolism to make new cellular materials.

Overall catabolic pathways are exergonic, that is, they yield energy, and this energy is often stored in new high-energy phosphate bonds. This addition of energy to adenosine diphosphate (ADP) and inorganic phosphate (Pi) in the presence of an adenosine triphosphate (ATP) synthase forms ATP. ATP is the universal molecule of energy transfer. Catabolic pathways are oxidative, in that some reactions remove hydrogens ($2H^+ + 2e^-$) from the nutrient energy source and save these energy-rich hydrogens for later use by giving them to hydrogen carriers such as the coenzymes NAD^+ or $NADP^+$. Catabolic pathways also produce intermediates (building blocks) for biosynthesis at many steps during the oxidation process.

Finally, when the cell can oxidize the carbon, energy source, or both no further, the product of the last reaction is excreted as waste including CO_2 (the most oxidized form of carbon), various organic acids or neutral compounds, and oxidized inorganic molecules.

Overall, anabolic pathways are endergonic, that is, they require energy, and this is frequently supplied by the hydrolysis of one of the high-energy phosphate bonds on ATP. Anabolic pathways are also reductive; some reactions use hydrogens ($2H^+ + 2e^-$) supplied by reduced NAD^+ and $NADP^+$ (NADH, NADPH). Anabolic pathways begin with intermediates produced by catabolism and then use these to form building blocks such as amino acids, fatty acids, sugars, purines, and pyrimidines. These building blocks are then polymerized into new cellular materials, such as proteins, lipids, polysaccharides, and nucleic acids. All of this synthesis (anabolism) requires a lot of energy.

The two major divisions of catabolism are respiration and fermentation. For purposes of general orientation, a schematic overview of the principal features of respiration and fermentation is provided in Fig. 3.1. This figure shows that both respiration and fermentation begin with glucose undergoing the process of glycolysis to produce pyruvate, which then follows the different pathways of respiration and fermentation. To understand the processes, one needs a basic understanding of carbohydrate metabolism. From this, discussions of respiration and fermentation will follow.

CARBOHYDRATE METABOLISM

Oxidation of carbohydrates is the primary source of cellular energy for most microorganisms. Although microorganisms can catabolize various proteins and lipids, glucose is by far their most common carbohydrate energy source. Glucose may be derived from polysaccharides and disaccharides. As shown in Fig. 3.1, the respiration of glucose takes place in three main stages:

- Glycolysis: Most microbes use this pathway for the catabolism of glucose. The product is pyruvate with the production of ATP and energy-containing NADH.
- The Krebs Cycle: Also known as the Citric Acid Cycle or Tricarboxylic Acid Cycle, following the conversion of pyruvate to acetyl coenzyme A (acetyl–CoA), the Krebs Cycle oxidizes the acetyl–CoA into carbon dioxide with the production of ATP, NADH, and the reduced electron carrier $FADH_2$.
- Electron Transport System (ETS): In this process, NADH and $FADH_2$ are oxidized and involved in a cascade of redox reactions using additional electron carriers. Considerable energy is generated from these reactions.

These three stages will be discussed separately.

Glycolysis (Embden–Meyerhof Pathway)

Most microbes use the glycolytic pathway for the breakdown of glucose. This multistep metabolic pathway takes place in the cytoplasm of microbes and many other living cells in the presence or absence of oxygen. Important features of glycolysis are that

- Glucose is split by enzymes into two three-carbon sugars that are oxidized, resulting in the release of

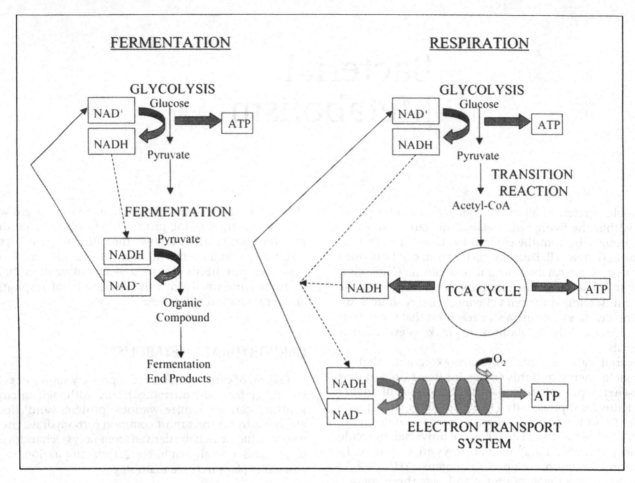

FIGURE 3.1   An overview of fermentation and respiration. Note that the sole purpose of the fermentation reactions is the regeneration of NAD$^+$; all of the adenosine triphosphate (ATP) was generated in the glycolysis portion of the reactions. In respiration, glycolysis and the tricarboxylic acid (TCA) cycle serve to generate NADH, which can donate its electrons to the electron transport system to generate large quantities of ATP.

energy and formation of two molecules of pyruvate.

- NAD$^+$ is reduced to NADH with production of two ATP molecules by substrate-level phosphorylation.
- The pathway consists of a series of chemical reactions, each of which is catalyzed by a different enzyme. The reactions involved are shown in Fig. 3.2.
- Two molecules of ATP are required to start glycolysis, and four molecules are generated in the process; thus, there is a gain of two molecules of ATP for each molecule of glucose that is oxidized.

Alternatives to Glycolysis

PENTOSE PHOSPHATE PATHWAY.   This pathway, which operates simultaneously with glycolysis, is an alternative to glycolysis for many bacteria. It produces NADPH and four- and five-carbon sugars that are required for many synthetic reactions. These four- and five-carbon sugars ultimately yield nucleic acids, carbohydrates for cell wall

synthesis, and amino acids. Among the bacteria that use this pathway are *Escherichia coli*, *Leuconostoc mesenteroides*, and *Enterococcus faecalis*. One molecule of ATP is obtained from one molecule of glucose in the pentose phosphate pathway.

ENTNER–DOUDOROFF PATHWAY.   Bacteria of the genera *Pseudomonas*, *Agrobacter*, and *Rhizobium* use the Entner–Doudoroff pathway instead of the glycolytic pathway for the oxidation of glucose to pyruvate. This pathway is not very efficient; from each molecule of glucose, two molecules of NADPH and one molecule of ATP are produced.

RESPIRATION

After glucose has been broken down by glycolysis to pyruvate, the pyruvate can be further used in respiration or fermentation (see Fig. 3.1). Respiration may be defined as the step-by-step oxidation of molecules via catabolic reactions that produce ATP, and the final electron acceptor in the process is usually an inorganic molecule. The final elec-

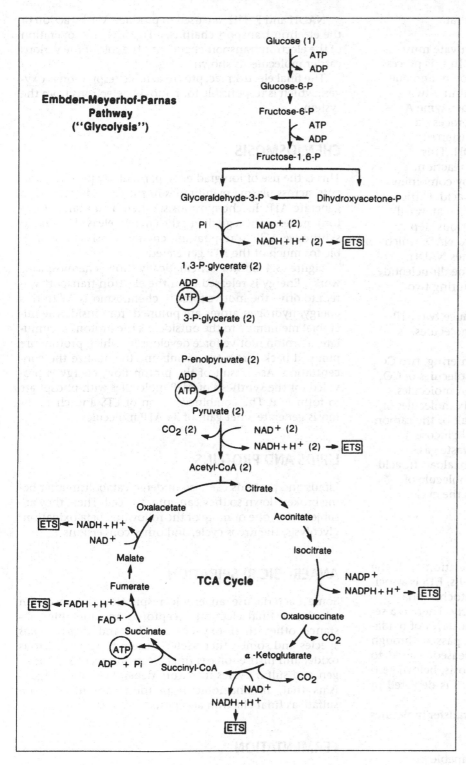

FIGURE 3.2 Respiratory catabolism of glucose to acetyl-CoA by the Embden-Meyerhof-Parnes (EMP) pathway, and further catabolism of acetyl-CoA to CO_2 by the tricarboxylic acid (TCA) cycle. Note how oxidation of glucose through the EMP pathway and TCA cycle illustrates the four characteristics common to all respiratory catabolism. ADP, adenosine diphosphate; Pi, inorganic phosphate; ATP, adenosine triphophate (ATP).

tron acceptor for aerobic respiration is O_2, and for anaerobic respiration is typically an inorganic molecule and only rarely an organic molecule.

An important feature of respiration is the electron transport chain (see Fig. 3.1). The following discussion of respiration, beginning with the Krebs Cycle, is that observed in aerobic bacteria.

KREBS CYCLE (CITRIC ACID CYCLE/TRICARBOXYLIC ACID CYCLE)

Energy is obtained from the breakdown of pyruvate by one of the previously discussed pathways, but a greater yield is obtained by the further oxidation of pyruvate in the presence of oxygen via the Krebs cycle (see Fig. 3.2).

Significant features of Krebs cycle are that

- Before entering the Krebs cycle, pyruvate must undergo conversion to acetyl–CoA. In this process, pyruvate is enzymatically broken down, and one carbon is released as CO_2. The remaining two carbon atoms are combined with coenzyme A, producing acetyl CoA. During the process, a hydrogen ion and electrons are transferred to NAD^+ to produce high-energy NADH. This reaction is known as the transition reaction.
- Acetyl–CoA enters the Krebs cycle by combining with oxaloacetic acid to form citric acid. Citric acid then undergoes a series of 10 enzyme-catalyzed conversions (see Fig. 3.1). In the various steps, high-energy electrons are released to NAD, which acquires a hydrogen ion and becomes NADH.
- In one reaction, FAD (flavine adenine dinucleotide) serves as the electron acceptor, acquiring two hydrogen ions to become $FADH_2$.
- Sufficient energy is released to produce two ATP molecules from the two pyruvate molecules entering the system.
- For each molecule of acetyl–CoA entering, two CO_2 molecules are formed; thus, four molecules of CO_2 are formed from the two acetyl–CoA molecules entering the Krebs cycle. Overall, six molecules of CO_2 are generated, accounting for all of the carbon molecules contained in the original glucose molecule. The CO_2 is given off as waste gas.
- The final product of Krebs cycle is oxaloacetic acid that, when combined with a new molecule of acetyl–CoA, begins another turn of the cycle.

ELECTRON TRANSPORT SYSTEM

In bacteria, the ETS takes place in association with the cell's plasma membrane. In eukaryotic cells, ETS is associated with the inner membrane of the mitochondria.

The chains of all ETS function similarly. There is a sequence of carrier molecules capable of a series of oxidation-reduction reactions. Electrons are passed through the chain stepwise, and the energy released is used to drive the chemiosmotic (see Chemiosmosis, below) generation of ATP. The operation of the ETS is depicted in Fig. 3.3.

There are three classes of carrier and transfer molecules in the ETS:

- Flavoproteins: Flavin coenzymes capable of performing oxidation-reduction reactions.
- Cytochromes: These proteins with an iron-containing group are capable of existing alternately as oxidized and reduced forms. The cytochromes include cytochrome b, cytochrome c_1, cytochrome c, cytochrome a, and cytochrome a_3.
- Ubiquinomes, or coenzyme Q, are small protein carriers.

NADH and $FADH_2$ are used to produce ATP by action of the electron transport chain (see Fig. 3.1). The operation of the electron transport chain with the role of the various carrier molecules is shown in Fig. 3.3.

The final electron receptor in aerobic respiration is oxygen, which is responsible for removing electrons from the system.

CHEMIOSMOSIS

This is the use of ion gradients, particularly proton gradients, across plasma membranes in the case of bacteria, to generate ATP. In chemiosmosis, when a substance (proton) moves along a gradient, the energy released is used to synthesize ATP. In respiration, chemiosmosis is responsible for much of the ATP generated.

Figure 3.4 shows schematically how chemiosmosis works. Energy is released from the electron transport system to drive the motive force in chemiosmosis. With this energy, hydrogen atoms are pumped from inside the microbial membrane to the outside. As the protons accumulate, a proton motive force develops by which protons are pumped back across the membrane to equalize the concentration. As a result of the proton flow, energy is provided for the synthesis of ADP molecules with phosphate to form ATP. The combined action of ETS and chemiosmosis generate a net gain of 34 ATP molecules.

LIPIDS AND PROTEINS

Lipids and proteins can also undergo catabolism after being broken down so they can enter the cell. There they are subjected to one or more of the following: beta oxidation, glycolysis, the Krebs cycle, and other conversions.

ANAEROBIC RESPIRATION

Some bacteria use anaerobic respiration, a process in which the final electron acceptor is an inorganic substance other than oxygen. *Bacillus* and *Pseudomonas* species and some other bacteria use nitrate gas, nitrous oxide, and nitrite ions as final electron acceptors. Nitrogen and sulfur cycles in nature depend on microorganisms that, in anaerobic respiration, use nitrate and sulfate as final electron acceptors.

FERMENTATION

As mentioned earlier, glucose is broken down by glycolysis to pyruvate. In fermentation, pyruvate is broken down, incompletely in the absence of oxygen, by specific enzymes to form alcohols, acids, and other end products. Other sugars, amino acids, organic acids, purines, and pyrimidines are also subject to fermentation.

Fermentation produces relatively small amounts of ATP. From each molecule of starting material, only one or

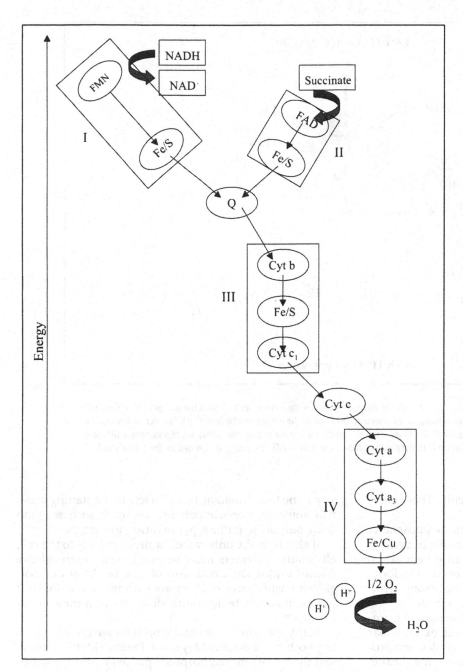

FIGURE 3.3 An electron transport chain. The electrons are passed to the electron carriers via oxidation-reduction reactions in a stepwise manner as indicated. The boxed-in electron carriers indicate complex I (NADH dehydrogenase), complex II (succinate dehydrogenase), complex III (cytochrome c reductase), and complex IV (cytochrome c oxidase). Ubiquinone (coenzyme Q or Q) and cytochrome c are not part of these complexes and, therefore, have more mobility within the membrane as a result. In addition, the succinate dehydrogenase enzyme (catalyzing the reaction converting succinate to fumarate) reduces the membrane-associated flavin adenine dinucleotide of complex II to $FADH_2$, which then transfers the electrons to the Fe/S center and, ultimately, to Q. Moving the electrons in this manner allows for release of energy in manageable quantities. Releasing it all at once would result in loss of the energy as heat, rather than conversion to ATP.

two ATP molecules are produced, depending on the fermentation pathway used.

Two of the more important fermentations are alcohol fermentation and lactic acid fermentation.

- Alcohol fermentation: This is carried out by yeasts and certain bacteria. Pyruvate is converted to ethanol and CO_2.
- Lactic acid fermentation: Some bacteria in the genera *Lactobacillus*, *Streptococcus*, and *Staphylococcus* use this type of fermentation in which pyruvate is converted to lactic acid.

The yield from respiration including the electron transport system and chemiosmosis is 34 ATP, compared with 2–3 ATP from fermentation.

A number of other types of fermentation, the microorganisms involved, and the products produced are given in Table 3.1.

LIPID AND PROTEIN CATABOLISM

Microbes can also derive energy from the oxidation of lipids. Some bacteria produce extracellular lipases that

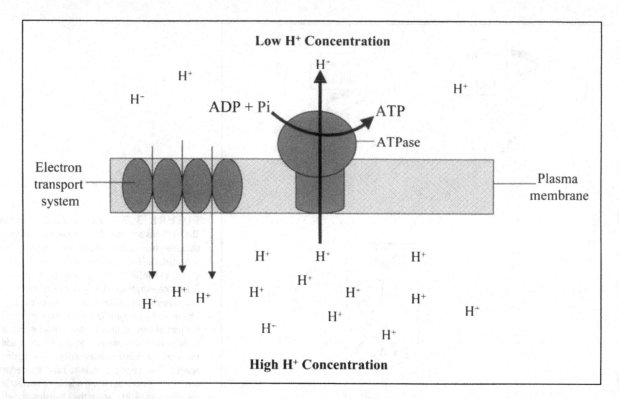

FIGURE 3.4   Chemiosmosis. The movement of electrons down the electron transport chain facilitates the pumping of protons (H$^+$) from inside the microbial membrane to outside the membrane. This accumulation results in the formation of a proton gradient across the membrane. A proton motive force then develops. The protons flow back to the inner side of the membrane through the adenosine triphophatase (ATPase) enzyme, which couples the movement of the proton with the production of a molecule of ATP. The energy is provided by the proton motive force in this case.

break down fats to glycerol and fatty acids. These compounds are then metabolized separately.

Glycerol is converted to dihydroxyacetone phosphate, which is metabolized by glycolysis and the Krebs cycle.

Fatty acids are oxidized by a process called beta oxidation, in which carbon fragments are removed from long-chain fatty acids and acetyl–CoA is formed from them. Acetyl–CoA is further oxidized in the Krebs cycle.

Proteins are too large to pass through the plasma membrane. Bacteria overcome this by producing extracellular peptidases and proteases. These enzymes break down proteins to amino acids that can cross the plasma membrane. Before being metabolized, amino acids must be converted to compounds that can enter the Krebs cycle. This is accomplished by processes that include deamination, decarboxylation, and dehydrogenation.

ANABOLISM (BIOSYNTHESIS)

Anabolism is the building up of reduced organic molecules, ultimately resulting in the formation of a new cell. Anabolism requires energy in the form of ATP and hydrogens (attached to reduced hydrogen carriers) that are generated in catabolic pathways. In addition, anabolism requires building blocks that are provided either extracellularly as nutrients or are formed intracellularly as intermediates of catabolic pathways. The term "building block" refers to the starting materials from which cellular polymers are made, such as amino acids, fatty acids, purines, pyrimidines, and sugars.

If glucose is the only carbon source available to the cell, all cellular polymers must be made from intermediates formed during the catabolism of glucose. Most microorganisms, whether or not they are pathogens, use similar if not identical catabolic intermediates to form these building blocks.

Many gram-negative enteric bacteria are capable of using both the Embden–Meyerhof–Parnas (EMP) pathway and the hexose monophosphate pathway (HMP) coupled with the Krebs cycle to carry out respiratory catabolism. In the absence of a terminal electron acceptor, the Krebs cycle enzymes no longer function as a cyclic pathway, but most of these enzymes continue to produce the catabolic intermediates that are essential for biosynthetic pathways. Figure 3.5 schematically shows the EMP and HMP pathways with the Krebs cycle and indicates which catabolic intermediates are commonly produced building blocks for each cellular polymer.

In an actively growing microorganism, pathways like EMP + Krebs cycle do not function solely for catabolism or energy production. One molecule of glucose may be entirely oxidized to CO_2, but the next molecule of glucose may be oxidized only as far as pyruvate, and from there the process may support synthesis of the amino acid alanine

T a b l e 3 . 1   End Products Excreted by Microorganisms Fermenting Sugars

Fermentation Type	Microorganisms*	Products Formed
Lactic acid	*Lactobacillus* *Streptococcus* *Leuconostoc* *Pedicoccus* *Sporalactobacillus* *Bifidobacterium*	Lactic, acetic, and formic acids, ethanol, glycerol, diacetyl, acetoin, butanediol, and CO_2
Ethanol	*Saccharomyces cerevisiae* *Zymomonas* *Sarcinia ventriculi* *Erwinia amylovora*	Mostly ethanol, CO_2
Butyric acid and acetone-butanol	*Clostridium butyricum* *Clostridium kluyveri* *Clostridium acetobutylicum* *Clostridium pasteurianum* *Clostridium perfringnes* *Neisseria* spp. *Bacteroides* spp. *Fusobacterium* spp. *Eubacterium* spp. *Butyrivibrio* spp.	Varying amounts of butyric and acetic acids, butanol, acetone, ethanol, isopropanol, H_2, and CO_2
Mixed acid	*Escherichia* *Salmonella* *Shigella* *Proteus* *Klebsiella*	Primarily lactic, acetic, and formic acids with little H_2, CO_2, and ethanol
Butanediol	*Enterobacter* *Serratia* *Erwinia* *Aeromonas* *Bacillus polymyxa* *Klebsiella*	Lots of butanediol, with some CO_2, H_2, and ethanol, and only slight amounts of mixed acids
Propionic acid	*Propionibacterium* *Clostridium propionicum* *Corynebacterium diphtheriae* *Veillonella* *Neisseria* spp.	Primarily propionic, acetic, and succinic acids and CO_2

*If the fermentation type appears to be characteristic of the entire genus, the genus name only is given; when characteristic of several species, the word "species" (spp.) is used; if characteristic of only one species, the entire species name is used.

and, ultimately, the synthesis of proteins. Thus, the "catabolism" of glucose appears to be a dynamic process that supports both the cell's need for energy and its need to produce building blocks for biosynthesis.

The ultimate function or consequence of biosynthesis is growth; for microorganisms, this means the production of new cells. All cells are composed of four types of polymers: protein, lipid, carbohydrates, and nucleic acids. Synthesis of the building blocks to support construction of these polymers, and the polymerization process itself, requires the expenditure of large quantities of energy. About 70% of the dry weight of the *E. coli* cell is protein, and it is estimated that about 88% of all energy obtained from glucose catabolism goes into making the cell's protein.

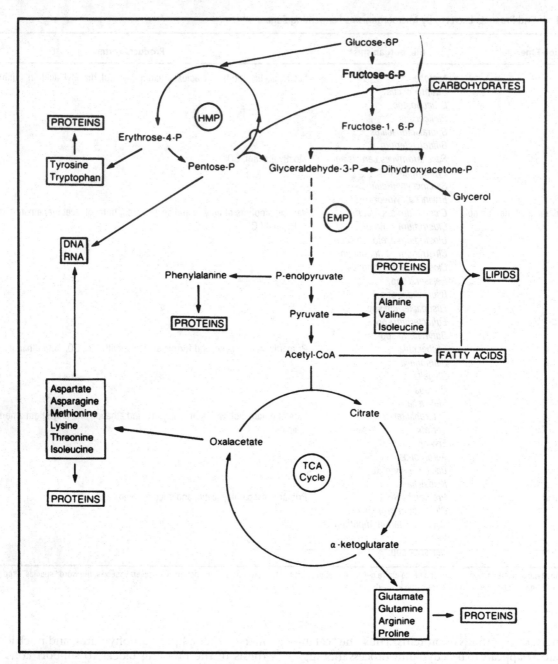

FIGURE 3.5 Common metabolic intermediates produced by respiratory catabolism and used as the starting point for anabolic (biosynthetic) pathways. Note that anabolism is often considered in two stages: first, pathways for the production of building blocks (e.g., amino acids) from catabolic intermediates, and second, mechanisms for the proper covalent binding of these building blocks into polymers (e.g., proteins). HMP, hexose monophosphate pathway; EMP, Embden-Meyerhof-Parnes pathway; DNA, deoxyribonucleic acid; RNA, ribonucleic acid.

4

Microbial Molecular Genetics

STRUCTURE AND FUNCTION OF THE BACTERIAL GENOME

Structure and Chemistry of the Bacterial Nuclear Region

The nucleus is defined as the membrane-bound organelle within a cell that contains chromosomes and nucleoli. Eukaryotic cells contain a nucleus, but prokaryotic cells (such as bacteria) do not. However, prokaryotes do contain genetic material, and its function is the same as that within the nucleus of eukaryotic cells. Where the genetic material is located inside a bacterium is called the nucleoid. Often the bacterial chromosome is referred to as the nuclear material or region to distinguish between it and any extrachromosomal genetic material, such as plasmids (see Fig. 1.2).

Investigators have isolated the nuclear region of *Escherichia coli* and many other bacteria, and the chemical analyses of all appear similar. Each is composed of about 80% deoxyribonucleic acid (DNA), 10% ribonucleic acid (RNA; mostly nascent), and 10% protein (mostly RNA polymerase).

In 1963, John Cairns developed a special technique that allowed him to isolate and spread out the chromosome of *E. coli* so its structure could be examined under an electron microscope. He found that the *E. coli* chromosome was circular and had the same width as one double-stranded DNA molecule and a circular length of about 1 mm. Because the chromosome's length was about 1000 times longer than the entire cell, it was immediately recognized that the molecular organization of the bacterial chromosome within the nucleoid must be very complex.

Realizing the DNA packaging problem for *E. coli*, based on Cairns work, further investigation revealed that the DNA molecule of the bacterial chromosome is supercoiled (twisted upon itself) and that this accounts for its efficient packing inside the cell. For the double-stranded helical DNA molecule to be supercoiled, one strand must first be broken (nicked) so that the helical molecule can be twisted upon itself (supercoiled). Studies suggest that there are 18–20 loops of DNA in the *E. coli* chromosome and that each loop is supercoiled, so that the entire molecule is reasonably compact.

Genetic Elements of Bacteria: Chromosomes and Plasmids

Microbiologists use the term genome to mean the complete set of genetic elements occurring within a cell or virus particle. Although the chromosome is the primary genetic element in bacteria, many bacteria also contain small pieces of extrachromosomal genetic material called plasmids. Therefore, the genomic material of bacteria comprises both the chromosomes and the extrachromosomal plasmids. For now, however, we will concentrate on the bacterial chromosome while remembering that much of what we say about chromosome structure and replication also applies to plasmids.

A gene is the basic unit of heredity that determines a particular characteristic or trait, such as height in pea plants. The physical location of that gene on the chromosome is the gene locus. Alleles are the alternative forms associated with that particular trait. In the case of height in peas, the alleles are dwarf and tall. Most nondividing eukaryotic cells are diploid; that is, they contain two copies of each chromosome per cell, one copy of each chromosome inherited from each parent. Eukaryotic chromosomes are structurally complex, and cells have a number of different types of chromosomes.

In contrast with eukaryotic cells, bacteria have relatively simple genetic systems. Bacterial chromosomes are single DNA molecules. Nongrowing cells are haploid; that is, they contain only one chromosome (DNA molecule) per cell (one set of genes). During growth, however, the bacterial cell contains at least one partial copy of its chromosome at any one time, because DNA synthesis must provide two complete copies just before cell division.

Prokaryotic Genomics

Recently, many prokaryotic genomes representing both the Eubacteria and the Archaea have been sequenced. The *Haemophilus influenzae* genome was, in 1995, the first genome to be completely sequenced. Since then, more than 50 bacterial genome sequences have been completed.

EUBACTERIA. Genomes of Eubacteria that have been sequenced have some common features. First, the eubacterial genome in general is small, typically less than 5 **Mb** in size, and circular. To date, several exceptions to the "small, circular genome" have been identified. These include *Bacillus megaterium*, which has a genome that is 30 Mb, and *Borrelia burgdorferi* and some *Streptomyces* spp. that possess linear genomes.

Second, eubacterial plasmids are small and contain relatively few genes. However, *Borrelia burgdorferi* carries approximately 17 plasmids that encode approximately 430 genes. Furthermore, *Vibrio cholerae* and other *Vibrio* spp. have two circular chromosomes. The second chromosome is thought to be derived from an ancestral plasmid that continued to add genetic material over time.

Last, gene density within the eubacterial genome is relatively high, approximately 1 gene per **kilobase** (kb) of DNA. For example, the *E. coli* genome is approximately 4.6 Mb in length and contains approximately 4288 protein coding regions. In addition, many of the genes are arranged in operons (described below).

ARCHAEA. Genomes of the Archaea are similar to those of the Eubacteria. The best-studied archaeal genome is that of *Methanococcus jannaschii*, which possesses three circular chromosomes, one large (1.66 Mb) and two small (58.4 and 16.5 kb). The entire genome is 1.7 Mb in size, encoding approximately 1738 proteins, and therefore, having a high gene density, as exemplified by the Eubacteria. Some of the genes are also arranged in operons.

In contrast with the Eubacteria, the Archaea share many features observed in eukaryotic genomes. Such similarities are found in genes associated with RNA synthesis, protein synthesis, and DNA synthesis; the presence of histone proteins associated with DNA packaging; and the presence of **introns** within the tRNA genes.

OVERVIEW OF MOLECULAR GENETICS

Genetic processes require at least three types of polymers: DNA, RNA, and proteins. During cell growth, all three types of macromolecules are made. Because the steps leading from DNA to RNA to newly synthesized protein require the transfer of information, DNA and RNA are often called informational macromolecules to distinguish them from other large molecules such as lipids and polysaccharides.

During the process of cell division, the DNA of the parent cell needs to be copied such that identical copies of the DNA are available for each of the daughter cells. The process of duplicating the DNA is called DNA replication, or simply replication. To preserve the information contained within the DNA molecule in the form of its sequence of nucleotides, each of the original DNA strands is used as a template for the manufacture of its complementary strand. This is called semiconservative DNA replication. In replication, the original DNA strand provides the template for the synthesis of the new, complementary DNA strand by the action of the enzyme DNA polymerase.

When we look at DNA and, ultimately, the protein products produced from information contained in the genes, we are looking at what is commonly called "infor-

mation flow" in a cell. The DNA molecule contains the information necessary to make various proteins. However, DNA cannot be directly used to make proteins. Instead, we find that the DNA provides a template that is transcribed into messenger RNA (mRNA) by the enzyme RNA polymerase. Messenger RNA can then be translated into protein, the amino acid sequence of the protein being determined by the sequence of nucleotides of the mRNA. The site of translation is the ribosome. This process, DNA →mRNA →protein, is referred to as the central dogma. There is one exception to the central dogma: the retroviruses. Retroviruses possess a unique enzyme known as reverse transcriptase, which is able to synthesize DNA from an RNA template.

DNA Structure and Synthesis

As DNA molecules are polymers of nucleotides, the basic structure of a nucleotide needs to be discussed. Each nucleotide in DNA comprises a phosphate group, deoxyribose sugar, and a nitrogenous base (Fig. 4.1). Each carbon within the deoxyribose is numbered and indicated by a prime (') to distinguish it from the carbons of the nitrogenous base. The phosphate group is covalently bound to both the 3' and the 5' position of adjacent deoxyribose molecules (ester linkages), forming what is commonly called the "sugar–phosphate backbone" of one DNA strand. Each DNA strand has a free 5' phosphate at one end and a free 3' hydroxyl at the other end. One of four possible nitrogenous bases is linked to the deoxyribose in the nucleotide molecule. These are either a purine (adenine, guanine) or pyrimidine (thymine, cytosine) base.

The single bacterial chromosome contains two complementary (not identical) DNA strands that are wound around one another in a helical fashion, with the ends covalently bonded together to form a circular macromolecule. Following Chargoff's rules, guanine forms hydrogen bonds with cytosine, and thymine forms hydrogen bonds with adenine (Fig. 4.2). Replication requires the unwinding the existing helix, followed by the incorporation of individual nucleotides, so that a new complementary DNA strand is built, using the original strand as a template (see bottom half of Fig. 4.2). This is known as semiconservative replication. Also note that replication of these two strands runs in opposite directions, which is known as antiparallelism (Fig. 4.3).

Replication always begins at the 5' end and progresses toward the 3' end of each DNA strand.

The region where the two strands unwind is called the replication fork, or the replicon. Replication begins with the double helix being unwound by the enzyme helicase. To stabilize the structure and maintain the replication fork, single-strand binding proteins bind the unwound DNA. An enzyme called primase then initiates the synthesis of a short RNA (primer), approximately 12–15 nucleotides in length. Once the primer is in place, DNA polymerase continues to covalently bond each additional nucleotide to the 3' hydroxyl end of the newly developing

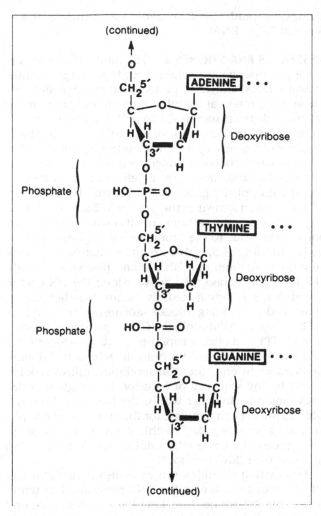

FIGURE 4.1   A small segment of deoxyribonucleic acid (DNA) showing alternating molecules of deoxyribose and phosphate covalently bonded together to form one strand of the double-stranded DNA molecule. Each purine or pyrimidine base is covalently bonded at the 1' position of the ribose and loosely associated by hydrogen bonding (···) to a complementary base on the adjacent strand (not shown).

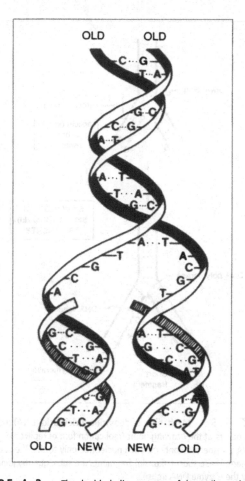

FIGURE 4.2   The double-helix structure of deoxyribonucleic acid during the replication process. At the top of this drawing, each sugar–phosphate strand is shown as a continuous band with the bases adenine (A), cytosine (C), guanine (G), or thymine (T) covalently bound to each sugar. The two strands are held together by hydrogen bonding (···) between each complementary base pair. During replication, the old strands separate, and one new strand is formed that is complementary to each of the old strands.

strand. As one molecule of DNA polymerase is responsible for the synthesis of both new complementary strands of DNA simultaneously, a logistic problem is created. One of the original strands can be replicated in the 5' to 3' direction. As this strand can be synthesized fairly quickly in a continuous manner, it is often called the continuous strand or the leading strand. In contrast, because of the antiparallel nature of the DNA helix, the strand oriented in the 3' to 5' direction appears to defy the polymerase law of synthesis in only the 5' to 3' direction. More recent work has uncovered that this strand of the DNA is wound around the DNA polymerase so that short stretches of the molecule are oriented in the 5' to 3' direction (see Fig. 4.4). As a result, for each new region of this strand wrapped around the DNA polymerase, primase must add a primer followed by DNA polymerase activity through this particular section. As a result, this strand is made up of many

small fragments and, therefore, takes longer to synthesize. We refer to this strand as the lagging strand, or the discontinuous strand. The short fragments of this strand are known as Okazaki fragments. The adjacent fragments are then covalently bonded together by an enzyme called DNA ligase. The RNA **primers** are eventually removed and replaced with DNA nucleotides, and any breaks in the backbone are sealed by DNA ligase. The end result of this synthesis is two double-stranded DNA molecules (two bacterial chromosomes).

Once replicated, each chromosome is then supercoiled. Supercoiling is believed to be an important factor in both the replication of DNA and its transcription. Enzymes called topoisomerases appear to regulate the degree of DNA supercoiling and, thus, its ease of replication and transcription. Each time that DNA is supercoiled, it is put under strain. Because it is under strain, it unwinds more easily than if it were not supercoiled. The topoisomerase that promotes DNA supercoiling in bacteria is DNA gyrase.

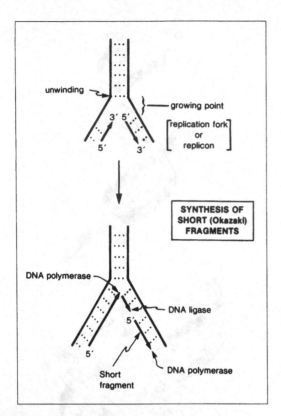

FIGURE 4.3 Mechanism of deoxyribonucleic acid (DNA) replication. Unwinding occurs at the growing point (replication fork or replicon). The enzyme DNA polymerase connects each nucleotide only to the 3' end of each short fragment. These short (Okazaki) fragments are subsequently joined together by the enzyme DNA ligase.

A highly schematic and oversimplified illustration of chromosome replication and the subsequent division of these two DNA macromolecules before cell division is shown in Fig. 4.5. The exact manner in which each chromosome finds itself in a new cell is not known, but it is believed that the site of attachment of the chromosome to the plasma membrane plays an important part in this partitioning process. Evidence also suggests that rapidly dividing cells have more than one growing point (site of replication), because the time between successive cell divisions is shorter than the time it takes to replicate an entire chromosome. If this is true, then at any one time during rapid growth, there may be at least one complete chromosome and several partial copies at various stages of completion.

RNA Structure and Synthesis

The bacterial cell's RNAs also play an important part in gene expression.

There are three major differences between the chemistry of RNA and that of DNA. First, molecules of RNA contain a sugar called ribose instead of deoxyribose. Second, RNA has a nitrogenous base called uracil instead of the base thymine. And finally, bacterial RNA is typically not a double-stranded molecule (some viral RNAs are double-stranded). Like all other cells, bacteria contain three major types of RNA: mRNA, transfer RNA (tRNA), and ribosomal RNA (rRNA).

MESSENGER RNA SYNTHESIS. The function of mRNA is to copy (transcribe) the genetic code from the gene (chromosomal DNA) and, thus, provide that message for translation into protein at the ribosome. Transcription of the genetic code refers specifically to mRNA synthesis.

To discuss transcription, one must look at the basic structure of a gene (Fig. 4.6). The portion of the gene that will ultimately encode a protein product following both transcription and translation is referred to as the structural portion of the gene. Upstream from the structural gene is a region known as the promoter. Each gene (or set of genes) on the chromosome has its own promoter. RNA polymerase binds to the promoter region, causing localized unwinding of the DNA strands so that the code may be transcribed from one DNA strand (the sense strand). The RNA polymerase then moves along the DNA sense strand while it simultaneously bonds together the ribonucleotide building blocks—adenosine triphosphate (ATP), cytosine triphosphate (CTP), guanosine triphosphate (GTP), and uridine triphosphate (UTP)—to form the new mRNA molecule. The order in which the ribonucleotides are inserted into the developing mRNA is determined by the sequence of bases on the single-stranded DNA molecule. In other words, the bases on the single DNA strand act as a template for the assembly of complementary ribonucleotides. In this manner, the transcription process transcribes the information from the DNA (gene) to the mRNA (message).

Termination of mRNA synthesis also occurs at a specific (termination) site on the DNA molecule. This termination site determines how long the mRNA will be, and this, in turn, determines how large the protein molecule will be. Several types of termination sites on the DNA molecule have been identified, and these effectively stop the action of RNA polymerase (and thus mRNA synthesis). The resulting complete, functional mRNA molecule is linear and single-stranded.

Not all mRNA molecules code for synthesis of a single protein molecule. In bacteria, some mRNAs code for synthesis of several related enzymatic proteins whose synthesis is coded on adjacent genes. For example, the genes that code for all of the enzymes needed in the synthetic pathway for formation of one amino acid may be sequentially arranged on the DNA. Instead of having one termination site at the end of the code for each enzyme, the DNA may have one termination site for the entire sequence of genes. Thus, one long mRNA molecule could be transcribed and encode the simultaneous synthesis of all enzymes required for that synthetic pathway. As shown later in this chapter, this mRNA arrangement allows for several mechanisms for regulation of the quantities of these gene products in the cell.

Several important antibiotics interfere with mRNA synthesis. Actinomycin inhibits mRNA synthesis by binding to the DNA molecule in such a way that it stops mRNA formation. Two groups of antibiotics, the rifamycins and the streptovaricins, are effective against bacteria because

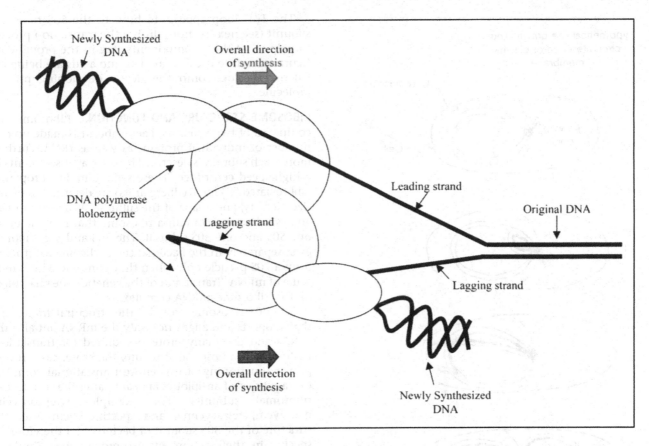

FIGURE 4.4   A simplified illustration of deoxyribonucleic acid (DNA) replication. Note that the original DNA of the lagging strand needs to "wrap around" the DNA polymerase holoenzyme (entire) to have small potions, as indicated by the grey box, that are in the appropriate orientation to facilitate polymerase activity in the 5' →3' direction. As a result, these pieces require the addition of a primer each time, followed by a short length of DNA polymerization. The result is commonly known as Okazaki fragments.

they appear to bind to the RNA polymerase molecule and inhibit its activity. The rifamycins seem to be highly specific for bacterial RNA polymerase.

TRANSFER RNA STRUCTURE AND FUNCTION.   tRNA is a single-stranded molecule that contains double-stranded regions as a result of the molecule folding back on itself. These folded regions have complementary bases across from each other, and hydrogen bonding holds these adjacent strands together. The structure of tRNA is generally drawn like a cloverleaf, with three distinct loops (of unpaired bases) and a stem that has two open ends.

To function properly, a molecule of tRNA (Fig. 4.7) must do four things: it must bind with an enzyme that activates amino acids, it must specifically bind with one type of amino acid, it must recognize a specific triplet code (codon) on the mRNA and hydrogen bond with the triplet bases on that codon, and it must nonspecifically bind with the ribosome to which an mRNA is bound. The structure of the tRNA molecule closely reflects how it functions in these ways during protein synthesis.

The D loop on tRNA selectively binds an enzyme called an aminoacyl–tRNA (AA-tRNA) synthetase. This enzyme does two things: first, it specifically activates one type of amino acid, and second, it binds that activated amino

acid to the acceptor stem of the tRNA. To activate the amino acid, AA-tRNA synthetase cleaves pyrophosphate from an ATP molecule and covalently bonds the remaining AMP to the amino acid. Thus, an activated amino acid is an amino acid–AMP complex. The specificity of the tRNAs toward only one type of AA-tRNA synthetase should be emphasized. It is extremely important that the correct AA-tRNA synthetase be attached to the tRNA molecule, because this enzyme determines which amino acid will be activated and bound to the tRNA. In turn, this determines which amino acid will be inserted in the developing protein during translation. Specific binding between a tRNA and an amino acid occurs in the **cytosol** of the cell. Once the amino acid has been activated and the amino acid–tRNA complex leaves the enzyme, the complex is available for integration into a polypeptide during translation.

The anticodon loop on tRNA contains three bases (the anticodon) that are complementary to three bases on mRNA (the codon). The function of the anticodon on this loop is to specifically recognize and bind an mRNA codon based on complementarity between the codon and the anticodon. As a result, the amino acid carried by this tRNA is brought in proper order to the site of translation based on the sequence of the mRNA, which in turn was determined by the information provided from the DNA.

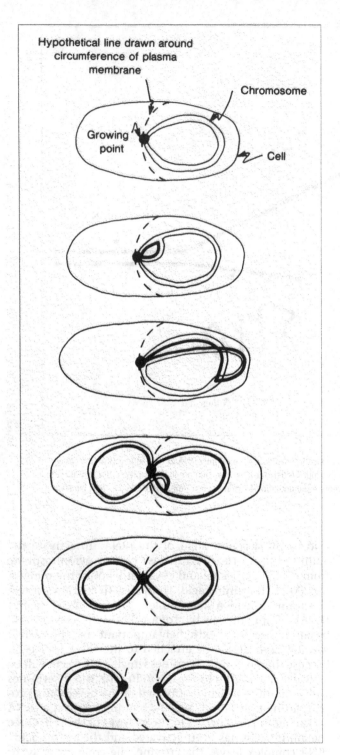

Hypothetical line drawn around
circumference of plasma
membrane

Chromosome

Growing
point

Cell

FIGURE 4.5   Replication of the bacterial chromosome. Each of the old strands of the chromosome is represented by a thin line, and the new strands are shown with heavy lines. Sites of attachment to the plasma membrane are also sites for deoxyribonucleic acid replication (growing point). Separation of growing points may allow for partitioning of each new chromosome before cell division.

In other words, the genomic message from the chromosome is transcribed into the mRNA, which comes into contact with the ribosome, where its message is translated by the tRNAs carrying the activated amino acids.

The TψC loop appears to bind to the 50S ribosome subunit (see next section) during the translation process to help all of these components stay in the proper configuration while the activated amino acids are being covalently bonded onto the newly developing protein molecule.

RIBOSOME STRUCTURE AND FUNCTION.   Ribosomes are composed of two subunits. Each subunit is made up of a number of individual proteins as well as rRNA. Furthermore, each subunit is described by the way it sediments in a high-speed centrifuge. These sedimentation properties (abbreviated "S" for Svedberg units) are determined by the size, density, and shape of the subunit. As a result of this analysis, bacteria contain a ribosome that is made up of one 50S and one 30S subunit. The 30S and 50S subunits exist separately in the bacterial cell and come together to form a 70S particle only when they combine with a molecule of mRNA. Translation of the genetic code takes place on this ribosome–mRNA complex.

The 70S ribosome provides the structural framework that supports and aligns not only the mRNA but also the tRNAs and the many proteins required for translation. Distortion of ribosomal structure, therefore, can prevent proper functioning of this entire translational complex. Certain types of antibiotics appear to alter the structure of ribosomal subunits. For example, streptomycin, neomycin, tetracycline, and spectinomycin alter the structure of the 30S subunit of bacteria and therefore are specific in their action against prokaryotes. Similarly, puromycin, chloramphenicol, erythromycin, and cycloheximide appear to alter the 50S prokaryotic subunits. Note, however, that this is not the only mode of action of these antibiotics. Most also affect other steps in protein synthesis.

THE GENETIC CODE

The information contained in the nucleotide sequence of the bacterial cell's chromosome (DNA) is ultimately translated into the sequence of amino acids that make up each protein. Thus, the genetic code is contained in the DNA. However, this code is transcribed from the DNA molecule to mRNA, and it is actually the mRNA that serves as a template for the assembly of amino acids during protein synthesis. Therefore, it is customary to speak of the genetic code in terms of nucleotide sequence of the mRNA molecules.

All RNAs contain four different nucleotide bases: adenine (A), guanine (G), cytosine (C), and uracil (U). Within the mRNA, three sequential nucleotide bases (triplets like CUA) are used to code for the positioning of an amino acid during translation. Each of the triplet nucleotide sequences on the mRNA strand is called a codon. Because there are four nucleotide bases and three bases in each codon, 64 different triplets (codons) are possible. However, there are only 20 different amino acids in nature. Therefore, many more codons are possible than are needed for translating genetic information from the mRNA to the developing protein. This is what is meant by the statement that the genetic code is redundant. There

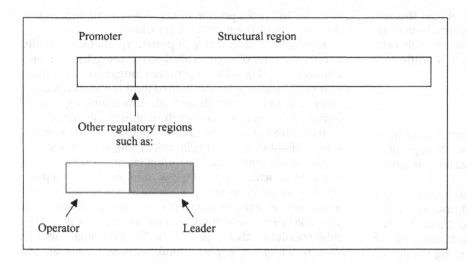

FIGURE 4.6 The basic structure of a gene includes a promoter region, where RNA polymerase binds to initiate transcription, and a structural region, encoding the sequence necessary to ultimately be translated into a polypeptide. Beyond the basic structure, located between the promoter and the structural region are additional regulatory regions, such as the operator and leader regions. Realize that these are only some of the regulatory regions associated with prokaryotic genes.

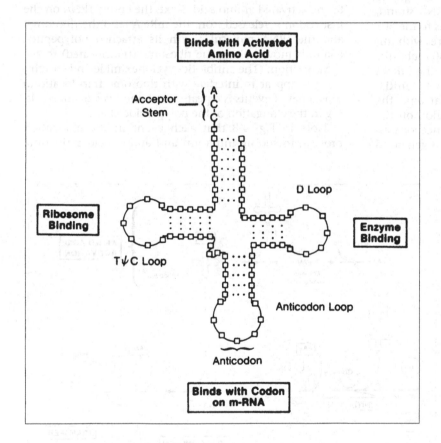

FIGURE 4.7 Molecular structure of a transfer ribonucleic acid (tRNA) molecule showing a cloverleaf arrangement. Nucleotides (boxes or letters) are covalently bound together (C) to form a long, single-stranded molecule that is folded back on itself. The folded tRNA is held together by hydrogen bonds (···) between adjacent complementary bases. Three loops are formed on folding, and each loop has a specific function. The two ends of this single strand form the stem of the molecule that will bind one type of amino acid. mRNA, messenger RNA.

are several codons coding for insertion of the same amino acid into the developing protein during protein synthesis. For example, UUA, UUG, CUU, CUC, CUA, and CUG all code for leucine insertion.

A few codons do not code for any amino acids (such as UGA, UAG, and UAA); these are called stop codons, as they serve as a signal to stop protein synthesis when the molecule is fully formed. Some evidence suggests that a few codons represent only starting points for new protein synthesis, such as AUG. These are called initiating codons. A distinct starting point is essential, so that translation begins at the proper location. Without a specific starting

point, the whole reading frame might be shifted and a completely different protein (or no protein at all) would be made, depending upon the extent of the reading frame shift. Interestingly, in bacteria, the AUG start allows the incorporation of a specially modified amino acid, N-formyl-methionine. Any other AUG within the polypeptide will have incorporated a methionine, but the first is always the N-formyl- form.

Errors in translating the message on mRNA are probably rare under normal circumstances. However, those antibiotics that act on the 30S or 50S ribosome subunits are thought to increase translation errors to such an extent that the newly formed protein is abnormal and the cell can no longer function properly. Drastic shifts from optimum pH, temperature, and cation concentration also appear to cause translation errors during protein synthesis.

Mechanism of Protein Synthesis (Expression of the Genetic Code)

Protein synthesis (translation of the genetic code from mRNA) is a continuous process that may be thought of as occurring in four steps: initiation, elongation, termination, and polypeptide folding.

Initiation (Fig. 4.8) requires the formation of a complex that contains mRNA, the 30S ribosome subunit, tRNA, the 50S subunit, and several proteins (called initiation factors). In bacteria, tRNA binds to the 30S subunit, and the 50S subunit binds to the 30S particle, forming the 70S ribosome. The anticodon on an activated tRNA recognizes and binds to the initiating codon on the mRNA strand, and the TψC loop of this same tRNA also binds to the 50S subunit of the ribosome. Streptomycin interferes with initiation, probably because of its effect on the 30S subunit.

In bacteria, the first (initiation) codon on the mRNA strand is typically AUG or GUG. Just preceding the initiation codon are three to nine nucleotides that bind the mRNA to the 30S ribosome subunit. This region on the mRNA is known as the Shine–Delgarno sequence, or simply the ribosome binding site. It is able to hydrogen bond with the 16S rRNA portion of the 30S subunit and, in this manner, orient the mRNA for translation.

Elongation, the next step in protein synthesis, is actually a repeated series of events called recognition, transfer, and translocation (Fig. 4.8). To achieve elongation, there must be a continual supply of activated amino acid–tRNA complexes. However, only those with anticodons capable of forming hydrogen bonds with the codon on the mRNA will be recognized and will bind to the mRNA at that position. (The antibiotics streptomycin, neomycin, and tetracycline appear to adversely affect this codon recognition.) Once the two amino acids are adjacent to one another, a peptide bond is formed between the amino group of the second amino acid and the carboxyl group of the first amino acid. This reaction is performed by a catalytic RNA called peptidyl transferase that is part of the 50S ribosomal subunit. As a result of the peptide bond formation between the amino acids, the first tRNA is no longer covalently bound to the activated amino acid. Next, the empty tRNA on the first codon is released from the mRNA (and the ribosome) and the tRNA molecule, with its attached polypeptide chain, is moved along the ribosome (translocated) to the next position. (The antibiotics cycloheximide and spectinomycin appear to interfere with ribosome translocation.) This series of events is repeated over and over again, resulting in the elongation of the polypeptide chain.

Note in Fig. 4.8 that each event in the elongation process, including initiation and amino acid activation,

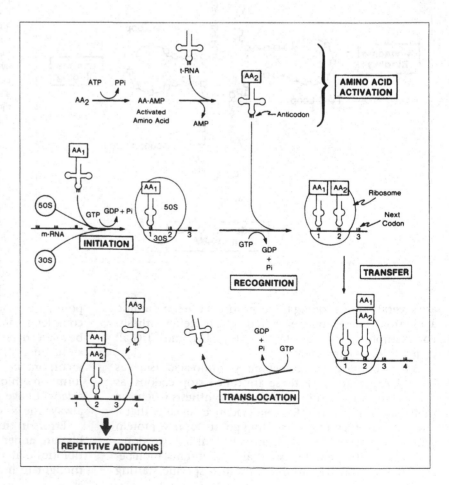

FIGURE 4.8   Translation of the genetic code from messenger ribonucleic acid (mRNA) molecule to the order of amino acids (AAs) on a protein molecule during synthesis. Once synthesis is initiated such that the mRNA–ribosome–AA$_1$ complex is formed, the addition of each additional amino acid (e.g., AA$_2$, AA$_3$, etc.) requires four events: amino acid activation, recognition, transfer, and translocation. These four events are continuously repeated in the elongation step of protein synthesis. ATP, adenosine triphophate; GTP, guanosine triphosphate; GDP, guanosine diphosphate; Pi, inorganic phosphate.

requires molecules that have high-energy phosphate bonds (ATP and GTP). For example, formation of the initiation complex (the initiation step) requires energy, and this is provided by the hydrolysis of one GTP molecule. High-energy compounds like GTP are supplied by catabolism of the cell's exogenous energy source. Catabolism (and anabolism too) is accomplished by enzymes (catalytically active proteins) that are made in the manner being described. Thus, catabolism of the energy source and synthesis of proteins are inseparably linked by the supply and demand for ATP and GTP.

Termination, the third step in protein synthesis, occurs when a mRNA codon is reached that does not code for the attachment of any AA-tRNA. These are called termination codons or stop codons. There are three termination codons that stop polypeptide synthesis in all cell types: UGA, UAG, and UAA. As a result, termination factors bind, stimulating dissociation of the ribosomal subunits and release of the polypeptide chain into the cytoplasm. In addition to their other activities, the tetracycline antibiotics also seem to interfere with the termination of protein synthesis.

Once released from the ribosome–mRNA complex, the polypeptide chain is free to fold into an active, three-dimensional protein structure that is held in this form by weak disulfide bridges and hydrogen bonding. This is the last step in protein synthesis, known as polypeptide folding. If everything has gone correctly, the result is a functionally active protein.

In bacteria, because there is no nucleus, the processes of transcription and translation are said to be coupled. Essentially, once RNA polymerase initiates transcription to the point where the ribosome-binding site has been transcribed and there is physically enough room, a ribosome will be able to initiate translation before transcription is even complete. Furthermore, once that ribosome-binding site is once again exposed as the first ribosome begins translating product, a second ribosome can begin translation before the first ribosome has completed translating the peptide. As a result, in electron microscopy one can often see a message covered with several ribosomes, all at different stages of translation of the mRNA; these are referred to as polyribosomes or simply polysomes.

Gene Regulation

Some gene products are always being made by the cell, so they are always present in relatively high concentration, and these are called constitutive genes. Others are only produced under certain conditions, and these are called inducible genes.

Three mechanisms of gene regulation will be briefly discussed here: the induction-repression mechanism, catabolite repression, and attenuation. Each of these control mechanisms acts at the transcription level, that is, on the gene (DNA), as its message is being transcribed to a new mRNA molecule. And each of these mechanisms functions to turn off gene expression (ultimately, protein synthesis) when the gene product is no longer needed for cellular metabolism. The function of repressing protein synthesis seems obvious, as it would be pointless for a cell to waste energy on making unneeded proteins.

The ability to repress protein synthesis is a valuable and widespread mechanism for energy conservation by all types of microorganisms. Regulating genetic expression in bacteria (prokaryotes), however, appears simpler than regulating expression in eukaryotic microorganisms. The following section deals only with genetic control mechanisms in prokaryotic cells.

INDUCTION AND REPRESSION. Control of protein synthesis by induction or repression usually involves not one, but a set of adjacent genes on the bacterial cell's chromosome. These structural genes are responsible for the synthesis of several enzymes that usually accomplish all or part of the catabolism of a specific energy source. This set of adjacent genes forms a functional genetic unit called an operon. The operon is located next to other parts of the DNA that regulate the expression of the structural genes and that include promoters, operators, and regulatory genes. The operon that has been most closely studied is the lactose (lac) operon from *E. coli*. The lac operon is responsible for the initial stages of lactose catabolism in this bacterium, and it contains three structural genes (Fig. 4.9): (1) the "Z" gene, which codes for production of an enzyme called β-galactosidase. This enzyme breaks apart disaccharide sugars that contain a galactoside molecule covalently joined by a β-glycosidic bond to another sugar; (2) the "Y" gene, which codes for galactoside permease production, an enzyme within the plasma membrane that transports galactoside molecules inside so that they can be cleaved into separate monosaccharide sugars by β-galactosidase; and (3) the "A" gene, which codes for production of galactoside acetylase, an enzyme whose function is not clearly understood.

Repression of the lac operon comes about in the following way. Transcription begins when RNA polymerase binds to the promoter region. The regulatory gene is the first part of the DNA sense strand transcribed. The function of the regulatory gene is to code for continuous production of repressor proteins (see Fig. 4.9).

If lactose (or another β-galactoside) is not present in the medium, then the repressor proteins are free to bind with the operator region of the DNA. In so doing, they also prevent the RNA polymerase from binding to the promoter and progressing to transcribe the structural genes of the lac operon. This alteration of the operator stops further transcription and effectively inhibits synthesis of the enzymes required for lactose use. Note that these enzymes are not needed in the absence of lactose, so this may be thought of as an energy-conservation mechanism.

For induction, a β-galactoside (such as lactose) must be present in the medium, and the β-galactoside itself serves as the inducer (Fig. 4.9). Cells probably always have a small number of galactoside transport proteins (permeases) in the membrane, even if transcription of the lac operon is repressed. Therefore, if lactose is added to the medium, a small amount of lactose is initially transported into the cell. The regulatory gene continues to code for synthesis of repressor proteins; however, lactose (the inducer) binds with these repressor proteins, so that the repressor proteins will no longer recognize and bind the operator region. Because the repressor proteins are now inactivated, transcription of the structural genes by RNA

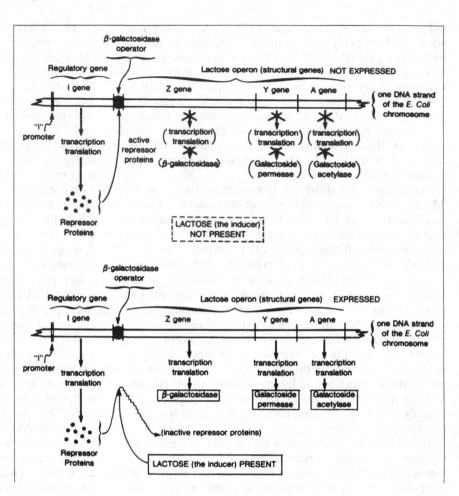

FIGURE 4.9   The lactose *(lac)* operon of *Escherichia coli. (Top)* In the absence of lactose, repressor proteins remain active and bind to the operator region, thereby preventing transcription of the structural genes that make up the *lac* operon. Because these genes are not transcribed, the unnecessary proteins are not made; thus, energy is conserved. *(Bottom)* However, when lactose is present, it binds to the repressor proteins, thereby making them unable to bind the operator region. This allows transcription and subsequent translation of the structural genes of the *lac* operon, so that all the enzymes necessary for lactose utilization are made. DNA, deoxyribonucleic acid.

polymerase can proceed. Thus, induction and repression both have the same underlying mechanism: control of the operator. Since induction actually interferes with the action of the repressor proteins, some microbiologists prefer to call the induction process derepression.

CATABOLITE REPRESSION.   Another mechanism for control of protein synthesis is called catabolite repression. To understand this mechanism, it is important to know that bacteria are often capable of growing on a variety of nutrient energy sources, but that some of these energy sources are used preferentially. For example, *E. coli* can catabolize either glucose or lactose to obtain energy for growth. If both are present, however, these bacteria will first use glucose until the supply is exhausted and then shift to lactose. As previously described, the enzymes responsible for lactose utilization are inducible, but the synthesis of these enzymes (transcription of the *lac* operon) is also subject to catabolite repression. When glucose is preferentially used in the presence of lactose, glucose is the catabolite (substrate for catabolism) that acts as a repressor on the *lac* operon. Once the glucose supply in the medium is exhausted, there is no catabolite to serve as the repressor, and catabolite repression is abolished. Lactose can then induce the *lac* operon, and lactose catabolism can begin after a short lag time.

The mechanism in which glucose acts as a catabolite repressor has been described, but it is first necessary to describe more fully how RNA polymerase binds to the sense strand of the DNA. In the previous section, it was stated that transcription (mRNA synthesis) begins when RNA polymerase binds at the promoter. However, with catabolite-repressible enzymes, binding appears to occur only if a catabolite-activator protein (CAP) has already bound to the promoter. When bound to the promoter, CAP facilitates RNA polymerase recognition of the promoter region. In order for CAP to bind, it must be in the proper three-dimensional structure, and this requires a molecule called cyclic AMP (cAMP) be bound to it. It appears that glucose either inhibits the synthesis of cAMP or causes cAMP to be broken down. Regardless of the reason, intracellular cAMP concentrations are low in the presence of glucose. The lack of sufficient cAMP prevents CAP binding to the promoter; thus, RNA polymerase does not bind, and transcription does not occur. Therefore, catabolite repression is really the result of a glucose-stimulated cAMP deficiency.

There is some evidence that glucose-controlled cAMP concentrations regulate enzyme synthesis for a number of other catabolic pathways in *E. coli*. This suggests that enzymes responsible for catabolism of energy sources other than glucose are not made in the presence of glucose (a preferred energy source for *E. coli*). This is because the enzymes associated with glycolysis are constitutively made and, therefore, always present in the cell. Thus, once again, the cell conserves energy by stopping synthesis of unneeded enzymes. Alternatively, when the preferred energy source (glucose) is depleted, the cell starts synthesis of other enzymes used for catabolism of other substrates. Perhaps cells capable of such feats are more adaptable to changing environments and thus more likely to survive than those that lack such regulation mechanisms.

ATTENUATION.   A third mechanism of regulation occurs in operons controlling synthesis of amino acids. The best studied of these is the tryptophan operon. This operon contains structural genes for the five enzymes required to convert catabolic intermediates to tryptophan. The adjacent regulatory sequence includes three major regions: the promoter, the operator, and a region that seems characteristic of attenuation-controlled regulatory sequences, called the leader sequence. Within the leader sequence is a region called the attenuator that codes for synthesis of a peptide (small–molecular weight protein) that is rich in tryptophan. If tryptophan is abundant in the medium and in the cell, then the leader can be assembled during translation of this region of the mRNA. With assembly of

the attenuator, translation halts, as translational termination signals are present. However, if intracellular tryptophan concentrations are low or absent, the ribosomes stall, waiting for charged tryptophan tRNAs for incorporation into the growing peptide. As a result, the attenuator does not form, and translation of the message of the structural genes progresses (Fig. 4.10).

The critical feature of this mechanism is that synthesis of the leader peptide causes transcription of the tryptophan structural genes to stop. However, if a tryptophan deficiency stops formation of the leader peptide, then transcription of the structural genes will take place, and tryptophan synthesis will occur inside the cell.

SUMMARY.   Although it may appear that much is known about how protein synthesis is regulated, there is much more detail to learn. For example, it is not known for sure whether anabolic and catabolic pathways are regulated in the same way. At this time, however, it appears that catabolic (energy yielding, degradative) pathways are controlled using either induction-repression or catabolite repression. Note that both of these mechanisms use the presence of the initial substrate (energy source) to "turn on" the synthesis of these catabolic enzymes. Alternatively,

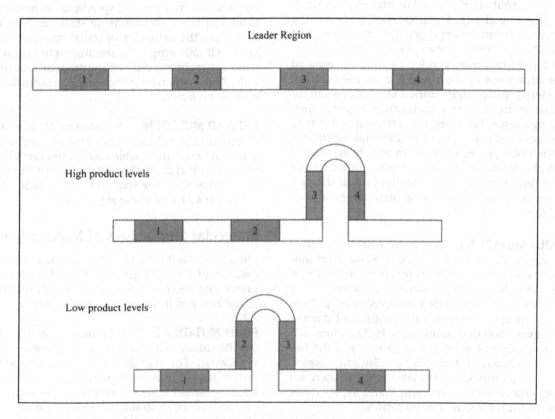

FIGURE 4.10   The attenuator regulatory region comprises four basic regions. Under conditions of high product concentration (such as tryptophan), there is no slow down in translation, facilitating the formation of a stem-loop structure in the mRNA. As region 4 is followed by eight Us, resembling a prokaryotic termination signal, causing the termination of translation of this message. In contrast, under low product concentrations, the ribosome stalls because of low amounts of tryptophan-charged tRNA molecules. This allows the formation of a stem-loop between regions 2 and 3. As this is not followed by a series of eight Us, translation of the message continues. The attenuation regulatory mechanism is unique to prokaryotes.

the attenuation mechanism appears to regulate anabolic (energy requiring, biosynthetic) pathways, and this mechanism uses the presence of the end product to "turn off" synthesis.

MUTATION

Introduction to Microbial Mutations

We previously examined the structure of the bacterial chromosome and how its genetic information is expressed and regulated under normal circumstances. Let us now shift attention to how infrequent but important changes occur in the nucleotide sequence of bacterial chromosomes.

A microbial strain (also called a clone) is a population of cells that are genetically identical. Pure culture techniques are extremely important for isolation and maintenance of microbial strains. The genotype of a strain refers to the genetic characteristics of the cell regardless of whether these genes are being expressed (transcribed and translated) at any given time. The phenotype of a strain is that set of genetic characteristics that can be seen or measured; in other words, phenotypic characteristics result from those genes that are expressed in that environment. If the environment is changed, genetic regulation may (by induction or repression) change genetic expression, and thereby also change the phenotype of that strain.

Microbiologists commonly refer to a strain isolated from the environment as the wild type. In the broadest sense of the term, mutation is defined as a sudden and inheritable change in the cell's chromosome (genotype). With microorganisms, however, it is often convenient to differentiate between two types of sudden and inheritable change in the DNA: recombination, in which the change is caused by the introduction of new genes from outside the cell, and mutation, in which changes occur that are not the result of introducing new genetic material from outside the cell.

SPONTANEOUS MUTATIONS. A spontaneous mutation is one that occurs without known cause. Spontaneous mutations result most commonly from errors made while copying the DNA during chromosome replication.

The accuracy with which DNA is copied during chromosome replication is very high (errors estimated at fewer than one in every 500,000 bases copied). Therefore, the rate of error in any one gene is very small, and the frequency of spontaneous mutation is rare. But microorganisms reproduce very quickly in the laboratory, so there are many chances for errors to occur, and therefore, microbes make excellent tools for studying mutation.

For any given gene, spontaneous mutation will occur at the frequency of only about one in every 10^5 to 10^9 cells. For example, an auxotroph (nutritionally deficient) mutant may arise spontaneously in a bacterial population in one out of every 10^7 cells; therefore, only 10 of these mutants could be found in every 10^8 cells examined. From these numbers, it should be apparent that detection of spontaneous mutation in the laboratory is difficult unless selection techniques are used.

Spontaneous mutation is one mechanism associated with antibiotic resistance. For example, exposure to an antibiotic such as streptomycin would result in only the growth of those cells with the spontaneous mutation that allowed only their growth. Such a mutation could arise as a result of modification of genes coding for ribosome synthesis. Because the ribosome is the target of streptomycin activity, a structurally modified ribosome would render the antibiotic ineffective.

Whether streptomycin-resistant mutants remain at the spontaneous level depends on the presence or absence of streptomycin. Continual prophylactic or therapeutic use of any single antibiotic encourages the selection of spontaneous mutants that are resistant to that antibiotic. The predominance of these mutants in the environment drastically decreases the effectiveness of this antibiotic in combating future infections.

Spontaneous mutation frequencies vary for different genes and also for the same gene in different microbial species. It is also important to realize that the frequency of spontaneous mutation for each gene is independent of all others. Thus, if the frequency of spontaneous mutation to streptomycin resistance in a bacterial strain is one in every 10^7, and the frequency of spontaneous mutation to penicillin resistance in that same strain is one in every 10^5 cells, then the frequency of mutation of two genes in the same cell (allowing both streptomycin and penicillin resistance) is the product of the two, or one in every 10^{12} cells. This is the reason that combined antibiotic therapy is often preferred.

INDUCED MUTATIONS. Induced mutations are the result of exposure to a chemical or physical agents, called mutagens. The most noticeable factor associated with induced mutations is that the frequency of mutation is considerably higher than the spontaneous mutation rate for that particular strain of microorganisms.

Molecular Mechanisms of Mutagenesis

Mutations result from alteration in the nucleotide base sequences of the cell's genes (DNA). There are two mechanisms that describe many (if not most) mutations: point mutations and insertion/deletion mutations.

POINT MUTATIONS. Point mutations result when one deoxyribonucleotide is substituted for another during DNA replication. For example, a deoxyadenosine may be inserted instead of a deoxyguanosine, and this means that adenine would replace guanine in the sequence of bases on the new DNA strand. Therefore, point mutations are alterations of only one base in the sequence of bases that make up a single structural or regulatory gene.

Whether or not a point mutation is phenotypically expressed depends on which base is substituted and where that substitution takes place on the gene. To explain this, let us consider a point mutation occurring in the DNA triplet that codes for the amino acid serine during translation. You may recall that the genetic code is redundant; for example, more than one triplet codes for the insertion of leucine during protein synthesis. If the point mutation causes a substitution that alters the DNA triplet such that the resulting mRNA codon will still code for leucine, then there will be no alteration in the amino acid sequence of the protein made by this gene. Because the same protein is made, it will function the same, and there will be no phenotypic expression of this point mutation. This is called a silent mutation, because the protein produced by that gene is identical to that made before the mutation.

Alternatively, the DNA-base substitution resulting from point mutation can alter the triplet such that the mRNA (produced during transcription) will code for the insertion of another amino acid during protein synthesis (translation). If this different amino acid is in a critical location, such as part of an enzyme's active site, then the function of that protein could be altered or even destroyed, resulting in a phenotypic change. If that protein were critical to the cell's survival, this point mutation could be lethal. However, if the substitution altered the amino acid sequence at a point on the protein not critical for its catalytic activity, then this mutation would not be phenotypically expressed. Note that this latter mutation is not silent because the amino acid sequence of the protein produced by that gene is altered.

Finally, such a substitution could occur anywhere within the protein, but the change results in a termination or stop codon, resulting in a truncated protein. This is known as a nonsense mutation. Nonsense mutations are frequently lethal to the cell.

INSERTION/DELETION MUTANTS. A deletion mutant is one in which a portion of one strand of the DNA is removed, and an insertion mutant is one in which nucleotides have been added. Anywhere from one to several hundred deoxyribonucleotides (bases) may be deleted or inserted. Deletion or insertion of a single base in a structural gene will probably result in a reading frame shift, known as a frameshift mutation. Deletion of large segments of the DNA can result in complete loss of genes.

REVERSIONS. A revertant is a strain in which a wild-type phenotypic characteristic, originally lost because of mutation, is restored regardless of the mechanism. Reversions are often called back mutations because a second mutation is required to restore the original characteristic. Many mutations are revertible, and the reversion may occur in one of several ways. For example, a back mutation may occur at the same site (or close to the same site) of the original mutation, such that a reading frame shift, originally caused by a small deletion, is corrected. Chemical or physical agents that increase the frequency of mutation (mutagens) also stimulate the frequency of reversion.

The ability to stimulate back mutation caused by mutagens has a very practical application in the use of the Ames test for determining the carcinogenic potential of chemical mutagens. The Ames test uses histidine auxotroph strains of *Salmonella typhimurium* that are very sensitive to reversion when subjected to chemical mutagens. This test is much more economical and takes far less time than using laboratory animals for initial screening of suspected carcinogens.

Mutagenesis and Carcinogenesis

It is now well known that a wide variety of chemical and physical agents induce (increase the frequency of) mutation by reacting directly with the cell's DNA. For example, some chemicals may cross-link adjacent DNA strands and cause either point mutations or deletions. Other chemicals, such as the dyes acridine orange and ethidium bromide, may insert between two base pairs during DNA replication and cause reading frameshift mutations. Physical agents (like nonionizing or ionizing radiation) may cause pyrimidine dimer formation or actually break the DNA strands. When the cell tries to repair these DNA alterations, errors may be introduced or actual deletions in the DNA strands may occur. These chemical or physical agents may increase the frequency of mutation from 10 to 100 times above the rate found with spontaneous mutation. Therefore, mutagens are frequently used in the laboratory to increase the possibility that certain mutants will be isolated.

There is good evidence that large numbers of animal cancers are caused by synthetic chemicals added to the environment. The variety of these chemicals that animals come in contact with each day is enormous. It is also important to note that good correlation exists between the mutagenic capability of a chemical and its carcinogenic ability. Therefore, laboratory procedures, like the Ames test, that assess mutagenic potential are helpful tools for screening large numbers of suspected chemical mutagens in a short period of time. It is not always true that mutagens are also carcinogens, but the correlation is quite high, and the knowledge that a chemical is mutagenic warns of a possible carcinogen. Also, if a chemical is not mutagenic for bacteria, this does not mean that it will not be carcinogenic for animals. Therefore, procedures like the Ames test should be used in conjunction with other tests for screening chemicals, and further confirmation of carcinogenic potential must be made with animal tests once the screening tests warn of the chemical's carcinogenic possibilities.

Veterinary Significance of Mutation

Even though spontaneous mutations are rare events, they may alter phenotypic characteristics that cause difficulties in identifying pathogenic microorganisms. The clinical microbiologist is very familiar with the isolation of strains that have all of the typical characteristics of a pathogen, varying perhaps in one or two. Indeed, clinical isolates commonly vary in one or more phenotypic characteristics from those described for a pathogen. It is assumed that these phenotypic variations between pathogenic strains are the result of altered environments that have allowed one or more mutants to overgrow the parental strain. A mutation may affect a wide variety of phenotypic characteristics.

One type of mutation commonly seen by the clinical microbiologist is the smooth-to-rough colony alteration. The smooth appearance of the colony is usually caused by the presence of an extracellular capsule that accumulates in the developing colony to such an extent that it makes the colony appear smooth and glistening. Smooth strains are often the more virulent strains because the presence of a capsule helps the cell resist phagocytosis; thus, it will be more evasive. Repeated cultivation on artificial media will often select for mutants that lack capsules and that appear dry and granular or rough. These rough strains are usually less virulent (pathogenic) than the smooth strains. However, when rough strains are placed back into the animal, the nonencapsulated cells are engulfed by phagocytes, and only the encapsulated mutants survive if present. Hence, animal passage selects for growth of encapsulated mutants, and this may result in the apparent restoration of a smooth strain. Some forms of antibiotic resistance occur in a similar fashion.

GLOSSARY

cytosol Fluid portion of cytoplasm that contains the organelles of a eukaryotic cell.

introns Portion of a gene that does not encode any part of the final gene and is removed by the process of splicing.

kilobase (kb) Measure of the length of a nucleic acid strand equal to 1000 nucleotides.

megabase (Mb) One million nucleotide bases.

primer Short, single-stranded oligonucleotide that anneals to a specific region on a RNA or DNA strand and that is employed by a polymerase as the location to begin synthesis of a complementary nucleotide strand.

5 Genetic Transfer, Recombination, and Genetic Engineering

In this chapter, we examine the events associated with the movement of genetic information between microorganisms. If the genetic information is moved from parent cells to daughter cells, it is known as vertical gene transfer. This occurs during the process of binary fission in microorganisms. However, if organisms are able to move genetic information from one cell to another (not an offspring), this is known as horizontal gene transfer. An example would be the transfer of a plasmid from one bacterial cell to another bacterial cell that did not previously contain the plasmid. These events are far-reaching with regard to our society, including human and veterinary medicine. They account for the transfer of antibiotic resistance genes and toxin genes and are exploited preferentially to "engineer" the manufacture of desired products or processes.

BASIC MECHANISMS OF GENE TRANSFER

There are three basic mechanisms of gene transfer between microorganisms: transformation, transduction, and conjugation. When the result of this genetic transfer is the integration of the DNA from two different cells, the resulting DNA is referred to as recombinant DNA and the resulting organism a recombinant. Recombination in bacteria involves the insertion of a genetically different piece of DNA from a donor cell into a recipient cell. Often, but not always, this foreign piece of DNA is inserted into the chromosome of the recipient cell and replicated along with the recipient's own chromosome, and the foreign genes are phenotypically expressed.

Transformation

Of the three known recombination mechanisms, transformation is the only one that appears to have evolved solely for the purpose of exchanging chromosomal DNA between bacterial cells. The other two accomplish an exchange of chromosomal DNA only as a consequence of errors in phage replication (transduction) or plasmid transfer (conjugation).

For transformation to take place, two things are essential: an appropriate source of free DNA (from a donor strain) and competent recipient cells. The long, continu-

ously closed, supercoiled, helix of double-stranded DNA (dsDNA) that serves as the chromosome within the bacterial cell does not stay in that form when the cell is lysed. Even with gentle lysis under laboratory conditions, the chromosome easily will break into 100 or more pieces. A competent cell will usually incorporate only a few of these DNA fragments, so that only a small portion of genes from a donor cell can be transferred to another cell by transformation. Competence in a cell is assessed by the recipient cell's ability to bind the DNA, translocate the DNA across the cell wall and plasma membrane, and ultimately integrate the DNA into its own chromosome.

NATURAL COMPETENCE AND TRANSFORMATION. Unaltered cells (recipients) that can take up free DNA fragments and be genetically altered (transformed) are said to be naturally competent. As will be discussed later, it is possible to force some cells to be competent by treating them with high concentrations of calcium ions and subjecting them to temperature shocks to increase the permeability of their wall and plasma membrane. This latter situation is part of a laboratory technique referred to as artificial transformation.

Natural transformation has been described with some gram-positive bacteria, including *Streptococcus pneumoniae*, *Streptococcus sanguis*, *Bacillus subtilis*, *Bacillus cereus*, and *Bacillus stearothermophilus*, as well as several gram-negative genera including *Neisseria*, *Acinetobacter*, *Moraxella*, *Haemophilus*, and *Pseudomonas*. The discovery of transformation involved the bacterium *S. pneumoniae* and was described in 1928 by Frederick Griffiths. One strain of this species was encapsulated (smooth) and virulent, and the other strain of the same species lacked the genetic information needed to produce a capsule (rough) and was avirulent. When heat-killed cells of the smooth strain were mixed with live rough cells and injected into mice, the mice died of pneumonia. When the bacteria were isolated from the dead mice, they were found to be of the smooth phenotype. We now know that DNA containing genes for capsule production were released from the heat-killed cells and that this DNA transformed competent cells in the live rough culture, changing the phenotype of the strain from rough to smooth and also increasing the virulence of the strain by its ability to produce a capsule.

Natural competence is affected by the physiologic state of the cells and the composition of the growth medium. For example, in the laboratory, the proportion of competent cells in a population of *S. pneumoniae* rises dramatically during the middle of exponential growth, then falls just as dramatically shortly thereafter. During the brief period when a large number of cells are competent, each competent cell produces and excretes a few molecules of a soluble protein called a competence factor, inducing cells to make about eight to 10 new proteins. During this period, the outer surface of the competent cells seems to change, so that dsDNA can bind at specific sites. When this excreted protein is added to noncompetent cells (of the same strain), these cells, too, become competent. These soluble protein competence factors have only been shown in gram-positive bacteria to date.

UPTAKE OF DONOR DNA BY COMPETENT CELLS. The dsDNA first binds to specific proteins on the surface of competent cells. In the case of the gram-positive bacterium *S. pneumoniae*, there are about 30–80 sites per cell, and only dsDNA will bind to these sites. Shortly after binding, one of the dsDNA strands is degraded by a cell-surface bound enzyme. The resulting single-stranded DNA (ssDNA) is then coated by a single, small–molecular weight polypeptide, and this complex enters the cell by an unknown mechanism.

In the case of the gram-negative *Haemophilus* and *Neisseria* species studied, dsDNA is not degraded to ssDNA before it enters the cell.

INTEGRATION OF DONOR ssDNA INTO THE CHROMOSOME. Once inside the cell, the donor ssDNA from *S. pneumoniae* tries to form base pairs with a homologous region on the host cell's chromosome. Once found, one strand of the host's dsDNA is opened up with an enzyme called an endonuclease, the dsDNA is unwound for a short distance, the opposite end of the host DNA (corresponding to the opposite end of the new donor DNA) is also cut with an endonuclease, the new donor strand is inserted, and enzymes called DNA ligases fuse both ends of the donor ssDNA with the adjacent host chromosomal DNA strand. As you might expect, many things can go wrong with this process, and thus the efficiency of natural transformation is usually quite low (from 0.1% to 1.0% of all cells present).

In the case of the gram-negative *Haemophilus* and *Neisseria* species studied, the dsDNA that enters the cell is closely associated with the host cell's chromosome before one strand is degraded. No free ssDNA intermediates seem to exist within the cell before incorporation of the donor DNA into the host chromosome. Once again, no single general mechanism appears to account for the way in which the transformed DNA is incorporated into the host chromosome in all bacteria. Interestingly, in the case of *Haemophilus*, only dsDNA of another *Haemophilus* species will be integrated into the genome.

ARTIFICIAL TRANSFORMATIONS. Many bacteria (including *Escherichia coli*) appear not to have evolved natural mechanisms for transformation, and attempts to emulate true transformation of open strands of ssDNA or dsDNA into the potential recipient cell's chromosome have generally failed. There seems to be no trouble in getting the linear pieces of ssDNA or dsDNA into the cell, but once inside, these DNA strands seem to be quickly destroyed by the host cell's own nucleases before they can be integrated into the chromosome.

In contrast, free, self-replicating forms of covalently closed strands of DNA (like plasmids and viral genomes) can be forced inside normally incompetent cells (e.g., by subjecting the cells to abnormally high concentrations of calcium ions at low temperatures, by **electroporation**, or with the use of **gene guns**), and the frequency of transformants in the survivors is high (about 20%). Apparently, these covalently closed circular forms of DNA are not attacked by the recipient cell's intracellular nucleases. The calcium and cold-shock treatment or electroporation are the most common methods for getting DNA into cells, but a freeze–thaw technique and treatment of protoplasts with polyethylene glycol also have been successfully used with some bacteria. Essentially, all of these techniques work by temporarily compromising the integrity of the cell wall and cell membrane in such a manner that transient pores are formed, allowing entry of the DNA into the host cell.

VIRAL LIFE CYCLES

To properly look at transduction, one must look at the life cycles of viruses in general. All viral life cycles, including that of bacteriophage, have four primary phases.

The first phase is attachment. The virus must interact with receptors on the surface of a target cell to gain entry. If these receptors are not present or are mutated in some form, then attachment, and ultimately infection, of that cell does not occur.

The second phase is penetration. This typically refers to the penetration of the virus genome into the target cell once attachment is complete. This allows entry of the virus genome into the cytoplasm of the target (now host) cell.

The phase following penetration is that of viral protein manufacture and assembly. Essentially, the viral genome allows for the host cell to become a virus "parts factory," dedicating the host cell specifically to this task. The timing of the third phase is dependent upon the life cycle of the individual virus.

The final phase of the life cycle is that of lysis. This is lysis of the host cell to allow release of the newly synthesized virus particles to infect new cells.

The portion of the life cycle that varies is what happens to the viral genetic information once penetration is complete. If the material remains in the cytoplasm of the host cell and is used very soon following entry to the cell, the life cycle is called the lytic cycle. Conversely, if the viral genome is integrated into the host cell genome and "activated" to a lytic cycle after a prolonged period of time, the life cycle is referred to as lysogeny. This is typically accomplished by lysogenic or temperate phages.

Transduction

Transduction is defined as the transfer of host genes between bacterial strains by bacterial viruses (called **bacteriophages** or simply **phages**). In the transfer of genetic material, transduction accomplishes the same function as transformation. Transduction appears to result from errors that occur during the replication of the virus. Although most commonly studied in *E. coli*, transduction has been demonstrated in a wide variety of bacteria, and it probably occurs widely in nature. In addition, some of these viruses contain bacterial genes, along with viral genes, resulting in new phenotypes expressed by infected cells.

During the assembly step in phage development, an occasional phage particle becomes filled with host chromosomal DNA or a mixture of both host and phage DNA rather than being filled only with phage DNA (Fig. 5.1). The resulting aberrant phage is often called a transducing phage or a transducing particle. It is a defective phage be-

cause it never seems to cause subsequent lysis of the newly infected host. After the transducing particle is absorbed to a new host, the phage DNA or donor-host DNA (or both) penetrate the cell wall and plasma membrane. The addition of donor-host DNA to the newly infected host's chromosome and the phenotypic expression of these new genes constitute completion of the transduction event.

Two types of errors in phage development lead to two types of transduction. The difference between these two types apparently depends on the site at which the phage genome is integrated into the chromosome of the host. The two types of transduction are specialized transduction and generalized transduction.

SPECIALIZED TRANSDUCTION. With specialized transduction, only a few host genes are transferred, and they are the same genes each time. Specialized transduction often occurs with a defective **temperate phage** (one

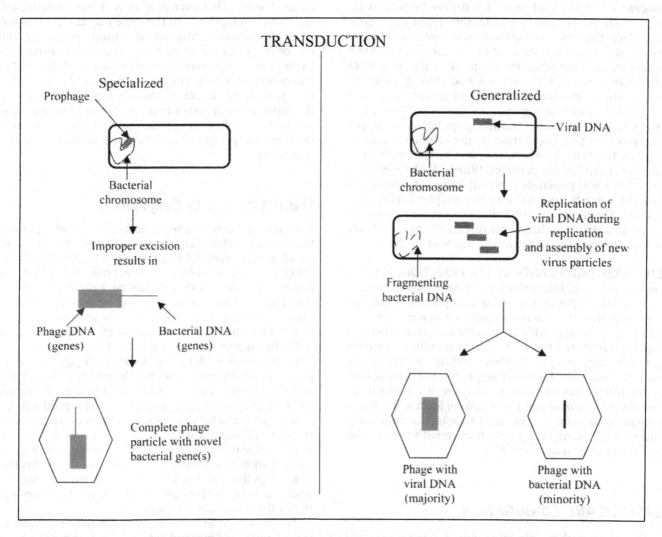

FIGURE 5.1   Comparison of specialized and generalized transduction. In specialized transduction, as incorporation of the prophage occurs at the same site in the bacterial genome, the bacterial gene(s) neighboring the prophage can be excised and packaged into the resulting phage particle. In generalized transduction, as the result of fragmentation of the bacterial chromosome during viral assembly, bacterial deoxyribonucleic acid of the proper size is packaged into the minority of capsids.

whose DNA is integrated into the host genome), specifically, those phages whose genomes always integrate into the host cell's chromosome at one specific site (Fig. 5.1).

The error occurs when something triggers (induces) the defective **prophage** to complete its replication cycle. Normally when this happens, only the prophage is cut from the chromosome and replicated. However, during specialized transduction, an error occurs during excision such that part of the adjacent bacterial chromosome is removed, along with part or all of the prophage.

GENERALIZED TRANSDUCTION.   With generalized transduction, almost any gene on the chromosome may be transferred from donor to recipient, but the frequency of transfer is often very low. For example, generalized transduction of genes from *Salmonella typhimurium* infected by phage P22 are usually about one in every 10^5 to 10^9 infected cells.

Unlike specialized transduction, generalized transduction seems to occur with either temperate or **lytic phages**. When a population of sensitive bacteria is infected with phage and the complete replication cycle takes place, the host DNA often breaks down into phage-genome sized pieces. If some of these chromosomal DNA pieces contain host DNA, then a piece of this host DNA may be incorporated inside a **capsid** during phage assembly. These defective particles are released along with the normal phage during lysis of the host. When this **lysate** is used to infect another population of similar cells, most of this population is infected with normal phage. A few cells, however, may be infected with these defective (transducing) particles. When that happens, the donor DNA will penetrate the recipient host, and donor DNA may then be inserted into the recipient cell's chromosome. The reason for the low transduction frequencies that occur with generalized transducing phage is probably the low numbers of phage containing host DNA.

VETERINARY SIGNIFICANCE OF TRANSDUCTION.   From a veterinary standpoint, perhaps the greatest significance of transduction is the ability of bacteriophages to transfer genes that allow for the bacterium to become more virulent or more invasive within the infected tissue. Examples of genes transferred from virulent to nonvirulent strains by transducing phage are those coding for botulinum toxin by *Clostridium botulinum* (types C and D), those coding for production of alpha-hemolysin or endotoxin by *Staphylococcus aureus*, and those coding for hyaluronidase in *Streptococcus equi*. At present, it appears that antibiotic-resistance genes are only rarely transferred to antibiotic-sensitive cells by transduction.

PLASMIDS AND CONJUGATION

As described earlier, plasmids are extrachromosomal pieces of DNA that store genetic information that may be phenotypically expressed. However, plasmids do not typically carry genes for essential metabolic activities; instead, the plasmid genes are for other, more specialized features. For example, plasmids may carry genes for the ability to mate and serve as a donor for genetic exchange; to be resistant to chemicals, such as heavy metals, that are normally toxic to microorganisms; and to degrade complex organic chemicals, such as aromatic hydrocarbons found in petroleum. Plasmids have veterinary significance, because some pathogens can transfer genes that code for virulence to normally nonpathogenic strains.

Plasmid Biology

Plasmids are typically covalently closed, circular, double-stranded molecules of DNA that probably exist inside the cell in a supercoiled state and seem to be present in almost all bacteria examined. However, the plasmids of some groups, such as *Borrelia* species, are linear DNA. Plasmids are usually less than one two-hundredth the size of the bacterial chromosome, although wide variation in plasmid sizes exists even within a single bacterial cell. Plasmid DNA replicates in the same way as chromosomal DNA; this involves initiation at a single point and bidirectional replication of each separate strand around the circle. However, plasmid and chromosomal DNA replicate independently of one another, and plasmid DNA replication is probably under a different type of control. Furthermore, there are often multiple copies of each plasmid in a bacterial cell, although the copy number seems to depend on the type of cell and the environment in which it is growing.

Plasmid Transfer by Conjugation

Conjugation between similar bacteria is a mating process that requires cell-to-cell contact and that results in transfer of genetic material from one cell (the donor) to another cell (the recipient), as illustrated in Fig. 5.2. The genetic material transferred may be a plasmid or part of the donor's chromosome that has been mobilized by a plasmid. Most of what is currently known about conjugation comes from studies of gram-negative bacteria, so the following applies only to this type of bacterial cell.

Cells capable of donating DNA via conjugation carry a plasmid that (in part) codes for the ability to be a donor, and this is called a conjugative plasmid. In gram-negative bacteria, the conjugative plasmid codes for production of a "sex" pilus and for some other proteins needed for DNA transfer. Although it is not clearly understood, it appears that the distal end of the sex pilus on the donor makes contact with an appropriate recipient cell. The pilus then retracts, pulling the two cells together until a conjugation bridge is formed, through which the DNA can pass between the donor and recipient cells.

For DNA transfer to occur, DNA synthesis must also occur. Current evidence indicates that this synthesis occurs at or near the conjugation bridge and that one of the DNA strands inserted into the recipient cell is from the donor and the other is newly made (Fig. 5.2). The "rolling circle"

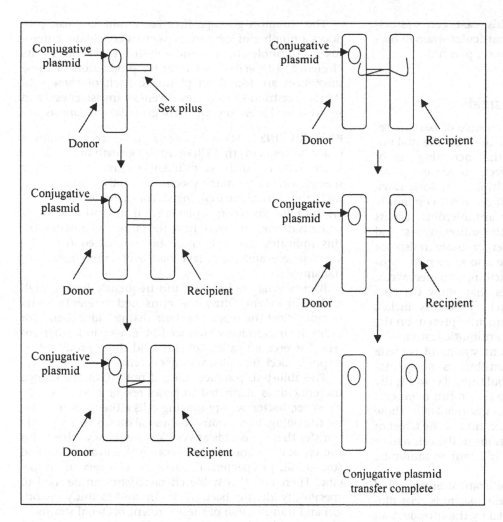

FIGURE 5.2 Gram-negative bacterial conjugation. The donor cell (containing the conjugative plasmid) attaches to the recipient cell via a sex pilus. The donor possesses the pilus, while the recipient possesses an attachment site for the pilus. Once the cells are attached, a single-stranded copy of the plasmid is transferred from the donor to the recipient. Following transfer, both cells replicate the plasmid to a double-stranded molecule. As both cells now contain a conjugative plasmid, they can no longer exchange DNA via conjugation. However, both are available to exchange information with other recipient cells.

model seems to best explain how this is accomplished. Initiation of plasmid DNA synthesis may be triggered by cell-to-cell contact, and this may open one strand on the donor's plasmid. As this opened strand (the 5' end) passes through the conjugation bridge, DNA synthesis simultaneously occurs at two places: along the newly unraveled strand, and along the closed complementary strand of the original plasmid. Once the new plasmid is made and fully transferred into the recipient cell, it is covalently closed (circularized) and supercoiled. With this mechanism, the donor cell duplicates its plasmid at the same time transfer occurs, so both the donor and recipient eventually have a complete copy of this plasmid.

Conjugative plasmids may contain not only genes that allow for conjugation to take place but other types of genetic information as well. Thus, each cell that receives a conjugative plasmid during conjugation not only becomes capable of donating genetic material but may also receive other genes (such as those that code for antibiotic resistance). This process is so efficient that almost every cell that forms a conjugating pair will acquire new genetic information, and this (along with indiscriminate use of antibiotics) helps to explain how bacterial populations can become resistant to antibiotics with such speed. Under proper conditions, the rate of spread of a conjugative

plasmid through bacterial culture can be exponential and resemble a bacterial growth curve.

Conjugative transfer of plasmids may occur between two strains of the same species, such as between a chloramphenicol-resistant strain of *E. coli* and a chloramphenicol-sensitive strain. Plasmids may also be transferred among different but related bacteria, such as those within the family Enterobacteriaceae (from *E. coli* to strains of *Shigella* or *Salmonella*).

Studies of conjugation in *Enterococcus faecalis* suggest that the mechanism of conjugation in gram-positive bacteria is different from that of the well-studied gram-negative bacteria. For example, conjugation between strains of *E. faecalis* does not require a sex pilus. Instead, potential recipient cells release soluble molecules (called **pheromones**), which stimulate plasmid-containing cells to produce a substance on their outer surface that allows donor and recipient cells to aggregate. It appears that plasmids are transferred from cell to cell within these aggregates.

There are various types of plasmids that may be transferred between cells, and these are often classified on the basis of the genes that the plasmid possesses. For example, the genes associated with the formation of a sex pilus are contained on F (fertility) plasmids. Plasmids with genes associated with heavy metal or antibiotic resistance are contained on R (resistance) plasmids. Last, genes associated with enhanced virulence of a particular strain of bacteria can be located on a Vir (virulence) plasmid.

Veterinary Significance of Plasmids

ANTIBIOTIC RESISTANCE. The emergence of bacteria resistant to several antibiotics is of considerable medical importance and is correlated with the increasing use of antibiotics for the treatment of infectious diseases. A variety of R plasmids can carry multiple antibiotic resistance genes on a single plasmid. Those most commonly observed carry resistance to four antimicrobial agents (chloramphenicol, streptomycin, the sulfonamides, and tetracycline), but some have fewer or more resistance genes on one plasmid. Plasmids are also known to transmit resistance to kanamycin, penicillin, and neomycin. Some plasmids also contain genes that allow the bacterium to be resistant to metals such as mercury, nickel, and cobalt, and these genes are frequently present on the same plasmids that carry genes for antibiotic resistance.

In some cases, antibiotic-resistant strains of bacteria arise by continual exposure to antibiotics or spontaneously arise within a bacterial population. Typically, the generation of antibiotic-resistant strains in this manner is the result of mutations within chromosomal DNA. These mutations often result in the modification of the target of antibiotic action, such as modifications in the cell wall or ribosome that make the mutants resistant to antibiotic attack.

However, the majority of drug-resistant strains isolated from patients contain drug-resistant plasmids. Plasmid-mediated resistance is usually caused by the introduction of new genes that code for the production of new enzymes that inactivate the drug itself. For example, cells having resistance to the aminoglycoside antibiotics (kanamycin, neomycin, streptomycin, and spectinomycin) make an enzyme that chemically modifies the antibiotic (by acetylation, adenylation, or phosphorylation), and as a result, the modified drug lacks antibiotic activity. In penicillin resistance, the plasmid codes for the production of penicillinase (a β-lactamase), an enzyme that cleaves the β-lactam ring of the penicillin molecule, thus rendering it inactive. In the case of chloramphenicol resistance, a gene on the plasmid codes for an enzyme that acetylates the antibiotic, thereby destroying its antibacterial activity.

TOXINS AND OTHER VIRULENCE FACTORS. Research with the gram-negative, enteropathogenic *E. coli* indicates that the ability of pathogenic bacteria to attach and grow at a specific site in the host and to produce toxins may be carried by genes on a plasmid. Specific recognition and attachment of *E. coli* to the epithelial lining of the intestine require that this bacterium produce a protein on its surface. In addition, the synthesis of two toxins (a hemolysin and an enterotoxin) is coded for by plasmid genes. At present, it is not clear why these virulence factors are plasmid coded and why others reside on the chromosome, nor is it understood how many other virulence factors are plasmid-related among the gram-negative bacteria.

The common gram-positive bacterium *S. aureus* produces a number of substances, such as coagulase, enterotoxin, fibrinolysin, and hemolysin, that add to its virulence. The genes that code for production of these substances are found on plasmids. Each of these substances contributes to the evasiveness, invasiveness, and survival, and therefore the pathogenicity, of *S. aureus*.

BACTERIOCINS. Many bacteria produce substances called bacteriocins that kill or inhibit growth of closely related bacteria, such as different strains of the same species. This very limited spectrum of activity can be useful to the clinical microbiologist. For example, if all of the *Proteus mirabilis* strains isolated from surgical wounds of patients in the same ward have the same bacteriocin type, this indicates that they probably originated from the same source and may have had a common means of transmission.

Bacteriocins are proteins and frequently have a high molecular weight. Often, the terms used to refer to bacteriocins reflect the type of bacteria that produce them. For example, bacteriocins produced by *E. coli* and other enteric bacteria are called colicins, and those produced by staphylococci are called staphylococcins.

The ability to produce most, if not all, of the known bacteriocins is attributed to genes residing on plasmids. However, bacteriocin-producing cells either lack the ability to conjugatively transfer these plasmids or they only transfer these plasmids at very low frequency. This helps the clinical microbiologist, because the production and susceptibility of bacteria to bacteriocins is very strain specific. Therefore, this stable characteristic can be used to specifically identify bacterial strains and to study the origin and transmission of these virulent bacterial strains.

TRANSPOSONS. Originally described by Barbara McClintock, transposons are mobile genetic elements that are capable of "moving" from one genetic location to another. The basic structure of a transposon includes an insertion sequence; a gene encoding an enzyme known as transposase to mediate the insertion of the element into either plasmid or chromosomal DNA; and at either end of the transposon, sections known as inverted repeats (9–41 nucleotides in length). To move itself, the sequence of the genetic element must copy itself using transposase and other host cellular enzymes. This copy will insert itself to another location within the genome in an essentially random manner. Note that the original copy remains in its original location. Sometimes, transposons include chromosomal genes in addition to those associated with transposition. These can include antibiotic resistance genes. Furthermore, viruses and plasmids are efficient vectors for the movement of transposons from one cell to another. In this manner, transposons can integrate within genes, disrupting their function and creating mutation or moving new genetic material into a cell.

GENETIC ENGINEERING AND BIOTECHNOLOGY

Genetic engineering refers to the application of basic principles of microbial genetics in the isolation, manipulation, and expression of genetic material. At present, genetically engineered bacteria are used in two rather different ways: to increase the quantity of microbial products, and to express inserted genes of animal or plant origin such that the bacterial cell produces a protein normally produced only by an animal or plant cell.

Increasing the Quantity of Microbial Products

The first and oldest application of genetic engineering uses genetic manipulation to increase the yields of desirable microbial products. This may be done by increasing the number of gene copies on the chromosome or by altering the gene such that production of the gene product is no longer tightly regulated by the cell.

Expressing Inserted Genes of Animal or Plant Origin

The second use of genetic engineering is more recent and has received more attention in the popular media. In that application, animal or plant genes are first removed from the chromosome. These genes are then inserted into a vector, such as a bacterial plasmid, and that genetically altered vector is placed back into the same bacterial cell. This altered bacterium will now produce a protein whose synthesis is directed by the animal or plant genes. Molecules of DNA that contain unrelated segments are referred to as "recombinant DNA." Hence, the phrase "recombinant DNA technology" is often used in place of "genetic engineering."

What follows is a brief introduction to the second application of genetic engineering and the ways in which genetic engineering may affect the future practicing veterinarian.

PLASMIDS AS CLONING VECTORS. The microbial geneticist frequently uses the word "clone" to refer to a population of identical bacteria having the same type of recombinant DNA. The term "cloning vector" is used to refer to the complete DNA molecule or virus that can bring about replication of a foreign DNA fragment in the cell. The "host" is the bacterium that contains the genetically reconstructed cloning vector.

A good cloning vector must have the following characteristics: first, it will self-replicate in the host; second, its DNA can be easily separated from the host and purified; and third, it must contain regions of the DNA that are not essential for vector replication and that can be removed from the vector and replaced with the foreign DNA fragment. In addition, it is very desirable that the cloning vector is a small piece of DNA that is able to enter the cell and replicate to a high copy number (many copies per cell). It is also desirable that the vector be stable in the host and that it direct a high product yield from the foreign gene. To date, the most useful cloning vectors are certain bacterial viruses and plasmids. However, the following discussion will be limited to the use of plasmids as cloning vectors.

The host for replication of the cloning vector must also be chosen with care. A desirable host is fast growing, ge-

netically stable, not pathogenic, and able to grow in an inexpensive culture medium. In addition, the desirable host must be transformable; that is, one must be able to make the potential host artificially competent so that it will take up the DNA used as the cloning vector. The methods used to accomplish the insertion of this DNA are the same as those discussed in the previous section on transformation.

Optimum expression of the foreign DNA on the cloning vector is extremely important. Therefore, the plasmid cloning vector must not only contain the proper foreign genes but should have adequate regulatory sequences, so that expression of the foreign genes is controlled. It is ideal to grow host cells to a high population density while the cloned genes on the plasmid are repressed and then add an inducer to allow maximum expression of the cloned foreign genes. For this reason, regulatory sequences are usually inserted along with and adjacent to the cloned genes. For example, constructing plasmid vectors that contain the regulatory components for the *lac* operon (promoter, regulator, and operator) to control synthesis of the foreign DNA is a common way to provide a suitable regulatory switch. When this is done, cells are grown in the absence of the inducer, which in this case is lactose (see Fig. 4.9), so that the switch regulating the adjacent foreign genes is turned off. When the cells reach maximum numbers, the inducer (lactose) is added to start expression of the foreign genes. Production of high levels of several mammalian proteins (up to 15,000 molecules of human interferon per *E. coli* cell) is achieved using this technique.

STEPS IN CONSTRUCTING A PLASMID CLONING VECTOR. The overall process of constructing a plasmid cloning vector is shown in Fig. 5.3. First, a plasmid (preferably one that already has a high copy number) is isolated from a bacterium that will later serve as an acceptable host. Cells are gently lysed, and the plasmid fraction is collected by ultracentrifugation. After separation of the various plasmids by size (molecular weight) and purification of a single plasmid type, this potential cloning vector is ready for gene manipulation. Alternatively, cloning vectors can be purchased commercially.

Second, the plasmid DNA is cut open using purified, site-specific enzymes called **restriction endonucleases**. These too may be obtained commercially.

Third, the animal or plant gene is either obtained (as shown in Fig. 5.3) or artificially constructed. If the gene is removed from the chromosome, the same types of restriction endonucleases are used, so that a similarly sized fragment is cut, having ends complementary to those on the cut plasmid. Alternatively, the eukaryotic gene may be artificially constructed in one of at least two ways: either the specific mRNA for that protein is isolated, and then an enzyme called **reverse transcriptase** is used to construct a DNA molecule from the sequence of bases on the mRNA; or with more difficulty, the desired gene product (protein) is purified, the amino acid sequence determined, an mRNA molecule constructed that will code for synthesis of this protein, and finally, reverse transcriptase used to construct the complementary DNA sequence (gene). Regardless of the method used, the foreign gene is now ready to be inserted into the cut plasmid.

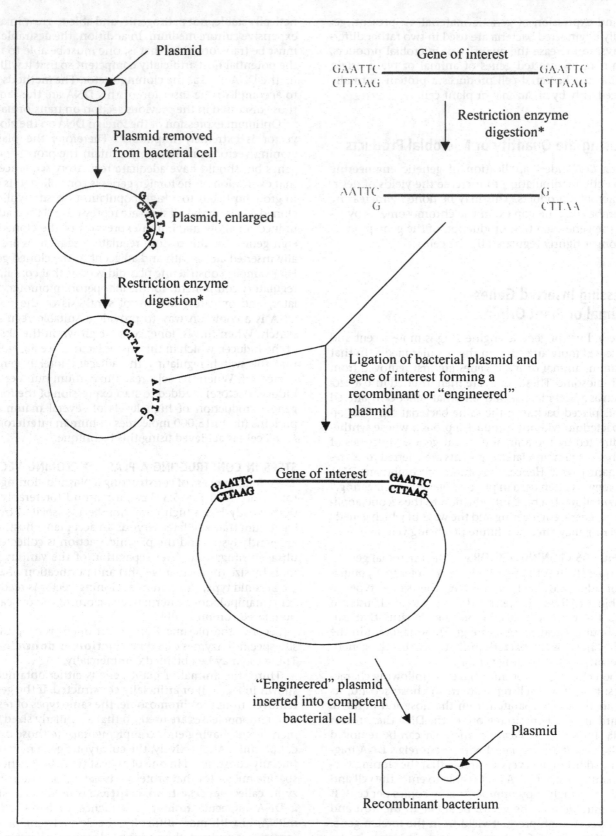

FIGURE 5.3 Steps in constructing a plasmid-cloning vector. This process is commonly called genetic engineering. An asterisk indicates that the same restriction enzyme must be used.

Fourth, the broken ends of the foreign DNA are attached to the homologous broken ends of the plasmid DNA with an enzyme called DNA ligase. This creates a recombinant plasmid that is part bacterial and part foreign (eukaryotic) DNA. Note that sometime during this process, the regulatory switch, such as that obtained from the *lac* operon, is also added to this recombinant plasmid.

Fifth, host bacteria are made artificially **competent** (by applying excessive calcium ions, by temperature-shock treatment, or by electroporation), and the DNA is forced into the cells. Unlike the transformation phenomenon, however, it appears that the entire double-stranded DNA molecule is taken in, and there is no subsequent integration into the cell's chromosome. This newly introduced, genetically engineered vector remains as an extrachromosomal self-replicating unit and now constitutes part of the host cell's genomic material. The information is now in a form that allows for vertical gene transfer.

Sixth, the host is now grown in such a way that the expression of the eukaryotic gene is regulated for maximum expression. Often, "**fusion proteins**" are made, either to make the protein more stable inside the cell, that is, to make it more resistant to the protein-degrading enzymes normally present inside the bacterial cell, or to allow the protein to be exported to the outside, where it can be more easily isolated and purified. Fusion proteins contain a short, prokaryotic, amino acid sequence at one end of the protein fused to the desired eukaryotic amino acid sequence at the other. Sometimes the intracellular accumulation of excessive quantities of fusion proteins is toxic to the cell, so additional genes must be added to the engineered plasmid to assure that this eukaryotic gene product can get out of the cell and be released into the medium. After the fusion protein is released from the cell, the prokaryotic portion may be removed and the eukaryotic part may be purified and readied for use.

Veterinary Significance of Genetically Engineered Plasmids

The potential application of genetically engineered prokaryotic cells for the production of animal proteins is staggering. Not only are these processes much less expensive and time-consuming than conventional methods of production, but the bacterially produced proteins are also easier to purify. Therefore, when administered to the animal, they cause fewer side reactions than proteins isolated from animal tissue. At present, genetically altered bacterial cells are producing human, porcine, and bovine growth hormone (for treatment of growth defects); human insulin (for the treatment of diabetes); human interferon (an antiviral agent); human serum albumin (for transfusion applications); parathyroid hormone (for calcium regulation); urokinase (for treating blood clotting disorders); and viral proteins (such as coat proteins from cytomegalovirus, hepatitis B virus, influenza virus, and foot-and-mouth disease [FMD] virus for vaccine production).

One of the most useful veterinary applications of genetically altered bacteria is the production of effective vaccine proteins. Effective vaccines may be made to protect the animal against prokaryotic, eukaryotic, or viral pathogens. For simplicity's sake, only virus vaccines will be discussed further.

Virus vaccines for animal use commonly contain either killed or live attenuated virus. With both types, there is a danger that the vaccine may contain virulent virus particles. This danger is the result of incompletely killed virus in a "killed" vaccine preparation or the reversion of some of the attenuated virus particles to a virulent state. In contrast, genetically engineered vaccines may contain only viral coat (capsid) proteins that serve as antigens to stimulate the immune response. Thus, it is desirable to produce the viral coat protein and use only this as the vaccine, so that the potentially dangerous use of live or killed suspensions may be avoided. Safe vaccines composed only of viral coat protein can be made by genetically altered bacteria that have been "engineered" to produce the viral coat protein. In general, viral DNA is isolated from purified viral suspensions and then fragmented with endonucleases. The fragments are then inserted into an appropriate vector (usually a plasmid) using DNA ligases, and the recombinant plasmid is artificially transferred into the host bacterium. The purified protein produced by these bacteria is then used as a vaccine.

In 1981, the U.S. Department of Agriculture announced the first vaccine produced by genetically altered bacteria (*E. coli*); this was the capsid protein for the virus causing FMD of cattle, sheep, hogs, and other animals. Although strict vigilance has prevented an outbreak in the U.S. since 1929, the disease is still a serious problem in Asia, Africa, South America, and southern Europe. The vaccines in use before the development of the *E. coli*–produced vaccine presented many problems. For example, the older vaccines had to be refrigerated, which presented problems with their use in developing countries. Also, each older vaccine protected against only one type of virus. Because the virus readily mutates, the usefulness of any one vaccine was limited. Nevertheless, an estimated 500 million doses were administered annually, which made it the most widely used antiviral vaccine.

From FMD data made available in 1981, it appears that the capsid protein was first made inside the genetically altered bacterial cell as a fusion protein that contained about equal parts of viral and bacterial protein. This fusion protein could be physically removed from the bacterial cell and cleaved by cyanogen bromide. This treatment released a small–molecular weight polypeptide (capsid protein) that protected steers from challenge with virulent FMD virus. The fusion protein was produced in large quantity by the genetically altered *E. coli* (about 10^6 molecules per cell).

Because of the economic advantages of using bacteria to produce pure viral proteins and the safety value of avoiding attenuated viral strains for vaccines, one might logically expect that genetically altered bacterial strains will soon be producing many other vaccines for veterinary use. It is also likely that proteins of animal origin will soon be produced for therapeutic use in domestic animals, as is now being done for use with humans.

TRANSGENIC ANIMALS. Similar techniques for the formation and insertion of recombinant DNA into bacteria can also be used in eukaryotic cells. Current research is investigating the use of animals, such as pigs, to express human proteins. These animals, although correctly called recombinants, have taken on the name transgenic. In some cases, eukaryotic genes expressed in bacteria (such as *E. coli*) do not yield an active protein. The reason for this is that some proteins need to undergo posttranslational processing (phosphorylation, glycosylation, acetylation, etc.) before they are active. Bacteria are generally unable to recognize the eukaryotic signals on the proteins, indicating modification sites. As a result, an inactive protein is made, even though the amino acid sequence of the protein is correct. To counter this problem, some eukaryotic genes, including some human genes, have been introduced into farm animals. Typically, these proteins are designed such that they are expressed in the mammary glands of the animals, so that the properly modified protein can be isolated from milk and be used as a pharmaceutical. For example, the genes for two different human blood clotting factors (VIII and IX) have been inserted into sheep and swine and expressed in mammary tissue, and the milk of these animals, containing vast quantities of human blood-clotting factors, has been purified and marketed.

POLYMERASE CHAIN REACTION

One of the most widely used DNA tools today is the polymerase chain reaction, or PCR. Discovered in 1985 by Cary Mullis, this technique capitalizes on DNA replication with a thermostable DNA polymerase that does not denature at 94°C, the temperature required to separate or melt the DNA strands. Essentially, large quantities of DNA are sometimes required for various DNA-based test procedures. Although cloning can increase the numbers of copies, it is not always practical in a variety of situations, such as when attempting to identify a corpse or a perpetrator of a crime.

An exploitation of DNA replication, PCR is basically artificial replication. It requires a DNA template (or source), deoxynucleotides, short pieces of DNA known as primers, a thermostable DNA polymerase (such as the one isolated from *Thermus aquaticus*, called *Taq* polymerase), and a machine known as a thermocycler that can change temperatures repeatedly. All the aforementioned ingredients are mixed together and placed in the thermocycler to undergo temperature cycling.

The initial phase of the cycle is heating at 94°C, which breaks the hydrogen bonds between the bases of the dsDNA making ssDNA (strand melting). The second phase is the decrease in temperature, typically to 60°C or less, which allows for the primers to bind the template DNA. This is known as annealing. The final phase of the cycle is an increase to 72°C, which is the optimum temperature for *Taq* polymerase activity.

These three phases make up what is called a cycle. When using PCR, the amplification (increase in numbers of copies of DNA) typically requires 35–40 cycles. Theoretically, a single copy of original DNA could result in millions of copies using this procedure.

The power of the procedure is the selection of the primers that one uses. For instance, in wanting specific identification of *Borrelia burgdorferi*—the causative agent of Lyme disease—one would want primers that annealed (complementary binding) specifically with *B. burgdorferi* and not other bacteria. Therefore, the primers would need to be designed to target amplification of a gene unique to *B. burgdorferi* to indicate its presence. In contrast, if you wanted to amplify all mammoth DNA from amber-bound mosquitoes, you would not want to target a specific region but, rather, random regions for amplification. One could later perform other tasks, such as DNA sequencing or even cloning, from these generated DNA fragments.

The primers also "define" the length of DNA produced by PCR, so scientists typically refer to, for example, a PCR product of 500 nucleotides in length. This means that from 5' to 3', including the primer lengths, is 500 nucleotides. As a fragment of this size becomes the greater in number with each successive cycle, when examined by gel electrophoresis, this is typically the only band observed. Figure 5.4 illustrates the process of PCR and the generation of specific product. Also shown is an example of a PCR product.

There are many variations of the "classical" PCR that have been developed for use. One example is RT-PCR (reverse transcriptase). This variation allows for the generation of DNA PCR products from RNA templates by using the viral enzyme reverse transcriptase. A second variation is consensus-PCR. In consensus-PCR, primers are designed to anneal at known regions that are conserved within a particular group of bacteria. The region amplified by PCR between two consensus regions is sequenced and differences are determined.

A technique similar to consensus-PCR is representational difference analysis, or RDA. RDA was described in 1993 and is used to detect differences between two complex sets of genomes. Its basis is to compare a baseline gene with one that is believed to be altered and to look at the DNA sequence differences between the two. Typically, the two genomes are from "normal" and "diseased" individuals. For example, the sequence for the human herpesvirus 8 was detected in Kaposi's sarcoma individuals by this technique. In addition, this technique can detect genetic changes associated with development, deletions, and rearrangements that may be associated with particular disorders.

PCR-based technologies are currently being designed specifically for use in the veterinary diagnostic laboratory. Such methodology will allow practitioners to identify diseases, such as that caused by the feline immunodeficiency virus (FIV), within 30 minutes.

DNA MICROARRAYS/DNA CHIPS

This technique involves the placement of oligonucleotide sequences of the genome of a microorganism in an array (typically 80 × 80) on a glass slide (other support sub-

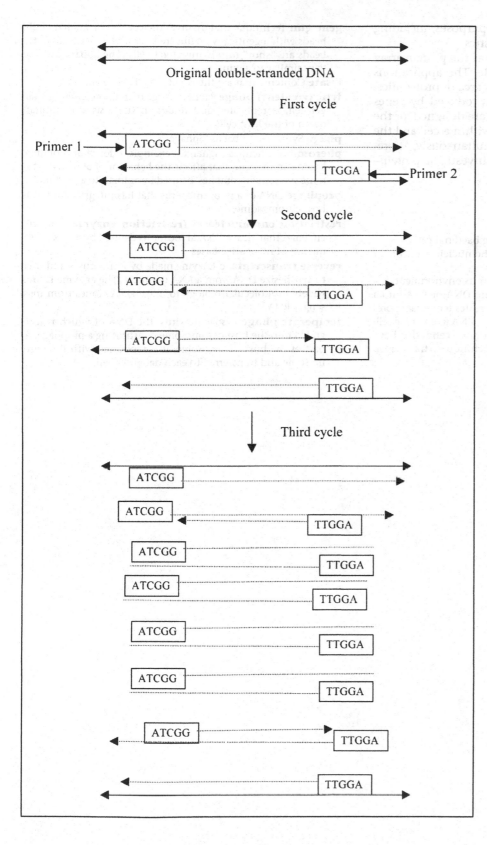

FIGURE 5.4   Diagram of the polymerase chain reaction through three cycles of the procedure. Note that following 30–35 cycles, the predominant one will be the short product.

stances can be used as well) or, alternatively, a silica chip. This technique is typically used to identify genes that have been induced or that are being produced at any time.

The basic principle of DNA microarrays is hybridization of complementary base pairs. Regions showing hy-

bridization are revealed by a laser and analyzed by computer software. The two major applications of the technique are sequence identification and expression level (number of copies of RNA) of a particular gene in a cell. Several companies distribute commercially available DNA microarrays for a variety of different purposes, including novel gene identification and diagnostics.

Recently, a new microarray known as the protein array or protein chips has become available. The applications for protein arrays are those of the new area of proteomics. Proteomics is the study of proteins produced by genes identified in genomics. Protein arrays are designed for the quantification of expressed proteins within a cell and the functional study of many proteins simultaneously. At present, protein arrays are being used to investigate protein–ligand interactions.

GLOSSARY

bacteriophage Virus capable of infecting bacterial cells.

capsid The protein coat that surrounds the nucleic acid core of a virus particle.

competent Cell able to take up DNA from its environment.

electroporation Technique for introducing DNA or RNA into a cell, using a pulsed electric field, which creates temporary pores in the cell membrane, allowing the DNA or RNA to enter the cell.

fusion protein Protein that is the result of two genes that have been put together via recombinant techniques, transcribed into mRNA, and then translated.

gene gun Technique that involves the coating of small metallic beads with a gentically engineered plasmid. Once coated, the beads are "shot" into living target cells. The apparatus looks very similar to a gun.

lysate Contents that are the result of lysis of a cell.

lytic (virulent) phage Bacteriophage that, upon entering a target cell, is replicated and results in the lysis and ultimate death of the host cell.

phage Synonym of bacteriophage.

pheromone Chemical signal, for example, odor, that is omitted by one animal and that affects the behavior of animals of the same species. Pheromones are used by animals to attract mates.

prophage DNA of a lysogenic virus that has integrated into the host chromosome.

restriction endonucleases (restriction enzyme) Bacterial enzymes that cleave DNA at locations defined by a specific sequence of nucleotide bases.

reverse transcriptase Enzyme made by retroviruses and used to synthesize DNA from a RNA template. The enzyme is used widely in molecular biology to make DNA clones from messenger RNA.

temperate phage Lysogenic virus, the DNA of which is integrated into the host chromosome constituting a prophage. As part of the host chromosome, it is replicated with the chromosome and transferred to each daughter cell.

6 Sources and Transmission of Infectious Agents

The microorganisms causing diseases in animals (including humans) are derived from the following sources: animals (including humans)—by far the most important source—and inanimate nature—relatively less important sources.

The various organisms that can cause disease have natural habitats to which they are well adapted. Most organisms that have the potential to cause disease in animals are associated with those animals. Some organisms will usually only grow and multiply in certain host species. Some disease-causing organisms are transmissible from animals to humans and vice versa.

There are a large number of microorganisms living in water, soil, and decaying vegetation. The great majority of these are incapable of causing disease in animals, but a few have the capacity to grow and multiply in animal tissue. Some only cause disease when the host's defenses are impaired. When disease is caused by organisms that ordinarily are considered nonpathogenic, the term opportunistic infection is frequently used.

ANIMAL SOURCES

Normal Flora

All animals have what is called a normal flora (microbiota). It consists of the bacteria, viruses, and fungi that live in or upon the normal animal without producing disease. Included in this normal flora are a number of potential pathogens. The study of germ-free animals contributed significantly to our understanding of the importance of the normal flora.

When considering the normal flora, it should be kept in mind that the kinds and numbers of bacteria and other organisms present in and on an animal species vary greatly with different individuals and different circumstances. The number of bacteria making up the normal flora of a human individual is estimated to be 10^{14}. The intestinal flora of the adult animal differs significantly from that of the young animal. The composition of the flora is influenced by climate, age, and geographic location of the animal and the pH, temperature, **redox potential**, availability of water, nutrients, and secreted immunoglobulins at the site.

The technical methods employed to recover **pathogenic** organisms may give a distorted idea of the kinds and numbers of organisms present. The anaerobic, gram-negative, non-spore-forming bacteria are the most populous in the large intestine, but this fact is often obscured because the methods used in the clinical laboratory do not necessarily support the growth of these bacteria.

The normal floras of the various domestic animal species have not been studied as thoroughly as those of humans and of the mouse. The little information available and first-hand experience in the veterinary diagnostic laboratory indicate a considerable similarity, in the broad sense, between the normal flora of humans and mice and that of domestic animals. However, it should be kept in mind that there are significant differences in the flora of the alimentary tract, depending on whether the animal is predominantly herbivorous, omnivorous, or carnivorous.

While considering the normal flora in general, it should be kept in mind that it plays an important role in the nutrition of animals, particularly in the herbivores. In some animals and in humans, *Escherichia coli* and other bacteria produce nutrients such as vitamin K, riboflavin, and vitamin B_{12}.

The normal microbial flora has a protective value in that it tends to exclude other nonresident bacteria from body surfaces, including those that are potentially pathogenic. The waste products of the normal flora may inhibit the growth of pathogens. The presence in the teat canal of *Corynebacterium bovis* may help protect the udder from bacterial infection. Disturbances in the normal flora caused by prolonged antibiotic administration may result in overgrowth and infection by various bacteria and fungi such as staphylococci and *Candida albicans*. Reduction of the gastrointestinal flora of experimental animals by treatment with streptomycin renders them more susceptible to *Salmonella* infection. The selective growth of *Clostridium difficile* in humans caused by antibiotic treatment may result in **pseudomembranous** colitis. The normal flora has also been shown to be important in immune stimulation of the individual.

Some of the kinds of bacteria that can be expected to occur normally in and upon domestic animals are as follows:

- **Mouth, Nasopharynx.** Micrococci, staphylococci, alpha- and beta-hemolytic streptococci, *Bacteroides*, lactobacilli, fusiform bacilli, *Actinomyces,* gram-negative cocci, coliforms and *Proteus* spp., spirochetes, mycoplasmas, *Pasteurella* spp., *Haemophilus*, diphtheroids, and yeasts, including *Candida albicans*.

- **Stomach.** In monogastric animals, the stomach is sterile or contains fewer than 10^3 organisms per milliliter. Most of the organisms that enter the stomach with food are killed by the hydrochloric acid or removed by forward peristalsis.
- **Duodenum, Jejunum, Ileum.** Only small numbers of bacteria are present in the duodenum and jejunum of humans. There are small numbers in the ileum, with increasing numbers toward its termination. The same probably applies to most of the domestic animals.
- **Large Intestine.** *Escherichia coli, Klebsiella, Enterobacter, Pseudomonas* spp., *Proteus* spp., enterococci, staphylococci, *Clostridium perfringens, Clostridium septicum*, and other clostridial spp.; many species of gram-negative anaerobes; spirochetes; and lactobacilli. The gram-negative non-spore-forming bacteria make up more than 90% of the fecal bacteria. One gram of feces contains about 10^{11} bacteria. Yeasts are present in small numbers.
- **Trachea, Bronchi, Lungs.** Few if any bacteria and fungi reside permanently in these structures.
- **Vulva.** Diphtheroids, micrococci, coliforms and *Proteus* spp., enterococci, yeasts, and gram-negative anaerobes. The same kinds of organisms and others can be recovered from the prepuce of the male.
- **Vagina.** The numbers and kinds of bacteria vary with the animal species, the reproductive cycle, and age. The cervix and anterior vagina of the healthy mare have few bacteria. Some of the organisms recovered from the vagina are alpha- and beta-hemolytic streptococci, coliforms, *Proteus* spp., diphtheroids, lactobacilli, mycoplasmas, yeasts, and fungi. Lactobacilli metabolize epithelial glycogen to produce lactic acid. The consequent low vaginal pH inhibits colonization by other bacteria.
- **Skin.** By virtue of their habits and environment, animals frequently possess a large and varied bacterial and fungal flora on their hair and skin. *Staphylococcus* spp. occur commonly, as do micrococci, diphtheroids, hemolytic and nonhemolytic streptococci, propionibacteria, clostridia, and nonpathogenic *Neisseria*. Among the fungi that occur are *Candida, Mucor, Absidia*, and *Malassezia*. Of the many organisms isolated, it may be difficult to determine which make up the resident flora and which are transients.
- **Milk.** Micrococci, staphylococci, nonhemolytic streptococci, mycoplasmas, and diphtheroids including *Corynebacterium bovis* are frequently shed from the apparently normal mammary gland. Some reside in the teat canal.

We have mentioned a number of **commensal** organisms that are potential pathogens. A number of organisms also exist that are not part of the normal flora and that, when present in or on an animal, almost always are associated with latent or overt disease. These organisms, for example, *Brucella* spp., certain *Mycobacterium* spp., and *Bacillus anthracis*, are sometimes called obligate pathogens.

SOURCES OF INFECTIOUS AGENTS

Animals Incubating a Disease

The incubation period is the period from the time of infection until clinical signs appear. During this period, the animal appears healthy but may be infectious, that is, capable of discharging or "shedding" disease-producing organisms. Examples are many of the respiratory diseases caused by viruses, *Pasteurella* spp., and *Haemophilus* spp., in which the organisms may be expelled in saliva or droplets. In intestinal diseases, pathogenic organisms may be shed in the feces in the incubative stage.

Animals with Overt Disease

Ordinarily, the largest numbers of organisms are shed when the animal displays clinical signs of disease. The route by which they are shed depends on the location of the disease. We have mentioned respiratory and intestinal routes of shedding of infectious organisms. They may also be released from the skin in such diseases as dermatophytosis (ringworm) and dermatophilosis and via the urine or genital secretions if infections involve these systems. The extent and duration of the shedding of organisms varies with different diseases. In the acute diseases such as anthrax, shedding is usually of short duration, whereas in chronic diseases such as tuberculosis, it may be long.

Some diseases such as actinomycosis are **sporadic** in their occurrence and are not considered transmissible. Sporadic, endogenous infections (those caused by the animal's own organisms) such as actinomycosis, bacterial endocarditis, and meningitis are often not transmissible to other animals.

Convalescent Carrier Animals

The causative organisms are usually shed for varying periods after clinical recovery from a disease. In respiratory infections, some of the causative organisms, such as *Pasteurella* spp. and mycoplasmas, may be shed by way of droplets during expiration for some time after apparent recovery. Likewise, in salmonellosis, the salmonella organisms may be shed for weeks in the feces, although the animal is clinically normal. These animals are referred to as convalescent carriers, and the state is often referred to as the carrier state. The number of organisms shed will diminish with time, but the period of "excretion" may range from a week to several months. Not all recovered animals are necessarily shedders.

In some diseases, such as salmonellosis and fowl cholera, a chronic carrier state tends to develop. In some severe diseases such as anthrax in cattle, there usually is no convalescent or chronic carrier state. In recovered strangles and hemorrhagic **septicemia**, the period of the carrier state is usually relatively short.

Contact Carriers and Subclinical Infections

Animals may acquire pathogenic organisms from other animals with infectious disease without contracting the disease themselves. In most groups of animals exposed to infectious disease, there will often be some that acquire the organisms but do not develop clinical disease. The number of such animals depends on the disease, the **virulence** of the microorganisms, and the animal's immune state. Such animals are referred to as contact or subclinical carriers. This carrier state may be temporary, lasting only a few days, or chronic, lasting weeks or months. Such contact carriers are associated with diseases such as strangles in horses and erysipelas and salmonellosis in swine. The term convalescent carrier is sometimes used for those recovered animals that still carry the pathogen.

Subclinical carriers represent a threat to other animals and are a means whereby the disease is perpetuated. Such states can only be detected, sometimes with difficulty, by demonstration of the organisms, usually by cultural procedures as in salmonellosis and Johne's disease. In bovine genital campylobacteriosis, "test mating" has been used to detect infected or carrier bulls. The suspected bulls are bred to susceptible heifers to see whether or not they infect them.

Inanimate Sources

Some species of *Clostridium, Proteus, Klebsiella,* and *Pseudomonas aeruginosa* exist in the free-living state in the soil, where they derive their sustenance from decaying vegetation. In addition, they may also inhabit the intestine as commensals and be shed in the feces. Less common free-living organisms such as species of *Acinetobacter, Aeromonas, Chromobacterium,* and *Flavobacterium* on rare occasions will cause disease in humans and animals. They ordinarily only cause disease under special circumstances. *Pseudomonas aeruginosa* may infect wounds and tissues damaged by burns. *Proteus* spp. can cause urinary tract infections, and *Klebsiella* strains can produce severe mastitis in cows. Impaired defenses and numbers of organisms (dosage) are important in such infections.

The spores of clostridia, which occur widely in soil and feces, gain entrance via wounds and cause tetanus and such gas gangrene-type diseases as blackleg and malignant edema. Other clostridia such as *C. botulinum,* which is also soil-borne, cause poisoning as a result of the production of a potent **exotoxin** in contaminated food. Certain toxin-producing strains of *C. perfringens,* which occur in soil and animal feces, produce toxins in the intestines that may result in severe toxemia.

A number of ordinarily saprophytic fungi have the capacity to produce disease in animals. They cause such usually sporadic diseases as sporotrichosis, histoplasmosis, blastomycosis and coccidioidomycosis. The occurrence of the latter three diseases is dependent to a large extent on the geographic distribution of the fungi in the soil.

TRANSMISSION

Infectious agents are most frequently transmitted to new hosts by direct or indirect contact. The direct process refers to spread by contact with the infecting organisms on the infected host; for example, contact with discharges on the animal that have emanated from the skin or various body openings. The other means of direct contact is by coitus.

In most diseases, the indirect process is involved. This means that the organisms shed or excreted by the host are carried in or on various vehicles such as water, milk, food, litter, air, or dust. Such contaminated inanimate objects as food, water, litter, bedding, mangers, and kennels are referred to collectively as fomites. Other indirect means of spread are contaminated medical, surgical, and dental instruments; syringes and needles (these may transmit equine infectious anemia and anaplasmosis); speculums; and dressings.

Various arthropods such as ticks, mites, lice, flies, and mosquitoes act as vectors of infectious diseases. Some agents are transmitted in a purely mechanical manner, whereas others are actually inoculated by biting insects, as with tularemia. In several diseases, the infecting agent may multiply in the vector. For example, *Yersinia pestis,* which causes plague, multiplies in the salivary gland of the flea.

Organisms enter the host by one of the following portals of entry:

- Inhalation and infection via the respiratory tract.
- Ingestion and infection via the alimentary tract.
- Inoculation or infection through the skin or mucous membranes by simple contact, injection (e.g., biting insect, contaminated hypodermic syringe or needle), or wound infection.
- Via the genital tract as a result of coitus. Also by means of contaminated instruments, catheters, and semen from artificial insemination centers.
- By transplacental infection.
- Via the umbilicus.

Most organisms produce infections only if they enter by way of a particular portal. For example, enteropathogenic *E. coli* gains entrance to the intestine through the upper digestive tract but not through the skin. *Staphylococcus aureus,* however, readily enters the skin but rarely causes infection as a result of ingestion. Some organisms such as *Brucella* spp. may enter the host through several portals: the skin and oral or genital tract mucous membranes. The lesions produced by the invading organism may involve tissues and organs remote from the site of entry. Although the mode of infection of the swine erysipelas organism may be ingestion, the lesions are not associated with the alimentary tract.

The terms vertical transmission and horizontal transmission are widely used. Vertical spread is from the female (dam, mare, etc.) to the fetus *in utero* or to the newborn during parturition or via ingestion of colostrum or milk. Vertical infection can also result from latent viruses in germ cells.

Horizontal spread is by the common direct and indirect means referred to above.

Infection via the Respiratory Tract

This is the common mode of infection in respiratory diseases, although these infections can also be acquired by direct contact and from fomites. The source of the organisms is generally the secretions of the respiratory tract of another animal. The infections are acquired by the inhalation of contaminated air. The organisms are trapped on the moist mucous membranes of the nasopharynx and lower respiratory tract. This is the way that diseases such as *Pasteurella* and *Mannheimia* pneumonias, viral pneumonias, and tuberculosis are transmitted. The spores of a number of fungi, such as *Histoplasma capsulatum*, that infect via the respiratory tract are acquired from the soil by inhalation.

Droplet Infection

Few or no organisms are shed into the air from the nose or mouth in normal breathing. However, large numbers of organisms are expelled during coughing and sneezing. Many of these organisms are derived from the mouth and oropharynx.

In coughing, the vast majority of particles emanate from the respiratory tract in the form of droplets. It is estimated that in humans, a vigorous cough may release 5000–6000 droplets, whereas a vigorous sneeze may liberate as many as a million droplets. The majority of the droplets expelled are less than 100 μm in diameter. These evaporate rapidly, leaving droplet nuclei suspended in the air for many hours. These consist of dried secretions that may contain organisms. Eventually, they fall to the ground or other surroundings, resulting in contamination. Droplets with a diameter of 100 μm or more have a very short trajectory and fall a very short distance from the host animal.

Of the droplets generated from saliva at the front of the mouth, many do not contain the infecting agent, and many are sterile. It should be kept in mind that only a small proportion of the droplet nuclei contain pathogens. However, it often takes only a few organisms to initiate some diseases.

Dust-Borne Infections

Many respiratory infections are probably acquired by the following indirect process: first, the infected animal contaminates itself and its environment with secretions and infected droplets, and second, the organisms dry on whatever they contaminate, subsequently to be dispersed into the air in the form of dust. The inhalation of these infectious dust particles constitutes an important mode of infection in respiratory diseases. The success of the method depends to a considerable extent on the capacity of the organisms to withstand the effects of drying. This mode of infection is responsible for the transmission of such diseases as psittacosis (transmitted through dried infectious feces) and tuberculosis.

Infection by Ingestion

Organisms causing intestinal diseases gain entrance to the alimentary tract after being swallowed, for example, salmonellas and enteropathogenic *E. coli; Mycobacterium bovis* also may enter by this route and cause disease involving the intestine. The preformed exotoxins of *Clostridium botulinum* and *Staphylococcus aureus* are conveyed to the intestine in food. *Clostridium perfringens* organisms that give rise to enterotoxemia may gain entrance to the body by ingestion. A number of infecting agents, such as *Brucella abortus*, enteroviruses, and *Coxiella burnetii*, may enter through the intestinal wall but produce their effects elsewhere. In intestinal disease, the feces are the principal source of the pathogens.

Animals may become infected with intestinal pathogens as a result of direct contact with the feces-contaminated host or, more commonly, by contact with fomites such as contaminated feed, milk, bedding, surroundings (stable, mangers), and water. Because of the habits of animals, with the consequent frequent exposure to feces, intestinal diseases usually spread rapidly.

Infection Resulting from Contact

Some diseases are spread by agents that can penetrate apparently undamaged skin or mucous membranes. *Brucella abortus, Bacillus anthracis*, and *Francisella tularensis* have this capacity. In animals, disease is spread in this manner most often by means of fomites such as infected litter and bedding, saddles, milker's hands, and milking machines rather than by direct contact. Included among the diseases that may be spread by these direct and indirect means are skin abscesses, pyoderma, poxvirus diseases, ringworm, the various viral papillomatoses, and dermatophilosis.

Infection Resulting from Inoculation

WOUNDS.   Many organisms gain entrance to the underlying tissues through breaks in the continuity of skin or mucous membranes. In animals, wounds have numerous causes, including accidents, surgical operations (especially docking and castration), calving, goring, biting, and wounds caused by nail punctures and bullets or shots. The sources of organisms that lodge in wounds are various. Tetanus results from the contamination of wounds by spores from the soil or feces. *Staphylococcus aureus* and *Arcanobacterium pyogenes*, which are carried in the nasopharynx of many animals, frequently infect wounds. Soil-borne nocardia introduced during non-aseptic treatment of the udder may produce a severe mastitis. Other soil- and fecal-borne organisms that infect wounds, resulting in gas gangrene, are *C. septicum* and *C. perfringens*. In surgery involving the stomach or intestine, incisions may become infected with such enteric organisms as *E. coli* and *Bacteroides* spp., sometimes leading to peritonitis.

INJECTION. As mentioned previously, infectious agents may be injected via the bites of arthropods or insects, or they may be injected mistakenly or carelessly by humans. Diseases such as equine infectious anemia and anaplasmosis, to mention only two, may be transmitted by contaminated hypodermic needles and surgical instruments. These two diseases are also spread by biting insects. The equine viral encephalitides are spread by mosquitoes, and Rocky Mountain spotted fever is initiated by the bite of an infected tick. Tularemia is spread mainly by ticks, and plague by fleas. The hog louse appears to be an important disseminator of swine pox virus.

Infection via the Genital Tract

Infectious agents may enter the genital tract to set up infections at various times but do so most frequently after parturition and at estrus. A number of important diseases are transmitted from male to female during coitus, including bovine genital campylobacteriosis, brucellosis, equine vesicular exanthema, and infectious pustular vulvovaginitis. *Corynebacterium renale*, a cause of bovine pyelonephritis, may gain entrance to the urinary tract from the genital tract.

Transplacental Infection

The fetuses of several animal species become infected and frequently are stillborn or aborted as a result of transplacental infection. In some diseases, such as brucellosis, *Campylobacter* abortion, and mycotic abortion, the disease process is primarily confined to the placenta, but the organisms can be recovered from the fetal stomach contents and various organs. Lesions within the fetus itself may be minimal. Abortion resulting from listeria infection occurs, and this organism may be recovered from the stomach contents and various organs. The fetus may be profoundly affected by the infecting agent; cerebellar **hypoplasia** may result from infection with the hog cholera virus, and extensive fetal damage occurs in chlamydial abortion of sheep and cattle.

Infection via the Umbilicus

Infection of the newborn may be prenatal, such as an extension of cervicitis or placentitis, or postnatal, in which the common modes of infection are ingestion, inhalation, or via the umbilicus. The umbilcus frequently becomes infected if the navel is not properly cared for immediately after birth. The young of all the domestic species are prone to infections that start from the umbilicus, but lambs are particularly susceptible. A variety of organisms enter via the umbilicus, including *Erysipelothrix rhu-*

siopathiae, *Salmonella*, *Klebsiella*, pyogenic streptococci, *Arcanobacterium pyogenes*, and *Actinobacillus equuli*.

The manifestations of these neonatal infections are variable, depending on the virulence of the organism and the resistance of the newborn. Most serious is **bacteremia**, which may proceed to septicemia and death. More often, however, the bacteremia results in organisms being disseminated to organs, lymph nodes, and joints, where disease processes develop.

Nosocomial Infections

These are hospital-acquired infections. A number of infectious agents, including bacteria, fungi, and viruses, may be transmitted within the veterinary hospital or clinic. Latent infections or carrier states may flare up into serious infections as a result of various stresses, and the agents involved may spread to and threaten other patients. In addition to stress, dosage of organisms, confinement, and immunosuppression may all contribute to occurrence and spread. Although most nosocomial infections result from frankly pathogenic organisms, some involve opportunistic microbes considered to be part of the normal flora. *Salmonella* infections are a major nosocomial problem in many large veterinary clinics, particularly in horses. Canine infectious tracheobronchitis (kennel cough) is a troublesome nosocomial infection in veterinary hospitals. Attempts are made to prevent and control these infections by careful attention to effective sanitation and management practices.

Iatrogenic disease is defined as disease induced inadvertently by medical treatment or procedures of a physician. Although rare, disease is sometimes induced as a result of veterinary treatment or procedures that are not always associated with the clinic or hospital.

GLOSSARY

bacteremia Presence of viable bacteria in the blood.
commensalism State in which one organism (e.g., a bacterium) lives on another organism (e.g., an animal), obtaining food and other benefits but imposing no damage on the latter.
exotoxin Toxic substance of a microorganism released into the surrounding medium during its growth.
hypoplasia Condition in which an organ or tissue does not fully develop or mature.
pathogenic Having the capacity to cause disease in a susceptible host.
pseudomembrane False membrane, sometimes called a diphtheritic membrane, composed mainly of fibrin and necrotic cells on the surface of an inflamed mucous membrane.
redox potential Oxidation-reduction potential.
septicemia Bacteria increasing in numbers in the blood, but also used as a synonym for bacteremia.
sporadic (infection or disease) Scattered in occurrence; usually individual cases.
virulence Degree of pathogenicity of a microorganism.

7

Host–Parasite Relationships

There are a variety of complex relationships whereby microorganisms can interact with other microorganisms and with eukaryotic organisms. Any organism that supports the survival and growth of microorganisms is referred to as a host. The types of relationship that microbes and their hosts can share include saprophytism, parasitism, and commensalism. A small number, such as species of *Candida*, *Proteus*, *Klebsiella*, and *Pseudomonas*, can exist as either saprophytes or parasites. In addition, commensal microorganisms, such as those associated with the gut, can become parasitic when present in another location within the host's body.

COMMON TERMS

Below is a list of common terms associated with the interaction of microorganisms and their host.

Saprophytism

Saprophytes are organisms that live on dead or decaying organic matter. They ordinarily are not parasites of animals, although on occasion they can cause disease. For example, brooder pneumonia is caused by the fungus *Aspergillus fumigatus*, which may be present in large numbers on food or litter. Some of the clostridia live in the soil as well as in the intestine.

Parasitism

This is a general term that denotes a state in which an organism lives on or within another living organism. The parasite does not necessarily harm the host; in fact, the most successful parasites achieve a balance with the host that ensures the survival of both. Among the parasites found on and within domestic animals and humans are bacteria, protozoans, fungi, mycoplasmas, rickettsia, and viruses. Those parasites that are capable of causing disease are called pathogens.

Commensalism

This is a parasitic state in which the organism lives in or on the host without causing disease. The organism benefits from this relationship, while the host may or may not.

Most of the bacteria in the alimentary tract, both aerobic and anaerobic, are commensals. Most commensals do not have the potential to cause disease. However, some may become pathogens under particular conditions within the host. For example, *Staphylococcus aureus* may cause bovine mastitis as a result of damage to the udder, and *Mannheimia haemolytica* may cause pneumonia in young cattle fatigued and weakened by shipment and extremes of weather.

Symbiosis

Symbiosis is the general term for a direct association between two or more species. It literally means "living together," and therefore refers to a range of interactions, including commensalism, parasitism, and saprophytism. Examples of symbiosis are the microfloras of the cecum of rabbits and of the rumen of ruminants, which are provided food and shelter while enabling the host through enzymatic processes to utilize cellulose.

Opportunistic Pathogen

This term describes organisms that are generally harmless commensals in their normal habitats but that can cause disease when they gain access to other sites or tissues. For example, non-enterotoxin-producing strains of *Escherichia coli* from the intestine can cause urinary tract infections when present in the urinary tract. As indicated below, many saprophytic bacteria and fungi can also cause opportunistic infections.

Impairment of the host's immune defenses is the principal factor leading to opportunistic infections caused by normally harmless commensals. Another contributing factor is the introduction of microorganisms to body sites where they are not normally found, such as from contaminated equipment or unclean hands. A final contributing factor is disturbances in the normal flora, such as those caused by antibiotic treatment.

A wide variety of ordinarily harmless bacteria and fungi have been incriminated in opportunistic infections. More than 200 species of saprophytic bacteria have been considered causes of opportunistic infections in humans. Among the fungi involved in infrequent opportunistic infections in animals are *Penicillium*, *Aspergillus*, *Absidia*, *Mucor*, *Candida* spp., and many other species that occur rarely. Bacteria, including *Pseudomonas aeruginosa*, *Acinetobacter* spp. and several species of enteric bacteria, are frequent opportunists in animals.

Obligate Pathogen

This denotes an organism that almost always causes disease when it encounters animals or humans. Examples include *Brucella abortus*, *Yersinia pestis*, *Mycobacterium bovis*, and *Bacillus anthracis*.

DEFINITION OF TERMS

The terms that follow are frequently used in the discussion of infectious diseases.

Pathogenicity

This is the capacity of the organism to produce disease. Variation in this capacity is referred to in terms of virulence.

Virulence

This is a measure of the degree of pathogenicity. For example, pathogenic strains of *Streptococcus equi* may vary in their capacity to produce disease in the horse. All strains may cause disease, but some may cause more severe disease than others.

Infectivity

This is the capacity of the organism to become established in the tissues of the host. It involves the ability to penetrate the tissues, to survive the host's defenses, and to multiply and disseminate within the animal.

Toxigenicity

This is the capacity of certain organisms to produce exotoxins. For example, there are both toxigenic and nontoxigenic strains of *Clostridium perfringens*; only the toxigenic form causes disease.

If the host–parasite relationship is kept in balance or equilibrium, no apparent disease results, and the infection is asymptomatic. In such diseases as tuberculosis and brucellosis, a delicate equilibrium may be established that is easily upset. Disease results when the parasite cannot be kept in check, and a combination of damage done to the host and the host's adaptive reactions results in the phenomenon we recognize as infectious disease.

The two principal determinants of the outcome of the host–parasite relationship are the virulence of the parasite and the resistance of the host. In the development of natural disease, the relative significance of each is difficult to estimate. For the sake of discussion, it is convenient to treat the roles of the parasite and the host separately.

PATHOGENIC PROPERTIES OF BACTERIA

Bacteria cause disease by two basic mechanisms: invasion of tissues and production of toxins. Those specific characteristics that contribute to the pathogenicity of microorganisms are frequently referred to as virulence factors. Some examples of virulence factors include bacterial structures such as pili or fimbriae for adhesion to cells or tissues, enzymes that allow the pathogen to hide from or circumvent host defenses, and the production of toxins directly associated with pathogenesis.

GENERAL COMMENTS

Great variation exists in the extent of invasiveness of microorganisms. At one end of the scale are the exotoxin producers, such as the tetanus bacillus, which are noninvasive. At the other end are organisms such as *Y. pestis* (plague) and *B. anthracis* (anthrax), which are highly invasive. Organisms such as some *Pasteurella* spp., streptococci, and *Haemophilus* spp. are in between and have only a moderate capacity to invade.

How do we know that a particular organism is pathogenic? The traditional criteria used are Koch's postulates:

1. The organism must be regularly isolated from cases of the disease.
2. It must be grown in vitro in pure culture.
3. Such a culture should produce the typical disease when inoculated into a susceptible animal species.
4. The same organism must be isolated from the experimentally induced disease.

Although these postulates have been met for many diseases, they have not been fulfilled for all, notably some human viral diseases (because viruses are frequently very host-specific), diseases such as leprosy and Tyzzer's disease (as the causal agent has not been grown on lifeless media) and diseases associated with stress and caused by primary and secondary agents.

Further investigation allows us to classify invasive bacteria as intracellular or extracellular parasites.

Intracellular Parasites

FACULTATIVE INTRACELLULAR PARASITES. These microorganisms are not confined to cells, but they can survive, and in some instances multiply, in phagocytic cells. The phagocytes may also destroy the parasite and prevent or ultimately eliminate an infection. For example, *B. abortus*, *Salmonella* spp., and *Mycobacterium bovis* may be eliminated by macrophages. When a balance is established between the bacterium and the phagocyte, usually macrophages, the bacteria may survive in this intracellular state of relative equilibrium for months or years.

OBLIGATE INTRACELLULAR PARASITES. Chlamydia, rickettsia, and viruses are obligate intracellular parasites in that they can only propagate within cells.

Extracellular Parasites

Extracellular organisms damage tissues while they are outside phagocytes and other cells. They do not have the capacity to survive for long periods in phagocytic cells. When phagocytized, these organisms, such as *Klebsiella* and *Pasteurella* spp., are readily destroyed.

Antiphagocytic Capsules

These surface structures are found principally on extracellular bacteria and protect the microorganisms from ingestion by phagocytic cells. Capsules are typically polysaccharides; however, the capsules of some organisms are composed of protein. Examples of polysaccharide capsules include those of mucoid forms of *Pasteurella multocida* and *Enterobacter aerogenes*. *Bacillus anthracis* and *Y. pestis* possess protein capsules.

Extracellular Enzymes

Some bacteria produce substances that are not toxic directly but that do play an important part in the development of disease:

- Coagulase, produced by *S. aureus*, clots fibrin that protects the bacteria.
- Hyaluronidases, produced by a number of bacteria, are thought to aid in the spread of organisms by breaking down the ground substance (hyaluronic acid) of tissues.
- Collagenase produced by some strains of *C. perfringens* aid in the spread of this organism by breaking down the collagen of tissues.

Other extracellular enzymes are streptokinase (a fibrinolysin) and streptodornase (a DNase [deoxyribonuclease]), produced by streptococci. Other extracellular enzymes will be described with specific pathogens.

Adherence to Surfaces

Most bacteria and fungi that live in or on their hosts adhere, at least temporarily, to host cells in order to colonize and grow. As a consequence, most of these organisms possess surface components called adhesins or ligands that enable them to adhere specifically to host cells via corresponding receptors on the surface of these cells. Microbial adhesins include components of outer membranes, capsules, and pili (fimbriae). Most adhesins of microorganisms thus far studied are glycoproteins or lipoproteins. The host cell receptors frequently are sugars such as mannose.

It has been shown that pili of enteropathogenic strains of *E. coli* are involved in adherence and colonization of the mucous membrane of the small intestine. Pili may also be involved in the adherence of *Moraxella bovis*, *Bordetella* spp., and many other gram-negative bacteria. Strains of *Mycoplasma pneumoniae* that have lost their capacity to adhere are also found to have lost their virulence. The adsorption of some bacteria to mucous membranes may be caused by a physicochemical attraction, particularly hydrophilicity or hydrophobicity, which depends on certain surface compounds associated with the capsules of virulent organisms. These compounds may be lost with in vitro cultivation.

The phenomenon of adherence of bacteria is now receiving a great deal of attention. Its study may have important practical implications, as suggested by the development of an *E. coli* pilus vaccine to prevent scours in swine.

Toxigenicity

EXOTOXINS.   Some properties of exotoxins are as follows:

- They are produced by almost all gram-positive bacteria and some gram-negative species, and they are released into the environment of the microorganism.
- They are typically proteins and are often easily denatured at temperatures above 60°C and by irradiation with ultraviolet light.
- They are among the most potent toxins known.
- They induce strong antibody production in the host. However, they induce little or no fever.
- They are highly specific; some act as neurotoxins, others as cardiac muscle toxins, and so forth.
- Following treatment of the toxin with chemicals such as formalin or heat, a toxoid is formed that can be used in immunization.

Most of the weakly or noninvasive bacteria that cause disease produce exotoxins. These are protein substances that are liberated from intact and lysed cells. They vary greatly in their toxicity, from the extremely potent botulinum toxin to the relatively weak toxin of *Arcanobacterium pyogenes*. They are almost all antigenic, eliciting specific protective antitoxic antibodies. The various disease-producing clostridia are notable for their production of exotoxins. Some of these toxins can be converted to nontoxic immunizing agents called toxoids by treatment with formalin.

Some of the bacteria other than clostridia that produce exotoxins are enteropathogenic *E. coli*, *Y. pestis*, several *Corynebacterium* species, the highly invasive *B. anthracis*, some strains of *P. multocida*, and *S. aureus*. It is of interest that the toxin of *Corynebacterium diphtheriae* and the erythrogenic toxins of *Streptococcus pyogenes* are only produced by lysogenic strains of these species. In these bacteria, the toxin-producing characteristic is coded for by bacteriophage DNA.

A number of exotoxins are encoded by plasmid genes. Examples are the tetanus neurotoxin, the enterototoxin of *E. coli*, and staphylococcal enterotoxin. Unlike endotoxins, the clinical and experimental effects of various exotoxins are associated with particular microorganisms and are therefore described in the discussions of the specific diseases.

ENDOTOXINS.   Some properties of endotoxins are as follows:

- They are produced by gram-negative bacteria, both pathogenic and nonpathogenic species, and they are released during growth and on lysis.
- They were originally described as phospholipid–polysaccharide–protein complexes (somatic O antigen). However, their biologic and immunologic properties reside with the lipopolysaccharide portion. As a result, the terms endotoxin and lipopolysaccharide are often used synonymously. Their chemical structure is described in Chapter 1.
- They are a major part of the cell wall of gram-negative bacteria.
- They are heat-stable, with molecular weights between 100,000 and 900,000.
- Their toxicity resides in the lipid portion, whereas their specific antigenic determinants are the sugars that constitute the side chains of the lipopolysaccharide. They do not form toxoids.
- They are less specific and potent in their cytotoxic effects than exotoxins.
- They are weak antigens, although they may have an adjuvant effect in combination with other antigens.
- They are responsible for a rapid rise in temperature and a variety of clinical manifestations referred to below.
- Potency differs among species.

Although many biologic effects have been ascribed to endotoxins, their role in the pathogenesis of bacterial diseases is poorly understood and largely conjectural. Part of their injurious effect is thought to be immunologic in nature. It is suggested that a state of immunologic sensitivity may be involved. It has been noted that germ-free animals are less susceptible to the toxic effects of endotoxins.

Among the effects of endotoxins observed clinically and experimentally are fever, leukopenia, hypoglycemia, hypotension and **shock**, intravascular coagulation, **Shwartzman reaction**, **adjuvancy**, and activation of complement components leading to acute inflammatory reactions. Endotoxins may have an effect on the clotting system leading to the kind of intravascular coagulation seen in gram-negative septicemias. Thrombocytopenia with lysis of platelets and the release of **histamine**, **serotonin**, and **bradykinin** may lead to the kind of cardiovascular changes that are seen in endotoxemia, including shock. The tumor necrosis factor-alpha (TNF-α) is produced by macrophages stimulated by endotoxin. TNF-α binds to various tissues and alters their metabolism. It may damage blood capillaries, resulting in increased permeability with loss of large amounts of fluids. Blood pressure may fall sufficiently to produce shock. Endotoxemia occurs in gram-negative **bacterial sepsis**, **hemorrhagic septicemia**, and other diseases caused by gram-negative bacteria.

The amount of endotoxin present can be determined by the limulus lysate assay. Endotoxin reacts with proteins from horseshoe crab amebocytes to produce a gel. It is a remarkably sensitive test that detects nanogram amounts of endotoxin.

NONSPECIFIC MECHANISMS OF HOST RESISTANCE

Nonspecific mechanisms of host resistance are sometimes referred to as innate immunity. It is well known that great differences in susceptibility to various infectious agents exist among domestic animal species. Some of the important features of innate resistance or immunity are discussed below.

The Skin

The skin provides a generally effective barrier. Some microorganisms, such as *B. abortus* and *Francisella tularensis*, can penetrate skin. Others enter and cause infections of sweat and sebaceous glands and hair follicles. The glands secrete acidic, antibacterial substances that contain fatty acids, which are both antibacterial and antifungal. Young animals are thought to be more susceptible to dermatophytes because they have a lower concentration of fatty acids on the skin than adult animals. Lysozyme, an enzyme that breaks down the cell walls of bacteria, is present on the skin. This mucolytic enzyme splits sugars off the glycopeptides of the cell wall of many gram-positive bacteria, leading to lysis.

Compromises in the integrity of the skin as a barrier, such as by a cut or wound, allow for entry of those microorganisms that would otherwise not have access to the body.

Mucous Membrane

Mucus covers the surface of the mucous membranes of the various tracts of the body. Bacteria are caught by the mucous film and are readily phagocytized. The phagocytes carry the bacteria to the lymph nodes, where specific immune responses to the bacteria can be generated. In addition, the cilia of the respiratory tract are constantly moving bacteria and mucus toward the oral and nasal openings. Both mucus and tears contain the protective enzyme lysozyme.

Hair in the nares is protective, as is the cough reflex. Saliva, stomach acid, and proteolytic enzymes have an antibacterial action. The acid pH of the vagina caused by lactobacilli has a limiting and stabilizing influence on the vaginal flora. The normal flora of mucous membranes is a rather stable ecosystem that resists the intrusion of alien bacteria. Disturbance of the flora by antibiotic therapy may allow establishment and multiplication of disease-producing organisms, such as staphylococci resulting in staphylococcal enteritis or *Candida albicans* resulting in mycotic stomatitis, gastritis, or enteritis.

Phagocytosis

Microorganisms entering organs and tissues such as the lungs, lymphatics, bone marrow, and bloodstream may be engulfed by various phagocytic cells. Among these are the polymorphonuclear leukocytes and the wandering and fixed macrophages. Phagocytosis may be nonspecific in the absence of antibody but specific when antibodies to the offending microorganism are available. Phagocytes may kill the engulfed microorganisms. However, some microorganisms may survive and, in some instances, actually multiply within the phagocytic cell (intracellular parasites).

The resulting phagocytic vacuole created by the engulfing of a microorganism is called the phagosome. The phagosome then fuses with a lysosome containing lysosomal granules providing the hydrolytic enzymes, including lysozyme, which aid in the destruction of microorganisms. Macrophages may be specifically activated by immunologically active T-lymphocytes to more readily engulf microorganisms, including extracellular bacteria and viruses.

Reticuloendothelial System

This system refers to the macrophages found in blood (monocytes) and the fixed macrophages (histiocytes) found in lymphoid tissue, spleen, liver, bone marrow, and other tissues. They engulf and remove particulate matter and microorganisms from the blood and lymph and from infected areas. Included in the system are the macrophages lining the blood sinuses of the liver (Kupffer cells), those lining the lymph sinuses, histiocytes found in tissues, and the alveolar macrophages in the lungs.

Resistance of Tissues

Various constituents of tissues have an inhibitory effect on microorganisms; thus, some tissues are more readily invaded than others. For example, the interferon produced by tissues in response to viral infection has antiviral properties.

Most healthy tissues inhibit the multiplication of microorganisms. This resistance can be impaired by depression of the inflammatory response by x-rays, corticosteroids, leukemic disease, and antineoplastic drugs. Injury resulting from foreign bodies, trauma, and disturbances in fluid and electrolyte balance may predispose to infection.

Natural Antibodies

These are immunoglobulins that react with a wide range of organisms and antigens to which the animal has not yet been exposed or immunized. Low levels are found in germ-free animals. Examples include ABO blood group system isohemagglutinins (associated with transfusion reactions) and **Forssman's antibodies.**

Inflammatory Response

Pathogenic microorganisms, like other damaging agents, elicit inflammatory responses of varying kinds and sever-

ity. The changes elicited are complex, and some of the phenomena involved include increased vascular permeability, edema, increased blood flow, infiltration of phagocytic cells, fluid exudation, fever, pain, and swelling. Many of these changes are brought about by the inflammatory mediators, serotonin, histamine, various kinins, **prostaglandins**, **leukotrienes**, **interleukin-1**, C3a and C5a (complement), platelet-activating factor, and products from fibrinogen breakdown.

Fever

Fever is frequently observed as a manifestation of the inflammatory response. It is the cardinal symptom or sign of infectious disease. Fever results from influences on the thermoregulatory centers in the brain.

The lipopolysaccharides released from phagocytes that have engulfed gram-negative bacteria cause macrophages to produce the cytokine interleukin-1. Interleukin-1 is carried by the blood to the hypothalamus, where it stimulates the temperature control center to release prostaglandins that reset the thermostat in the hypothalamus to a higher temperature, thus causing a fever. Aspirin reduces fever by inhibiting the production of prostaglandins.

In fevers of unknown origin in animals, the most frequent causes are probably undetected infections and neoplasms. Other causes may be endocrine disturbances and hypersensitivity reactions.

CONDITIONS AND FACTORS INFLUENCING INFECTIONS

Species, Sex, and Age

There are great differences in susceptibility to infectious agents among animal species. Likewise, there are differences in susceptibility among individual animals and between males and females of the same species. Age is also an important factor. Generally speaking, infectious diseases in both animals and humans are more severe at the extremes of life. The importance of species, sex, and age as they relate to particular infections is discussed later under specific infectious agents.

Stress

The term stress is frequently used to summarize various factors and circumstances that contribute to the development of an infectious disease or diseases. Although both mental and physical disturbances lead to the stress reaction, the latter are probably most important in animals.

Among the more common disturbances leading to stress are fatigue, exposure to extremes of cold and heat, crowding, wounds, transport, change in feed, and weaning. The stress of transport may activate latent infection, such as that caused by *Chlamydia psittaci* in birds. A number of physical disturbances contribute to the development of "shipping fever." For example, viral or mycoplasmal infection of the respiratory tract may seriously damage the epithelium and ciliary activity, thus predisposing the animal to bacterial colonization and infection.

If the disturbances are severe enough, a coordinated response originating in the cortex and hypothalamus is initiated that involves either the autonomic nervous system or the pituitary–adrenal axis. Corticosteroids and **catecholamines** are released in an effort to counter the deleterious effects of the disturbance. Corticosteroids in large amounts depress the inflammatory response and have pronounced effects on lymphoid tissues, causing lymphocyte destruction and thymic involution with possible aggravation of infection.

Circulatory Disturbances

Such disturbances may be local, causing **ischemia** or congestion and edema, or general, as in shock. They interfere with the mobilization and functioning of phagocytic cells. Mechanical obstruction of the biliary or urinary tracts can have similar effects, thus contributing to infections.

Nutritional Deficiency

There has long been an association between famine and pestilence. Poorly fed animals are more susceptible to a variety of infections. Vitamin A deficiency results in the loss of integrity of epithelium. Other nutritional deficiencies may lead to diminished phagocytic capacity, reduction of the efficiency of the reticuloendothelial system, weakened antibody response, lowered production of lysozyme and interferon, undesirable changes in microbial flora, and alterations of the endocrine system.

Extremes of Temperature and Humidity

There is experimental evidence that animals are less resistant to bacterial infections if they are maintained at a low temperature for extended periods. Environmental stresses, including cold and intemperate weather, no doubt contribute to the occurrence of bovine pneumonia caused by *M. haemolytica*. High humidity, with an increase in infectious droplets, may contribute to an increase in respiratory disease in groups of animals. Production of corticosteroids by stressed animals is anti-inflammatory and immunosuppressive, thus contributing to or aggravating the infectious process.

Genetic Effects

There is evidence of genetic resistance to bovine mastitis. Leghorns are more resistant to Marek's disease than some other breeds. Some varieties of rabbits are more resistant to myxomatosis, and as a consequence, the highly susceptible strains have been eliminated by the disease. Defects in the immune system frequently have a genetic basis, including combined T- and B-cell deficiencies contributing to fatal adenoviral infections in Arabian foals, disseminated histoplasmosis in dogs with thymic hypoplasia, and greater susceptibility to bacterial infections in humans and animals with agammaglobulinemia.

Chronic Infections

Chronic, low-grade infections may predispose animals to more severe infections often caused by opportunistic microorganisms, such as sporadic pneumonias in many animal species. Some viral infections such as influenza and feline leukemia may suppress resistance to certain bacterial infections.

Other Factors

It is widely held that extreme physical fatigue predisposes animals to infection, presumably because it contributes to stress.

Diabetics and animals receiving adrenal steroids are known to be abnormally prone to infections.

Acute radiation injury may result in damage to the bone marrow with consequent granulocytopenia and, thus, a lowering of the host's resistance.

Prolonged antibiotic administration can lead to alteration, suppression, or elimination of normal microbial flora. The term superinfection is frequently used for infections caused by nonresident organisms that replace the normal flora as a result of prolonged chemotherapy. An example is staphylococcal enteritis.

SPECIFIC MECHANISMS OF HOST RESISTANCE

Nonspecific resistance has already been discussed. Immunity is classified as follows:

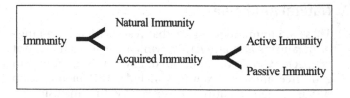

Immunology is of such importance in veterinary medicine that it is taught as a separate discipline. It involves the study of the immune responses to foreign material (antigens). The essential function of the immune system

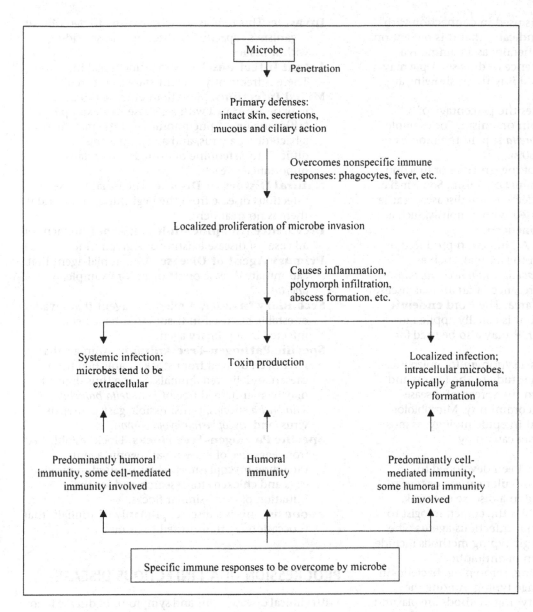

Microbe

↓ Penetration

Primary defenses:
intact skin, secretions,
mucous and ciliary action

↓ Overcomes nonspecific immune
responses: phagocytes, fever, etc.

Localized proliferation of microbe invasion

↓ Causes inflammation,
polymorph infiltration,
abscess formation, etc.

Systemic infection;
microbes tend to be
extracellular

Toxin production

Localized infection;
intracellular microbes,
typically granuloma
formation

↑

Predominantly humoral
immunity, some cell-mediated
immunity involved

Humoral
immunity

Predominantly cell-
mediated immunity,
some humoral immunity
involved

↑

Specific immune responses to be overcome by microbe

FIGURE 7.1 Host–pathogen interactions in the production of disease. Note that the pathogen must evade both natural and specific immune responses of the host to achieve infection. Pathogens possess a variety of mechanisms by which they attempt to circumvent the immune responses of the host. Reproduced with permission from Wise, DJ, and Carter, GR. *Immunology: A Comprehensive Review*, Ames, IA: Iowa State Press, 2002.

(but not the only one) is defense against infectious agents. The immune system is of paramount importance in this regard.

For purposes of general orientation, the progress of infection as it relates to immunological defense mechanisms is summarized in the outline in Fig. 7.1.

Acquired immunity consists of passive immunity and active immunity. Passive immunity, which lasts for only a few weeks, results from the acquisition of antibodies that have been produced in another animal or acquired by the fetus or the newborn from the mother.

Active immunity results from the immune response mounted by the host. It consists of cell-mediated immunity and humoral immunity. The cell-mediated immune response is dependent on certain cells, whereas humoral immunity is mediated by antibodies. The three important features of cell-mediated and humoral responses are recognition of foreign material or "non-self," specificity, and memory.

SOME TERMS USED IN THE DISCUSSION OF INFECTIOUS DISEASES

Axenic. This term is used to denote animals that have been raised in a germ-free atmosphere and that are consequently germ-free. These animals are remarkably susceptible to infectious agents. They have a retarded development of antibody-producing organs and are consequently deficient in immunoglobulins. The absence of normal flora influences the responsiveness of the host to infectious agents.

Carrier. When this term is used in connection with an infectious agent, it indicates that it is present on or within an animal, generally as a commensal. There is usually no evidence of disease. A pig may carry *Salmonella choleraesuis* without showing any clinical signs of disease.

Carrier Rate. This denotes the percentage of animals carrying a certain organism. For example, the carrier rate of *Pasteurella* spp. in the mouths of cats may be as high as 60%.

Disease. Any disturbance of the structure or function of constituents of the animal organism. Some make a distinction between infection and disease. Because these terms are mostly used synonymously, such a distinction is not recommended.

Endogenous Infection. An infection produced or originating from within the animal, such as infections caused by *Fusobacterium necrophorum*.

Enzootic. The habitual presence of an animal disease in a certain geographic area. The word **endemic** has the same meaning but is usually applied to human beings; however, it may also be used for animals.

Epidemic may be used as a synonym for epizootic.

Epidemiology. This is the study of the factors and mechanisms that govern the spread of disease within a population or community. Microbiology is particularly important in epidemiology, as most of the diseases studied are caused by microorganisms.

Special methods have been developed to identify precisely the particular variety or type of microorganism involved in a disease outbreak. Such identification enables the epidemiologist to trace the spread of various infectious agents. The well-known epidemiologic typing methods include the antibiogram (pattern of antibiotic susceptibilities), biotyping, serotyping, bacteriocin typing, and bacteriophage typing. Among the more recent molecular typing methods are plasmid analysis, restriction endonuclease analysis of chromosomal DNA, ribotyping, and electrophoresis of various proteins.

Epizootic. A disease attacking a large number of animals within a short time span and usually spreading rapidly, such as foot-and-mouth disease.

Exogenous Infection. An infection produced or originating external to the animal; for example, anthrax.

Gnotobiotic. This term is used to describe animals whose flora and fauna are known because they have previously been defined and established. To maintain their gnotobiotic status, they must be kept in isolation to prevent the addition of exogenous organisms.

Incidence (in Epidemiology). A measurement of only the new cases of a disease occurring during a given period.

Infectivity. The capacity to become established in the tissues of the host.

Invasive. This term is sometimes used to describe an organism's capacity for entering and spreading within tissues.

Latent Infections. Persisting subclinical infections. There is frequently a latent state in tuberculosis.

Mixed Infections. More than one microbial agent may be associated with a disease. For example, "shipping fever" pneumonia in cattle may involve a bacterium, a virus, and a mycoplasma. It may be difficult to determine or estimate the relative importance of each.

Natural History of Disease. The usual course of infectious disease from the beginning to the end if there is no treatment.

Prevalence (in Epidemiology). A measurement of all cases of disease existing at a given time.

Primary Agent of Disease. A microbial agent that can initiate disease on its own; for example, *B. abortus*.

Secondary Invader. A microbial agent that invades or establishes itself in tissues that have been infected by a primary agent.

Specific Pathogen–Free Animals. Animals that have been derived from stock established from caesarian-delivered animals. Swine thus derived may be maintained free of *Bordetella bronchiseptica*, *Salmonella* species, transmissible gastroenteritis virus, and *Mycoplasma hyopneumoniae*.

Specific Pathogen–Free Flocks. Flocks established from eggs free of known pathogenic agents, including mycoplasmas. They are used to provide eggs and chickens for research and for the initiation of other similar flocks.

Zoonosis. This is a disease, primarily of animals, that is occasionally transmitted to humans.

PROGRESSION OF AN INFECTIOUS DISEASE

With clinical disease, signs and symptoms of disease follow a particular course from the initial symptoms to signs of recovery. These clinical signs often give the clinician some indication as to the pathogen involved. The phases of disease progression can be generalized to give an overview of the development of most diseases. Even with treatment, the disease typically follows essentially the same progression.

Incubation Phase

This is the first phase of the progression of disease. It is defined as the period of time beginning with the initial infection through to the point where the individual presents with clinical signs. The disease agent has entered the body, localized to a particular region, and begun replication. Although this phase is asymptomatic, the individual is capable of transmitting the disease agent to others. The duration of the incubation phase varies based on the nature of the disease agent, numbers of organisms present, and virulence. For example, in canine rabies the incubation phase is 21 days to 2 months.

Prodromal Phase

This phase in disease progression is relatively short in comparison to the others. It is characterized by nonspecific, mild signs. These may include, for instance, local redness and swelling, depression, and anorexia. Some diseases do not have a prodromal phase but, rather, have a sudden onset of more specific signs, such as fever.

Invasive Phase

This is the phase in which the characteristic signs of a particular disease are apparent. Individuals are contagious during this phase. Signs of the invasive phase include cough, fever, swollen regional lymph nodes, skin rashes, nasal congestion, nausea, vomiting, and diarrhea. During the invasive phase, a point is reached when the signs are at the greatest intensity. This is known as acme, the point in disease progression when the pathogen has invaded and damaged host tissues. An acme can be sudden and severe or chronic, depending upon the characteristic of the pathogen. It is during this time that host–pathogen interactions are at their most intense and the disease outcome is decided. If the host "wins," the result is recovery. If the pathogen "wins," the result is potentially death or some other impairment.

Decline Phase

This phase is characterized by the decline in signs associated with the disease. This is the result of a "win" for the host defenses or may be the result of the combined efforts of treatment and the host immune response. Secondary infections may occur at this time, as the immune system has been compromised during the interaction with the original pathogen.

Convalescent Phase

This is the period in which the host begins to repair the damage caused by the presence of the pathogen, and the host recovers. This phase is sometimes marked by the presence of circulating antibodies—these can be obtained from the individual and are referred to as convalescent serum. Even in this phase, some individuals can be infectious if the disease is characterized by some type of scab or accessible lesion.

CONSEQUENCES OF THE HOST–PARASITE INTERACTION

- **No infection.** The organism for reasons of insufficient numbers or virulence or the defenses of the host are unable to establish an infection and is eliminated.
- **Colonization.** The organism infects the body and colonizes but is unable to spread because of the body's defenses; for example, a local *S. aureus* infection.
- **Unapparent or subclinical infection.** The host becomes infected, often generally, but the specific immune response prevents the organism causing overt clinical disease. The organism, for example, a *Salmonella* species, may infect several tissues, and the host is said to be a carrier.
- **Clinical disease.** This results as the organisms multiply and the defenses of the body attempt to control the infection. The results may be recovery with specific immunity and elimination of the pathogen, a carrier state, or death.
- **Death.** Usually the result of the infection, but underlying illness is involved.

GLOSSARY

adjuvant Substance that increases the potency (immunogenicity) of an antigen or immunogen.

bacterial sepsis Presence of bacteria and their toxins in the blood or tissues.

bradykinin Composed of a chain of nine amino acid residues that is formed in injured tissues and acts in the inflammatory process by dilating small vessels.

catecholamines Substances that act as hormones or neurotransmitters or both.

Forssman's antibodies Antibodies to glycolipid antigens that are found on the tissue cells of many species including the dog, cat, horse, and sheep, but not humans, rabbit, rat, pig, or cow.

hemorrhagic septicemia Specifically, an acute disease of mainly cattle and water buffalo, caused by a variety of the bacterial species *P. multocida*.

histamine Vasodilator and smooth muscle constrictor widely distributed in tissues and in high concentrations in mast cells. It is released when cell-bound IgE (an antibody) reacts with antigen.

interleukin-1 One of a number of interleukins that mainly function in the regulation of the immune system. They are produced by lymphocytes and monocytes.

ischemia Deficiency of blood in tissue caused by obstruction or functional constriction of a blood vessel.

leukotrienes Group of metabolites of arachidonic acid that have a number of pharmacological effects. They may be released from mast cells, leukocytes, and platelets.

prostaglandins Number of hormone-like compounds that have a variety of functions as inflammatory mediators.

serotonin Found in platelets and mast cells, this compound is a neurotransmitter and causes smooth muscle contraction, increased vascular permeability, and vasoconstriction of larger vessels.

shock In general, a state of circulatory failure associated with reduced total blood volume and low blood pressure. It has various causes including endotoxin.

Shwartzman reaction Follows the second of two doses of lipopolysaccaride. It is characterized by local skin necrosis or generalized disease of kidneys, liver, heart, and lungs.

8   Antimicrobial Agents

Chemotherapy, a term that originated with Paul Ehrlich, refers to the treatment of infectious diseases by administering drugs that are inhibitory or lethal to the infecting agents. Such a drug must exhibit a selective toxicity directed at the causative organism rather than the host. Drugs that are highly toxic to both organism and host are obviously unsatisfactory.

Although chemotherapeutic drugs were known before Ehrlich's time, he was the first to deliberately seek new antimicrobial compounds. When he found a compound that showed at least limited activity for an organism, he would synthesize closely related compounds to find more effective ones. Organic chemists are still using this approach. In 1907, after trying many compounds for their activity against the spirochetes of syphilis, Ehrlich found that the arsenical compound arsphenamine was selectively toxic for *Treponema pallidum*. This was the first of a long series of drugs to be synthesized in the laboratory.

A number of years later, Domagk (1935) showed that the red dye Prontosil was effective in the treatment of streptococcal infections. Later, it was shown that the treatment's antibacterial activity was the result of sulfanilamide derived from Prontosil. The success of this drug stimulated a search for related compounds and resulted in the synthesis of a host of effective compounds of the sulfonamide group. Although Ehrlich is rightly considered the father of modern chemotherapy, a number of drugs were developed for various diseases before his time. Paracelsus (sixteenth century) used mercury compounds for the treatment of syphilis. By the nineteenth century, the natives of South America had found that quinine was an effective treatment for malaria.

ANTIBIOTICS

An antibiotic is defined as an antimicrobial substance produced by a living microorganism. Pasteur and Joubert (1877) first reported that some common airborne contaminants had a lethal effect on a culture of *Bacillus anthracis*. Similar observations were made over the years, and Fleming (1929) observed that a fungus, *Penicillium notatum*, when present on a culture plate, strongly inhibited the growth of staphylococci. In fact, he carried out a crude plate susceptibility test. This discovery was not exploited until 1940, when Chain, Florey, and associates succeeded in obtaining preparations from *Penicillium* that had high antibacterial activity but low toxicity for humans and animals. The remarkable therapeutic efficacy of penicillin against a variety of diseases was soon demonstrated.

After the discovery of penicillin, an extensive search for antibiotics began. The richest source of these drugs was found to be species of *Streptomyces*. Other sources of useful antibiotics have been bacteria, particularly actinomycetes, and certain fungi.

Mechanism of Action of Antimicrobial Drugs

Antimicrobial drugs are divided into two classes, based on their general effects on bacterial populations. Bactericidal drugs have a rapid lethal action. Examples are penicillin, streptomycin, the cephalosporins, polymyxin, and neomycin. In high concentrations, erythromycin may be bactericidal. Bacteriostatic drugs inhibit the growth of organisms. Examples are tetracyclines, sulfonamides, and chloramphenicol. They depend upon the immune system to kill and remove the bacteria.

In practice, this classification is not always clear-cut. Most drugs are, in varying degrees, both bactericidal and bacteriostatic. The way in which they act depends on the drug, its concentration, and factors such as the type, quantity, and growth state of the organism. For example, penicillin is strongly bactericidal against rapidly growing organisms but has little effect on organisms in a stationary state. Intracellular bacteria may be dormant in macrophages and, thus, are not destroyed by antimicrobial drugs.

Major antimicrobial drugs of veterinary importance are grouped here according to their mechanism of action (Table 8.1).

The sites of action of major groups of antimicrobial agents are shown schematically in Fig. 8.1.

INHIBITION OF GROWTH BY ANTIMETABOLITES (MOLECULAR MIMICRY)

Sulfonamides

As mentioned earlier, sulfonamides are bacteriostatic; that is, they inhibit growth but do not kill. They are effective against growing and proliferating bacteria but not against

Table 8.1   Major Antimicrobial Drugs of Veterinary Importance Based on Mechanism of Action

Mechanism of Action	Antimicrobial Agent
Inhibition of growth by antimetabolites (molecular mimicry)	Sulfamides; sulfones
Inhibition of cell wall synthesis	Penicillins; cephalosporins; bacitracin; vancomycin; carbapenems
Inhibition of protein synthesis	Aminoglycosides; streptomycin; neomycin; kanamycin; gentamycin; tobramycin; spectinomycin; amikacin; tetracyclines; chloramphenicol; florphenicol; erythromycin; tylosin; tilmicosin; azithromycin; roxithromycin; clarithromycin; clindamycin; lincomycin; tiamulin; valnemulin; pirlimycin; mupiricin; virginiamycin; linezolid
Impairment of membrane function	Polymyxin
Inhibition of nucleic acid synthesis	Quinolones; fluoroquinolones; nitrofurans; nitroimidazoles; rifampin; novobiocin
Additional chemotherapeutic agents with various modes of action	Mandelamine; arsenicals; ethambutol; isoniazid

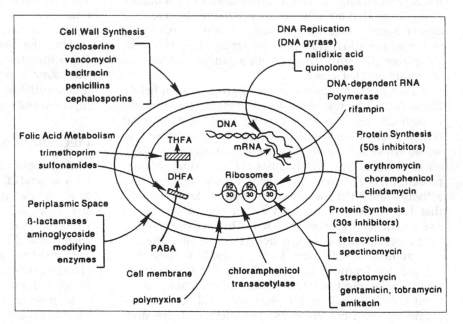

FIGURE 8.1   Sites of action of various antimicrobial agents. DNA, deoxyribonucleic acid; mRNA, messenger ribonucleic acid; tRNA, transfer RNA; PABA, para-aminobenzoic acid; DHFA, dihydrofolic acid; THFA, tetra-hydrofolic acid. (Courtesy of H. C. Neu, *Science*, 257: 1064, 1992.)

dormant ones. Unlike animal cells, for many bacteria, para-aminobenzoic acid (PABA) is an essential metabolite in the synthesis of folic acid, which is subsequently required in the synthesis of purines. Sulfonamides are structural analogues of PABA and thus can compete with it, resulting in the formation of nonfunctional analogues of folic acid. Some bacteria, like some animal cells, cannot synthesize folic acid but require it for growth. These organisms are not inhibited by sulfonamides.

An excess of PABA, such as that released during extensive tissue destruction, counteracts the inhibiting action of sulfonamides. For this reason, PABA may be added to culture media when attempting to isolate bacteria from animals that have been treated with sulfonamides.

Sulfonamides may be combined with a diaminopyrimidine (trimethoprim, ormetoprim, and others) to produce sequential blocking that results in enhanced activity with bactericidal consequences. Trimethoprim, which is most commonly used, blocks the formation of folic acid by inhibiting the action of dihydrofolic acid reductase. This reductase is essential for the formation of tetrahydrofolate from dihydrofolate.

The susceptibility of some groups of bacteria to diaminopyrimidine–sulfonamide combinations, such as trimethoprim + sulfadiazine (Tribrissen), is as follows:

- **Very susceptible:** *Escherichia, Proteus, Salmonella, Pasteurella,* and *Streptococcus.*
- **Susceptible:** *Staphylococcus, Corynebacterium, Clostridium, Neisseria, Bordetella, Klebsiella,* and *Fusiformis.*
- **Moderately susceptible:** *Nocardia, Moraxella,* and *Brucella.*
- **Not susceptible:** *Mycobacterium, Erysipetothrix, Pseudomonas,* and *Leptospira.*

Trimethoprim is combined with various sulfonamides, including sulfadiazine, sulfadoxine, and sulfamethoxazole. The combination ormetoprim–sulfadimethoxine is used widely in dogs and cats.

Many sulfonamides are available, and their use depends to some extent on their physicochemical characteristics, particularly their solubility. Among the sulfonamides most frequently used in veterinary practice are sulfamethazine, sulfadimethoxine, and sulfachlorpyridazine.

Although mutant resistance occurs with sulfonamides, most resistance is caused by an R factor (plasmid; see Chapter 5).

Sulfones

The sulfones are also structural analogues of PABA, and their mode of action is similar to the sulfonamides. The sulfones are relatively toxic and have a limited antimicrobial spectrum. Their actions include suppression of non-specific inflammation.

Dapsone is the most widely used sulfone. It is used in the treatment of human leprosy and mycobacterial infections in dogs and cats, including feline leprosy.

INHIBITION OF CELL WALL SYNTHESIS

The peptidoglycan of bacterial cell walls is unique. Thus, it is not surprising that a number of antimicrobial drugs that inhibit the synthesis of glycopeptides are effective clinically. Synthesis of peptidoglycan is inhibited at several points, depending on the drug administered.

Penicillins

Penicillin inhibits the synthesis of cell walls of growing, susceptible bacteria. The bacterial protoplasm increases and eventually bursts the cytoplasmic membrane, resulting in lysis and death. If the bacteria are growing in a medium of high osmotic tension, cell wall–deficient forms called protoplasts (gram-positive) or spheroplasts (gram-negative) with intact cytoplasmic membranes are formed. Penicillin inhibits the enzyme responsible for the cross-linking between the layers of peptidoglycan. Although penicillins are most active against the gram-positive organisms, they are also active against a number of gram-negative ones.

Of the many different penicillins derived from *Penicillium*, only several are of value in treatment. Two that are widely used are penicillin G (benzyl penicillin), which is administered intramuscularly, and penicillin V (phenoxymethyl penicillin), which is resistant to acid decomposition and can therefore be given orally. Procaine is used in penicillin preparations to delay absorption.

Some penicillinase-resistant, semisynthetic penicillins, including methicillin, oxacillin, cloxacillin, and nafcillin, have been obtained by adding side chains to naturally occurring 6-amino penicillanic acid. The addition of these side chains prevents, by steric interference, degradation of the β-lactam ring by penicillinase (β-lactamases). The hydrolysis of the β-lactam ring by β-lactamase is illustrated in Fig. 8.2.

Penicillin Groups

The penicillins can be grouped in several ways. Below they are grouped primarily on the basis of differences in their antibacterial activity. Only some of the more important penicillins are included.

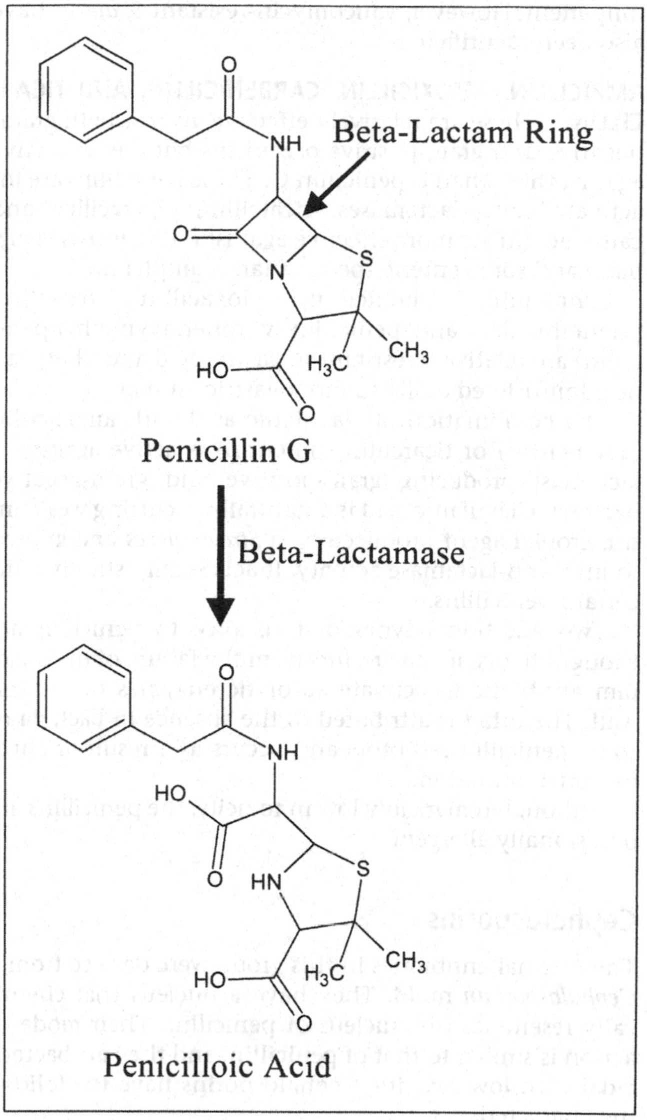

FIGURE 8.2 Hydrolysis of the beta-lactam ring of penicillin (active) by beta-lactamase into penicilloic acid (inactive).

PENICILLIN G (BENZYL PENICILLIN). This penicillin has the greatest activity against gram-positive organisms and is active against some gram-negative species. It is susceptible to β-lactamase (penicillinase) inactivation and acid hydrolysis.

OXACILLIN, METHICILLIN, CLOXACILLIN, AND NAFCILLIN. These penicillins are less active against gram-positive organisms than penicillin G. They are inactive against almost all gram-negative bacteria and are relatively resistant to staphylococcal β-lactamases.

Recently, there has been an emergence of methicillin-resistant *Staphylococcus aureus* (MRSA), which is often nosocomially acquired. The Centers for Disease Control and Prevention estimate that as many as 80,000 patients a year acquire MRSA infections after they enter the hospital. At present, treatment is limited to vancomycin and imipenem. However, vancomycin-resistant *S. aureus* have also been identified.

AMPICILLIN, AMOXICILLIN, CARBENICILLIN, AND TICAR-CILLIN. These are relatively effective against both gram-negative and gram-positive organisms but are less active against these than is penicillin G. These penicillins are inactivated by β-lactamases. Ticarcillin, piperacillin, and carbenicillin are more effective against *Pseudomonas aeruginosa* and some enteric species than is ampicillin.

Ampicillin, amoxicillin, cloxacillin, oxacillin, phenethicillin, and penicillin V (phenoxymethyl-penicillin) are relatively resistant to gastric acid and, thus, can be administered orally to monogastric animals.

The combination of clavulanic acid with amoxicillin (augmentin) or ticarcillin (timentin) is active against β-lactamase–producing gram-positive and gram-negative bacteria. Clavulanic acid is a naturally occurring weak antimicrobial agent produced by a *Streptomyces* and known to inhibit β-lactamase activity. It acts synergistically with certain penicillins.

Two additional types of resistance to penicillin are thought to occur. One results from the failure of the β-lactam antibiotic to activate autolytic enzymes in the cell wall. The other is attributed to the absence in bacteria of some penicillin receptors and occurs as a result of chromosomal mutation.

Although remarkably low in toxicity, the penicillins are occasionally allergenic.

Cephalosporins

The original antibiotics in this group were derived from a *Cephalosporium* mold. They have a nucleus that chemically resembles the nucleus of penicillin. Their mode of action is similar to that of penicillin, and they are bactericidal with low toxicity. Cephalosporins have the following characteristics:

- Resistance to penicillinase in varying degrees.
- Not as allergenic as penicillin.
- A broad spectrum of activity and can be used against staphylococci (including penicillin-resistant strains), streptococci (although enterococci are resistant), and a wide range of gram-negative bacteria.

Some of the oral cephalosporins in use are cephradine, cephaloglycin, cephalexin, and cefadroxil. The parenteral cephalosporins include cephaloridine, cephalothin, cephapirin, cephalonidine, cephradine, cefadroxil, cefoxitin, and cefamandole.

Many cephalosporins have been developed, a number of which are not available in the United States. The older cephalosporins (cephalothin, cefazolin, cephapirin, cephradine, cephadroxil, and cephalexin) are referred to as first-generation cephalosporins. These are active against most gram-positive bacteria but have limited activity against gram-negative bacteria.

The second-generation cephalosporins (cefamadole, cefonicid, ceforanide, cefotiam, cefuroxime, cefotitan, cefoxitin, and cefaclor) are active against most gram-positive bacteria and have a broader spectrum of activity against gram-negative organisms than the first-generation agents.

The third-generation cephalosporins (cefotaxime, ceftiofur, moxalactan, cefixime, cefatazidime, ceftizoxime, cefoperazone, and cefmenoxine) have limited activity against gram-positive bacteria but are effective against most gram-negative organisms. Not all of the cephalosporins have been listed above.

Some cephalosporins used in susceptibility tests in veterinary laboratories are ceftiofur, cephalothin, cefazolin, ceftazidine, and cefositin.

Bacitracin

This is a polypeptide produced by a strain of *Bacillus subtilis*. It interacts with the bacterial cell membrane to prevent the transfer of structural cell wall units. It is bactericidal and acts principally against gram-positive organisms. High toxicity precludes its systemic use, but it is useful for topical application and is often combined with such drugs as polymyxin and neomycin.

Vancomycin

This antibiotic is derived from a streptomycete. Its mode of action and spectrum of activity are similar to those of bacitracin. Although rather toxic (it may cause nerve deafness, thrombophlebitis, and kidney damage), it is used in emergencies to treat staphylococcal infections caused by multidrug-resistant *S. aureus*. However, some strains of *S. aureus* have developed vancomycin resistance, and linezolid and synercid have been used as last-resort drugs.

Carbapenems

Imipenem was the first carbapenem developed for clinical use. This broad-spectrum, semisynthetic antibiotic is a derivative of thienamycin, which is produced by *Streptomyces* spp. Imipenem is given with cilastatin; the latter is a peptidase inhibitor that counteracts inactivation by dihydropeptidases in the renal tubules. Other carbapenems are meropenem and biapenem. They are structurally related to the β-lactam antibiotics.

The carbapenems work by inhibiting cell wall synthesis. They have a very wide spectrum of activity against many gram-negative and gram-positive organisms, and thus, their use may lead to superinfections. They are resistant to most plasmid- or chromosome-mediated β-lactamases. Imipenim is the most frequently use carbapenem in veterinary practice.

INHIBITION OF PROTEIN SYNTHESIS

Aminoglycosides (Aminocyclitols)

All drugs in this group of antibiotics, derived from *Micromonospora* spp. (gentamicin, sisomicin, and netilmicin) or from *Streptomyces* spp. (streptomycin, neomycin, tobramycin, spectinomycin, and kanamycin), have similar structures and modes of action. They bind to the smaller (30S) of the two ribosomal subunits, resulting in the miscoding of proteins and inhibition of peptide elongation.

STREPTOMYCIN. This drug is bactericidal and is active against gram-negative bacteria, mycobacteria, and some gram-positive organisms. Resistance to streptomycin is encountered frequently and may be caused by mutation or R factors. It is not absorbed from the gut and is normally administered intramuscularly. When combined with tetracycline it is very useful in the treatment of brucellosis and plague.

Streptomycin sulfate has replaced the more toxic dihydrostreptomycin. Prolonged high blood levels of streptomycin can result in severe disturbances of hearing and vestibular function.

NEOMYCIN AND KANAMYCIN. These drugs are closely related structurally and have similar activity and complete cross-resistance. They are stable, and both are poorly absorbed from the intestinal tract but readily absorbed if given intramuscularly. Both are excreted in the urine. Kanamycin is less toxic than neomycin and, consequently, is used systemically.

Both drugs are bactericidal for many gram-negative species. In animals, neomycin is used most frequently to treat intestinal infections, metritis, and bovine mastitis. Neomycin also is used with other drugs in topical preparations.

Both drugs may cause renal damage and nerve deafness.

GENTAMICIN. Gentamicin resembles neomycin and is mainly active against many gram-negative organisms, including *P. aeruginosa*, and some gram-positive species. It is included in topical preparations with other drugs.

TOBRAMYCIN. Tobramycin resembles gentamicin chemically and pharmacologically.

SPECTINOMYCIN. This drug somewhat resembles the aminoglycosides in structure and site of action. It has been used mainly to treat infections caused by gram-negative bacteria and mycoplasmas.

AMIKACIN. Amikacin is a derivative of kanamycin and resembles gentamicin. It is active against many gram-negative organisms that are resistant to tobramycin and gentamicin. It is mainly used in horses and dogs.

RESISTANCE TO AMINOGLYCOSIDES. There are several mechanisms of resistance to aminoglycoside antibiotics:

- **Impaired ribosomal binding:** For example, in some *Escherichia coli* and *P. aeruginosa* strains, a single step mutation prevents the binding of the aminoglycoside to the ribosome. This is not considered an important mechanism of resistance.
- **Impaired transport:** This involves impairment of transport across the cell membrane. Because transport is oxygen dependent, this nonplasmid-mediated resistance occurs more frequently with anaerobes.
- **Aminoglycoside-altering enzymes:** This type of resistance may be either plasmid or chromosome mediated and is encountered with both gram-negative and gram-positive bacteria. Three different enzymes may be involved in the inactivation of the drug.

Several other mechanisms of resistance of minor importance have been described.

Tetracyclines

Drugs in this group are derived from streptomycetes. The three naturally occurring tetracyclines are chlortetracycline, oxytetracycline, and demethylchlortetracycline. A number of antibiotics have been derived semisynthetically from these; for example, tetracycline, methacycline, doxycycline, and minocycline. They act by binding to the 30S ribosomal subunit, causing inhibition of the function of tRNA. They are bacteriostatic, and their mode of action is reversible. Trade names of the more common tetracyclines are Achromycin (tetracycline), Aureomycin (chlortetracycline), and Terramycin (oxytetracycline).

The tetracyclines are broad-spectrum antibiotics that are active against a wide range of gram-positive and gram-negative organisms, including rickettsiae, chlamydiae, and mycoplasmas. Organisms that are resistant to penicillin are often susceptible to the tetracyclines. Also, they are often of value in treating mixed infections. In animals, they may be conveniently administered in feed or water.

Superinfection with *Candida albicans* or *S. aureus* can be a complication after treatment with the tetracyclines. Although they are of relatively low toxicity, liver damage has been encountered in pregnant women receiving the drugs. In addition, tetracyclines may inhibit the growth of bones and teeth in the fetus and in infants. Long-term administration should be avoided in children and, presumably, in young animals.

Other drugs in this group include doxycycline and minocycline, which have greater anti-inflammatory activity than other tetracyclines. The antibacterial activity of drugs among the tetracycline group is similar, but they differ slightly in their duration of action and rates of absorption and excretion.

Resistance to the tetracyclines depends for the most part on decreased penetration of the drug into bacteria that were previously susceptible. Plasmid-mediated resistance (R factor) is widespread and results in either reduced uptake or efflux of the drug from bacteria. General cross-resistance exists among the tetracyclines.

Chloramphenicol (Chloromycetin)

This is a broad-spectrum drug derived from a streptomycete. It is bacteriostatic and acts by specifically binding to the larger 50S ribosomal subunit, thus inhibiting protein synthesis. It is a very effective drug in animals, although its use in food-producing animals is restricted in the United States and Canada.

In rare instances, prolonged administration results in severe or even fatal depression of bone marrow function, leading to aplastic anaemia. Because of this, its use in humans is reserved for very serious infections, such as typhoid fever. Veterinarians have found chloramphenicol to be a relatively safe drug for a variety of infections in companion animals.

Chloramphenicol resistance, which is plasmid-mediated, is caused by the inactivation of the antibiotic by the bacterial enzyme chloramphenicol acetyltransferase.

Florfenicol, a thiamphenicol derivative of chloramphenicol, is more active in vitro than is chloramphenicol against the same bacterial pathogens. Florfenicol has been approved for use in cattle and is sometimes administered to other animals.

Macrolides

ERYTHROMYCIN, TYLOSIN, AND TILMICOSIN. The macrolide antibiotics contain a macrocyclic lactone ring to which one or more sugars are attached. These antibiotics are derived from streptomycetes and inhibit protein synthesis by binding to the 50S ribosomal subunit. Erythromycin, tylosin, and tilmicosin are the most useful of the macrolides from a veterinary standpoint. Related drugs are spiramycin and oleandomycin.

The macrolides are effective against gram-positive bacteria including staphylococci, streptococci, clostridia, corynebacteria, and *Listeria*. Some gram-negative bacteria, including *Pasteurella*, *Campylobacter*, and *Haemophilus*, are susceptible, as well as mycoplasmas, chlamydia, and rickettsia. The macrolides are used as substitutes for penicillin in the treatment of staphylococcal and streptococcal infections. Other indications are bronchopneumonia, upper respiratory tract infections, pyoderma, metritis, enteritis, urinary tract infections, and bovine mastitis. Except for tilmicosin, toxic reactions and side effects from macrolide use are uncommon.

Resistance may be plasmid-mediated or chromosomal mutation in origin. With gram-negative bacteria, resistance involves the inability to penetrate the cell, and with gram-positive bacteria, it involves alteration of the receptor site on the ribosome. The resistance caused by modified ribosomes crosses to clindamycin and lincomycin, suggesting that the site of action of these two nonmacrolide drugs is similar to that of erythromycin.

Tylosin inhibits protein synthesis by preventing the translocation of the aminoacyl-tRNA on the 50S ribosomal subunit. It displays partial or complete cross-resistance with erythromycin. Tylosin is relatively water insoluble and is administered in feed to treat intestinal infections and systemically for some gram-positive, gram-negative, and mycoplasmal infections; for example, various pneumonias, chronic respiratory disease of chickens, and infectious sinusitis of turkeys. Tylosin has been widely used as a feed additive for promoting growth in poultry and in livestock.

Tilmicosin is derived from tylosin and is active against some gram-negative and gram-positive bacteria. It has been used to treat bovine and ovine respiratory disease caused mainly by *Mannheimia haemolytica*. It is used orally in swine to treat infections caused by *Actinobacillus* spp. and *Pasteurella multocida*.

ADVANCED-GENERATION MACROLIDES. Included in this category are azithromycin, roxithromycin, and clarithromycin. They have much the same antibacterial spectrum as the other macrolides but are more effective against intracellular bacteria. To date, they have had limited veterinary use. Advantages are a once-daily oral administration for a shorter time than the well-known macrolides and fewer adverse effects. A disadvantage is their high cost.

CLINDAMYCIN AND LINCOMYCIN (LINCOSAMIDES). Lincomycin is derived from a streptomycete, and clindamycin is a chlorine-substituted derivative of lincomycin. They resemble erythromycin in mechanism of action, spectrum of activity, and possession of ribosomal receptors. They are active against a number of gram-positive species and several gram-negative bacteria that are penicillin resistant. Clindamycin is useful in the treatment of some infections caused by *Bacteroides* and other anaerobes.

Clindamycin has been implicated in human antibiotic-associated colitis caused by *Clostridium difficile*. This clindamycin-resistant organism gains prominence in the colon when other members of the colonic flora are diminished. The pseudomembranous colitis caused by the necrotizing toxin of *C. difficile* can be fatal. Clindamycin is widely used in veterinary practice.

TIAMULIN. Tiamulin is a semisynthetic derivative of the fungal-derived **diterpene** antibiotic pleuromutilin. It inhibits protein synthesis by binding to the 50S ribosomal subunit. Its antimicrobial spectrum is similar to the macrolide tylosin, and it has similar applications, although it is used much less frequently. It is effective against a number of porcine diseases including swine dysentery, enzootic pneumonia, swine pleuropneumonia, and *Streptococcus suis* infections.

PIRLIMYCIN. The spectrum of activity of this amide against aerobes and anaerobes is similar to that of clindamycin. Probably because of its concentration and retention in tissues, it is useful in the treatment of bovine mastitis caused by gram-positive bacteria.

MUPIROCIN. This recently derived antibiotic is obtained from *Pseudomonas fluorescens* by fermentation. It is a strong inhibitor of bacterial isoleucyl transfer RNA synthetase and, thus, stops protein synthesis. It is bactericidal and most active against staphylococci and streptococci. Although it may have limited veterinary application, it has been used effectively in the topical treatment of feline acne.

VIRGINIAMYCIN. This is an antibiotic mixture (virginiamycin M and S) derived from a streptomycete, which acts by interfering with protein synthesis. It is active against gram-positive aerobic and anaerobic bacteria; most gram-negative organisms are resistant. Virginiamycin is mainly used as a feed additive in poultry. It is closely related to the drug synercid, which is used to treat humans infected with multidrug-resistant enterococci.

LINEZOLID. This drug is one of a group of synthetic antimicrobial agents called oxazolidinones. It acts by inhibiting protein synthesis by preventing the formation of the *f*met-tRNA:mRNA:30S subunit complex. It also binds to the 50S ribosomal subunit, similar to chloramphenicol. However, the oxazolidinones are not inhibitors of the enzyme peptidyl transferase. The group is mainly active against gram-positive bacteria and mycobacteria with a lack of useful activity against gram-negative bacteria. Linezolid is used in human medicine to treat both drug-resistant staphylococcal and enterococcal infections in particular.

IMPAIRMENT OF MEMBRANE FUNCTION

An example of antibiotics that impair membrane function are the polymyxins. These polypeptide antibiotics are derived from *Bacillus polymyxa*. They damage the membranes of gram-negative species in particular, resulting in a loss of osmotic control, which in turn causes leakage of potassium ions and other vital bacterial components and, ultimately, death. Polymyxin is poorly absorbed from the intestinal tract and is nephrotoxic and neurotoxic. Unlike most other bactericidal drugs, it kills resting as well as multiplying cells. It is occasionally used in intrauterine infusions in cattle and to treat bovine mastitis and other serious infections caused by *P. aeruginosa* and resistant (to other drugs) enteric bacteria. At present, it is mainly used with other antibiotics in topical preparations.

Polymyxins are large molecules that diffuse poorly in agar media and, therefore, result in small inhibition zones in disc susceptibility tests. The tube dilution test shows greater susceptibility.

INHIBITION OF NUCLEIC ACID FUNCTION

Quinolones/Fluoroquinolones

Quinolones are synthetic analogs of nalidixic acid that possess activity against a wide range of gram-positive and gram-negative aerobic bacteria. The earlier quinolones, such as nalidixic acid, cinoxacin, and oxolinic acid, did not achieve effective systemic levels when given orally and, thus, were only useful as urinary antiseptics. The fluorinated derivatives, enrofloxacin, ciprofloxacin, enoxicin, norfloxacin, and others, have low toxicity and greater antibacterial activity and achieve effective levels in tissues and blood. They are particularly effective against the Enterobacteriaceae and other gram-negative bacteria but less so against streptococci, some other gram-positive organisms, and obligate anaerobes. Ciprofloxacin is used in the prophylaxis of human anthrax and in the treatment of human inhalation or pulmonary anthrax.

Quinolones inhibit bacterial **DNA-gyrase**, leading to a reduction in supercoiling of chromosomal DNA around an RNA core. The loosely coiled DNA then is degraded quickly into small, nonfunctional fragments by the action of exonucleases. The quinolones, which are bactericidal,

often have significant antibacterial activity at very low concentrations when compared with other classes of antimicrobial agents with similar spectra of activity.

Bacterial resistance to quinolones has been observed during therapy. Chromosomal resistance involves two mechanisms: a change in outer membrane permeability resulting in a decrease of the amount of the drug in the bacterium; and an alteration in the A subunit of DNA-gyrase. Although injectable forms are available, quinolones are commonly administered orally. The quinolones used most frequently in veterinary practice are enrofloxacin and ciprofloxacin.

Nitrofuran Derivatives

These synthetic compounds are strongly bactericidal in vitro for many gram-positive and gram-negative bacteria. Most are very insoluble, and some, such as nitrofurazone, are used in topical preparations. The nitrofurans are thought to inhibit a variety of enzyme systems of bacteria and also to damage DNA, but their precise mechanism of action is not known.

Because of toxicity and a low concentration in tissues, the nitrofurans have limited veterinary use.

Nitrofurantoin is used to treat urinary tract infections in dogs and cats. Furazolidone and nifuraldezone are employed to treat intestinal infections caused by *Salmonella* and *E. coli*. Other nitrofurans are incorporated in antibacterial topical preparations.

Nitromidazoles

Metromidazole, dimetridazole, and other nitromidazoles are active against anaerobic bacteria and some gram-positive bacteria. These drugs are taken into susceptible cells and reduced to a cytotoxic factor. The activated cytotoxic factor interacts with DNA, causing mutations that interfere with DNA synthesis. The drugs are bactericidal with a spectrum of activity similar to the nitrofurans. They are administered orally and have good tissue penetration and distribution. In veterinary medicine, they are mainly used to treat anaerobic infections.

Although chromosomal resistance occurs, it is of a low order; plasmid-coded resistance appears to be infrequent.

Rifampin

This is a semisynthetic derivative of the *Streptomyces*-derived antibiotic rifamycin. It inhibits DNA-dependent RNA polymerase activity, which is responsible for the synthesis of cellular RNA. Rifampin is given orally and is active against a wide range of gram-positive organisms and some gram-negative bacteria, chlamydiae, and poxviruses. It is notable for its activity against intracellular bacteria. It has been used effectively in combination with other drugs in the treatment of human tuberculosis. Thus far, it has had little veterinary use.

Novobiocin

This drug, derived from a streptomycete, is readily absorbed from the intestinal tract, but its effectiveness is limited because it binds to protein. It is bacteriostatic and acts by inhibiting the synthesis of DNA and teichoic acid at the cell membrane. Although active against gram-positive cocci and some gram-negative organisms in vitro, it is only used in combination with other drugs in the treatment of serious staphylococcal infections.

Side effects, such as impaired renal function, vomiting, and jaundice, are frequently encountered in humans. It is has very limited veterinary use.

ADDITIONAL CHEMOTHERAPEUTIC AGENTS

Mandelamine (Methenamine Mandelate)

Like nalidixic acid, this drug is used as a urinary antiseptic. It is most useful for suppressing bacteria in the urine of animals and humans with chronic urinary tract infections. It requires a urinary pH lower than 5.5 to be effective. At this pH and below, it is hydrolyzed to ammonia and formaldehyde. This compound has no antibacterial activity by itself.

Arsenicals

The arsenic-containing compounds sodium arsanilate, arsanilic acid, and 3-nitro-4-hydroxyphenylarsonic acid are used to treat swine dysentery and diarrhea of unknown origin in swine. They are also used to promote growth in poultry and swine. There is little data on the efficacy of these compounds in the treatment of diarrhea and dysentery in swine.

All three compounds, and particularly the 3-nitro derivative, are toxic if administered at a therapeutic level to swine for more than a week.

Ethambutol

This synthetic, complex alcohol is sometimes used in combination with other drugs in the treatment of infections caused by atypical mycobacteria. The mechanism of action is thought to be inhibition of the incorporation of mycolic acid into the cell wall.

Isoniazid (Isonicotinic Acid Hydrazide)

This inexpensive, relatively nontoxic compound, when used with other drugs, is very effective in the treatment of human tuberculosis. Resistance develops readily, which is the reason for combinatorial treatment. There is some evidence that it may also be of value in the treatment of bovine nocardial mastitis, bovine actinomycosis, and actinobacillosis. It acts by inhibiting the synthesis of mycolic acids.

SUSEPTIBILITY TESTS

Two kinds of tests are carried out in the diagnostic laboratory: disc susceptibility and tube susceptibility.

Disc Susceptibility Test

Resistant strains are now so prevalent that it is recommended that all clinical isolates considered significant be tested for susceptibility.

The plate or disc procedure is routinely used in veterinary diagnostic laboratories (Fig. 8.3). It involves the uniform inoculation of a plate containing a suitable medium with a standardized amount of organism of the culture to be tested. Paper discs impregnated with the various antimicrobial drugs are then applied, appropriately spaced, with a dispenser. After incubation, usually 24 hours, the size of the zones of inhibition is measured, and based on values that have been established, a culture is reported as being susceptible or resistant. Some laboratories report zones between susceptible and resistant as intermediate.

Because different antimicrobial agents are used for different animal species, diagnostic laboratories have dispensers loaded with the discs required for various categories, e.g., cattle, swine, horses, dogs and cats, poultry, exotic mammals, etc. Discs for each dispenser are selected based on current clinical usage for the organism in question.

Most laboratories now use the Kirby-Bauer procedure, which employs high-potency discs and Mueller-Hinton agar in large Petri dishes. The zones of inhibition described as susceptible, intermediate, and resistant relate to blood concentration and therapeutic efficacy in humans. Mueller-Hinton agar is free of PABA. If PABA is present in the medium, it will inactivate or inhibit the activity of the sulfonamide disc, thus yielding an erroneous result. PABA should only be used in media for isolation purposes if the animal had been treated with a sulfonamide.

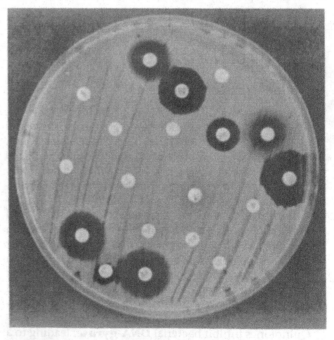

FIGURE 8.3 Disc susceptibility test. The antimicrobial agents incorporated in the discs diffuse into the agar, inhibiting the bacterial growth (clear zones).

Direct susceptibility tests employing clinical material such as pus and urine as inocula are not recommended. The inoculum is not standardized and may contain several different organisms.

Appropriate modifications in the routine Kirby-Bauer procedure are made for fastidious organisms and anaerobes. Blood, serum, and nicotinamide adenine dinucleotide or yeast extract have to be added to grow such organisms as *Haemophilus* species, *Actinobacillus pleuropneumoniae*, *Arcanobacterium pyogenes*, and some streptococci.

Tube Susceptibility Test

This procedure is more complicated than the disc susceptibility test and is infrequently carried out in veterinary diagnostic laboratories. The aim of the test is to determine the minimum inhibitory concentration (MIC) of the drug. This is accomplished by adding a standardized inoculum of organisms (pure culture) to a series of tubes containing increasing concentrations of the drug being tested (Fig. 8.4). After incubation, the results are recorded. The MIC is defined as the highest dilution (the least amount of the drug) that prevents growth. For the drug to be effective clinically, the MIC must be well below the peak blood concentration of the drug expected under recommended dosage schemes.

The minimum bactericidal concentration (MBC) can be determined by plating loopfuls of bacteria from the three successive tubes not showing evidence of growth onto a suitable agar medium. The plate showing no growth indicates the tube in which the concentration of antibiotic being tested has been bacteriocidal and, thus, the MBC.

MICs are not commonly conducted in veterinary diagnostic laboratories, but the availability of automated instruments for the performance of MICs may hasten their use in the larger laboratories.

Serum Bactericidal Test

This is essentially the same as the MIC test except that the drug is present in the patient's serum. This test is rarely carried out in veterinary laboratories. The standardized inoculum of organisms is added to the dilutions of serum. After incubation, the test is read and the serum bactericidal concentration is defined as the highest dilution of serum that prevents growth.

E-Test

The E-test, a variant of the disc susceptibility test, allows the qualitative determination of MICs. The test system consists of a plastic strip containing a gradient of antimicrobial agent on one side and an interpretive scale on the other side. The strip is placed on the surface of an agar plate containing a uniform lawn of the test organism. The strip is incubated at 37°C for 24 hours. The MIC is determined by reading the scale at the point where the zone of inhibition intersects the strip. Results of these tests appear to agree well with the standard agar dilution method.

The cost of the E-test limits its use in veterinary laboratories. It is of particular value in testing the susceptibility of yeasts, fastidious anaerobes, and some mycoplasmas.

Automated Systems

A variety of new automated and semiautomated systems have been introduced in recent years for susceptibility testing of bacteria. Some contain components for rapid identification of bacteria. These systems are capable of providing qualitative (susceptible, intermediate, or resistant) and quantitative (MIC) information in a relatively short period of time. These same-day procedures are more expensive to perform than the traditional tests, and the

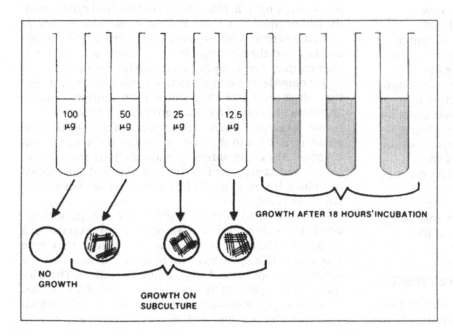

FIGURE 8.4 Tube susceptibility test for determining the minimum inhibitory concentration. Those tubes without evidence of growth (turbidity) are plated out to determine the minimum bactericidal concentration. Note: minimum inhibitory concentration = 12.5 μg/mL; minimum bactericidal concentration = 100 μg/mL.

automated equipment required is too expensive for many diagnostic laboratories.

DRUG RESISTANCE

Many organisms have the ability to produce mutants that are resistant to most of the antimicrobial compounds to which they would ordinarily be susceptible in the wild state. The use of subinhibitory or subtherapeutic levels of antimicrobial compounds in livestock and poultry feeds for growth promotion may contribute to the survival and multiplication of resistant mutants. The degree of resistance, and the time it takes to develop, depends on the organism and the antimicrobial agent.

It is of interest that group A *Streptococcus pyogenes* has not yet developed resistance to penicillin. The development of resistance by *S. aureus* in response to penicillin and the tetracyclines has been typically slow, occurring in small steps over a considerable period of time and exposure. However, after a number of years, many resistant strains now exist. In contrast, resistance of the tubercle bacillus to streptomycin may develop to a high level in a single-step manner.

Resistance is specific, in that an organism will become resistant to a particular antibiotic. Cross-resistance occurs among closely related drugs such as the different tetracyclines, aminoglycosides, macrolides, and fluroquinilones. Resistance to one drug may be followed by resistance to another drug, and thus strains emerge that are resistant to a number of drugs. In addition to this type of chromosomal resistance, multidrug resistance caused by R factors is encountered. This is referred to briefly here, and in detail in Chapter 5.

Mechanisms of Drug Resistance

Some of the mechanisms of drug resistance are as follows:

1. Adoption by the organism of an alternative metabolic pathway to bypass the inhibited reaction; for example, those bacteria resistant to sulfonamides adapt to using preformed folic acid.
2. Production of an enzyme that destroys the antibiotic, such as penicillinase (β-lactamase) from *S. aureus* and other bacteria, or production of enzymes by some bacteria that inactivate drugs by acetylation, adenylation, or phosphorylation.
3. Change in permeability or decreased uptake of the drug by the cell or some special part of the cell, such as occurs in bacteria resistant to tetracyclines and polymyxins.
4. Altered structural target(s) for the drug; for instance, erythromycin-resistant organisms have an altered protein on the 5OS subunit of the bacterial ribosome.

Development of Resistance During Treatment

MUTATION. Resistant mutants may emerge during treatment. The occurrence and establishment of resistant mutants varies with different drugs. Selection of mutants is favored by underdosage, prolonged administration, and the presence of a "closed" focus of infection, such an abscess.

The drugs listed below are grouped roughly according to the likelihood that resistant mutants will emerge during treatment.

- **Frequent:** Sulfonamides, streptomycin, nalidixic acid, and rifamycin.
- **Less frequent:** Erythromycin.
- **Infrequent:** Tetracyclines, penicillin, cephalosporins, and chloramphenicol.

SUPERINFECTION. This term is frequently used to describe the infection that is caused by "alien" organisms such as *C. albicans* as a result of the alteration or suppression of the normal flora by prolonged antibiotic administration. The disturbance of the normal flora in animals does not ordinarily cause more than occasional intestinal upsets and diarrhea. However, prolonged administration of antibiotics affecting gram-negative intestinal organisms may cause a deficiency or diminution in the amounts of vitamin K, biotin, riboflavin, pantothenate, and pyridoxine available to the host. Supplementation with vitamins, particularly vitamin B complex, is used in humans during prolonged administration of certain antibiotics.

Superinfection is also used to describe the replacement of the original infecting agent with a new strain of the same species that is resistant, or a resistant strain of another species. *Pseudomonas aeruginosa* and *Acinetobacter* are frequently encountered as "replacement" strains.

Infectious Drug Resistance

Transferable multiple drug resistance caused by R factors occurs most commonly in members of the Enterobacteriaceae. This type of resistance, that is, the whole multiple pattern, is transferable among strains of the same species and among strains of closely related species, such as from a *Salmonella* to an *E. coli*. Transfer of this kind can be readily demonstrated in vitro and no doubt also occurs in vivo. It is now very widespread, and strains are commonly encountered that are resistant to as many as four drugs; for example, streptomycin, a tetracycline, penicillin, and a sulfonamide. It seems likely that some increase in infectious drug resistance has resulted from routinely adding antibiotics to animal feeds for growth promotion.

For example, there are three main mechanisms whereby *E. coli* can develop or acquire resistance to antibiotics. These are intrinsic (natural) resistance, mutational resistance, and extrachromosomal (acquired) resistance. Instances of all of these can be found in various strains of *E. coli*.

With regard to intrinsic resistance, *E. coli* possess the *acrAB–tolC* operon system. This operon is an example of a multidrug efflux system. The combined action of the gene products of this operon system result in the secretion of a variety of lipophilic and amphiphilic inhibitors. These inhibitors are capable of neutralizing a variety of antibiotics.

An example of mutational resistance in *E. coli* is associated with the development of resistance to cefoxitin. In this case, it is observed that cefoxitin-resistant strains possessed mutations predominantly in the attenuator and or promoters of a variety of genes. Another mutational resistance mechanism of *E. coli* is known as translational stress-induced mutagenesis. Under stress, these *E. coli* produce a mutant glycine tRNA, which may interfere with those drugs (such as streptomycin) whose mode of action is to cause translational misreading.

The most common mode of antibiotic resistance in *E. coli* is via the acquired route. Typically, this is plasmid-based (R plasmids) from organism to organism. In addition, resistance can be acquired by natural transduction (infection by bacteriophages containing resistance genes that become integrated) or by transposition.

Many antibacterial resistance genes have been identified. For example, at least 10 resistance genes have been identified in different bacteria for resistance to aminoglycosides, seven for β-lactam drugs, 11 for tetracyclines, and so on. Although seldom used in veterinary laboratories, DNA probes and PCR primers are available for the identification of resistance genes in many bacteria of significance in human infections.

The genetics of drug resistance is discussed in Chapter 5.

SUGGESTIONS ON THE USE OF ANTIMICROBIAL DRUGS

1. When selecting and using antimicrobial drugs, the possibility of the emergence of resistant organisms should always be kept in mind.
2. Antimicrobial agents should not be employed for mild, inconsequential infections. The harm done through possibly selecting out resistant organisms may outweigh the benefit derived from treatment.
3. Agents should only be used prophylactically for exposed and in-contact animals if a real risk of severe infection exists, as, for example, in blackleg in cattle or fowl cholera.
4. Although treatment may have to be started before the laboratory report is received, it should be modified if indicated.
5. The laboratory report should not necessarily be considered a mandatory directive for treatment. The choice of the best drug to use should be made after considering a number of factors. In general, it is poor practice to use a broad-spectrum antibiotic if the infecting agent is susceptible to a more specific one. It should be remembered that all antimicrobial drugs are potentially toxic and that some may have serious side effects.
6. In general, when antimicrobial drugs are administered, they should be given in full therapeutic doses for an adequate length of time. This will vary with the disease and the drug. The period ordinarily should not be less than 3–5 days. In some diseases such as nocardiosis, atypical mycobacterial infections and fungal diseases, treatment will have to be continued for weeks.
7. Because of the danger of superinfection, the use of some drugs, such as the tetracyclines, should not be unnecessarily prolonged. If there is no response or poor response to treatment, it is possible that a resistant population of organisms has developed. In such cases, specimens should be forwarded to the laboratory for additional susceptibility testing. Special attention may have to be given to animals with abscesses (poor penetration) and mixed infections.
8. In some instances, it is advisable to consider the simultaneous use of two drugs. Only drugs that act synergistically should be given together.
9. There are regulations that set withdrawal times for various microbial drugs prior to slaughter. These range from 24 hours to 30 days and must be taken into account in the selection of drugs for treatment of food animals.

COMBINATIONS OF ANTIMICROBIAL AGENTS

In some circumstances, such as the inaccessibility of the infecting agent, mixed infections, and very serious unresponsive infections, it may be advantageous to use a combination of two drugs that act synergistically. Prompt combination therapy may sometimes be indicated in very serious infections.

The combinations that are generally synergistic consist of pairs of drugs that are bactericidal. Antagonism is usually observed when a bactericidal drug such as penicillin, which kills rapidly multiplying organisms, is used with a bacteriostatic drug such as a tetracycline. Although they are bacteriostatic, the sulfonamides do not appear to antagonize penicillin, perhaps because their action is slow. Because the bactericidal action of polymyxin is exerted on resting cells as well as on multiplying cells, it is not antagonized by bacteriostatic drugs.

In treating mixed infections with two drugs, it is advisable to select drugs that have rather different spectra of activity, thus broadening the overall antibacterial spectrum. The simultaneous use of two drugs has the following theoretical advantage: Considering the rate of mutation of bacteria to resistance, the probability of an organism becoming resistant to two antimicrobial drugs being used for treatment is very low. When three drugs are used, as in, for example, the treatment of tuberculosis, the probability of a mutant emerging that is resistant to all three drugs is extremely low.

Sometimes the combination of two drugs permits a reduction in the dose of a drug that might be toxic at a higher dose.

ANTIBIOTICS AND GROWTH PROMOTION

Antibiotics have been administered to cattle, swine, and poultry for growth promotion for many years. A number of effects have been attributed to antibiotics as feed additives in livestock and poultry and are summarized as follows

(Prescott, J.F., Baggot, J.D., Walker, R.D., Editors. 2000. Antimicrobial Therapy in Veterinary Medicine, 3rd ed. Iowa State University Press, Ames, Iowa):

- Inhibit the growth or metabolism of harmful gut bacteria.
- Decrease elaboration of toxic substances, including bacterial toxins.
- Reduce bacterial destruction of essential nutrients.
- Increase synthesis of vitamins and other growth factors.
- Improve efficiency of nutrient absorption by modifying the gut wall.
- Reduce intestinal mucosal epithelium cell turnover.
- Reduce intestinal motility.

Over the years, there has been serious concern that the widespread use of antibiotics as feed additives may contribute to antibiotic resistance among bacterial pathogens that may infect humans.

Other public health concerns are the following:

- The presence of antibiotic residues in milk. For example, they may produce allergic reactions.
- The elimination of competitive bacteria may increase the *Salmonella* reservoir.
- Antibiotic resistance in food-borne bacteria; for example, *Campylobacter*, enterococci and *Salmonella*.
- Environmental contamination via animal wastes resulting in human exposure to resistant bacterial pathogens.

Among the antibiotics approved as feed additives in cattle, swine, and poultry in the United States are bacitracin, tetracyclines, lincomycin, penicillin, tiamulin, virginiamycin, and tylosin. Catfish, salmon, and trout on fish farms receive antibiotics, as do honey bees in hives.

The continued use of antibiotics as feed additives has resulted in much controversy over the years. Although it has been difficult to demonstrate the adverse effects on public health, there is evidence that increases in antibiotic resistance in human pathogens is related to the use of antibiotics as feed additives. Human enterococci are considered to have acquired drug resistance to synercid from chicken enterococci that are resistant to virginiamycin, a poultry-feed additive. Virginiamycin is closely related to synercid, a last-resort human antibiotic. Antibiotics in cattle feed are thought to account for the presence of multidrug-resistant *Salmonella typhimurium*, a food-borne pathogen that has caused serious human infections. Several reports, including Britain's Swann report, as early as 1969 recommended the phasing out of the use of certain antibiotics as feed additives in livestock and poultry.

GLOSSARY

diterpene Terpene containing twice as many atoms in a molecule as a monoterpene. Terpenes are present in essential oils and used as organic solvents.

DNA-gyrase Enzyme that catalyzes the conversion of double-helical DNA to the superhelix form.

9 Sterilization, Disinfection, and Antisepsis

Sterilization and disinfection are of great importance to the practicing veterinarian. The sterilization of dressings, surgical instruments, and syringes is commonplace procedure, as is the disinfection of kennels, infected premises, and contaminated footwear. So that such operations can be carried out effectively, an understanding of the general principles of sterilization, disinfection, and antisepsis is necessary.

STERILIZATION

This is the process whereby all viable microorganisms are eliminated or destroyed. The criterion of sterilization is the failure of the organisms to grow if a growth-supporting medium is supplied. The limiting requirement of sterilization is destruction of the bacterial spore, the most resistant form of microbial life.

DISINFECTION

Disinfection involves the destruction of pathogenic organisms associated with inanimate objects, usually by physical or chemical means. All disinfectants are effective against the vegetative (growing) forms of organisms but not necessarily against their spores.

ANTISEPSIS

Antisepsis involves the inactivation or destruction by chemical means of microbes associated with the animal. Antiseptic agents may be bactericidal or bacteriostatic. Bacteriostatic means the inhibition of multiplication or growth, which, unlike the bactericidal effect, may be reversible. For ordinary purposes, the terms disinfectant and antiseptic are used synonymously.

PHYSICAL METHODS

Moist Heat

Moist heat is used to destroy microorganisms in three different ways described below.

BOILING. Steam or boiling water (common instrument, sterilizer) at 100°C is widely used in veterinary practice for preparing syringes, needles, and instruments for minor surgery. This process kills vegetative forms of microorganisms and viruses in 5 minutes. Many spores are also killed at 100°C in this same period, but many of the more resistant spores, like those of *Clostridium tetani* and the common *Bacillus* species, can survive boiling for as long as several hours. Thus, although boiling kills most pathogenic bacteria, boiling is not sterilization as the term is defined.

Boiling water for as long as 30 minutes damages the cutting edge of instruments.

STEAM UNDER PRESSURE (AUTOCLAVE). The most resistant spores are killed by a temperature of 121°C for 15 minutes. This temperature is obtained at sea level by steam at a pressure at 15 lb/in^2 in excess of atmospheric pressure. The autoclave, which is a metal cylinder designed to contain steam under pressure, is an essential piece of equipment in microbiology laboratories and operating rooms. Many veterinarians have small autoclaves for the sterilization of instruments, dressings, solutions, and surgical packs. To obtain a temperature of 121°C, all air must first be blown out. In the large, modem, high-vacuum autoclaves, 98% of the air is removed by a powerful pump. Air is removed in two stages in the downward-displacement autoclaves. Steam is admitted at the top of the chamber, and residual air is driven out at the bottom.

The killing power of steam is attributable to the fact that when it condenses on the item being sterilized, it liberates a large amount of latent heat. The shrinkage resulting from condensation, a thin film of moisture on the surface of the load, draws in fresh steam and thus more heat. As this process continues, the steam penetrates and surrounds the various items, producing a high uniform temperature.

The following points should be kept in mind when using the office autoclave:

- Air and condensate must be removed for effective sterilization.
- The required temperature of 121°C must be maintained.

- All mechanisms, such as gauges and timers, must be in proper working order.
- Packs should be properly prepared. They should not be too large, nor should the wrappings be impervious. Volumes of fluid should not be too large. The load should be arranged to allow for penetration of steam.
- The effectiveness of the autoclave can be tested by affixing heat-sensitive tape to the packs being sterilized. Paper strips impregnated with spores of *Bacillus stearothemophilus* also can be used to test the autoclave. If the autoclave is functioning effectively, the spores will be killed.

The high-vacuum autoclaves used in clinics and hospitals should be operated strictly according to directions provided by the manufacturer. Pressures, temperatures, and times of each sterilization cycle must be recorded, and routine checks must be made of temperatures and sterilizing effectiveness.

PASTEURIZATION.   This process, which involves the heating of milk, milk products, and some other foods (liquid) to the point that all potential human pathogens are killed, has greatly reduced the incidence of brucellosis and tuberculosis in humans over the years. The occasional outbreaks of group A (*Streptococcus pyogenes*) streptococcal disease spread by milk also have been eliminated.

In the slow method of pasteurization, milk is held at 62.78°C for 30 minutes, and in the flash method, at 71.67°C for 15 seconds. A few heat-resistant vegetative bacteria (thermoduric) and spores survive. The milk is rapidly cooled after pasteurization to discourage growth of the remaining viable organisms.

Ultraviolet Light

Direct sunlight kills unprotected vegetative organisms fairly rapidly, but spores are resistant. The bactericidal activity of sunlight is caused by the ultraviolet portion of the spectrum. Glass is impervious to this radiation. Sunshine is, no doubt, of great importance in the destruction of pathogenic organisms contaminating fields, pastures, and other areas used by livestock.

Ultraviolet (UV) light is a nonionizing or low-energy radiation with a wavelength in the range of 2500 Å. UV light is absorbed by DNA, resulting in the formation of pyrimidine dimers that interfere with base pairing. DNA synthesis is inhibited, and the bacteria are inactivated. The DNA can be repaired by some organisms so that normal synthesis can proceed. The mutagenic activity of UV light on living cells is well known.

Ultraviolet light from mercury vapor lamps is widely used in inoculating hoods, operating theaters, animal quarters, and other areas to reduce airborne infections. It acts most efficiently at temperatures from 27° to 40°C.

Ionizing Radiation

This form of radiation (x and gamma rays) has an energy content much higher than that of ultraviolet light and, consequently, has a strong disinfectant action. The water within cells is ionized, resulting in free radicals that recombine to form peroxides that damage the DNA. Gamma rays emitted from cobalt-60 are used commercially to sterilize disposable syringes, needles, pipettes, surgical sutures, dressings, bone grafts, plastic arterial prostheses, catheters, plastic Petri dishes, and other heat-sensitive items. Unfortunately, when ionizing radiation is used on foods, flavors may be affected, and when it is used on such items as drugs, hormones, and enzymes, potency may be reduced.

Filtration

Filtration has been used for decades to sterilize bacteriologic media, serum, injection solutions, and other solutions containing heat-sensitive substances. A pore size of 0.45 μm or less removes almost all bacteria from solutions. Membrane filters composed of cellulose esters and plastic polymers have largely supplanted other kinds of filters in the microbiology laboratory. The porosities of these membrane filters range from 0.1 to 10 μm. The coarse sizes are used for clarification (removal of large particles) before using the smaller pore sizes. Those filters commonly used to remove bacteria do not hold back viruses or mycoplasmas. Filters with a porosity of about 0.3 μm are used to filter air in rooms and operating theaters.

Laminar flow systems of the kind used for biological containment hoods and operating rooms use filtered air pumped into the space at a pressure needed to displace the regular circulating air.

Microwaves

Microwaves, a form of radiation, have by themselves minimal effect on microorganisms. They induce water molecules to vibrate at a high rate and, thus, produce heat. The heat, if sufficient, and not the microwaves, kills microorganisms.

FACTORS INFLUENCING THE ACTIVITY OF DISINFECTANTS

Disinfectants and antiseptics act more selectively on microorganisms than do the physical methods, such as heat and radiation. Some of the factors and considerations relating to the activity and efficacy of disinfectants are summarized as follows.

Type of Microorganism

Spores are highly resistant compared with vegetative forms, and only a few disinfectants, such as halogens, mercuric chloride, formalin, and ethylene oxide, are effective in the concentrations usually used. Mycobacteria are more resistant than most other vegetative organisms. Phenolic and alcoholic compounds are recommended for this group. Generally speaking, viruses are more resistant than vegetative bacteria. Halogens, oxidizing agents, formalin, and sodium hypochlorite are active against many viruses; quaternary ammonium compounds are not.

Organisms Inhibited

Growing and multiplying cells are more readily poisoned than are those in a resting or stationary state. It is preferable that organisms be killed rather than merely inhibited. The quaternary compounds employed in high dilutions are bacteriostatic rather than bactericidal. Such agents as formaldehyde, ethylene oxide, and chlorine are clearly bactericidal.

Exposure Time

The time required for inactivation of the microorganism depends on the organism and the antimicrobial agent. The rate of action differs greatly among the various chemical agents. Some act rapidly, whereas others are completely effective only after some minutes or even hours.

Temperature

The temperature required for inactivation depends on the mechanism of action and the chemical nature of the antimicrobial agent. All are more active at higher temperatures. In general, it is considered that the rate of inactivation doubles with each increase in 10°C.

pH

Each disinfectant has an optimum pH range.

Inhibitory Considerations

All disinfectants are to some extent inhibited in their activity by organic matter, such as feces, pus, exudates, discharges, and blood. Halogens and quaternaries are especially inhibited by organic matter. In the disinfection of premises, stables, and kennels, the ability to penetrate dirt, grease, and organic matter is important. Soaps and surface-active agents assist penetration.

Side Effects

Other limiting considerations are toxicity, possession of an irritating vapor, undesirable staining properties, and destructive effects on instruments and fabrics. Antiseptics or disinfectants used on or around animals should be relatively nontoxic to tissues.

EVALUATING DISINFECTANTS

Phenol Coefficient

This value expresses the capacity of a disinfectant to kill bacteria when compared with phenol. In the official test, a broth culture is diluted 1:10 with different concentrations of the test compound. The end point is the lowest concen-

tration that yields sterile loopful samples following incubation for 10 minutes at 20°C. The compound is generally recommended for use at five times this concentration. For example, a phenol coefficient may be stated to be 40, which means its killing power is 40 times that of phenol. The three organisms used in the official test are *Salmonella typhi* (gram-negative), *Staphylococcus aureus* (gram-positive), and *Pseudomonas aeruginosa* (gram-negative).

Although of some value, the phenol coefficient does not take into account such considerations as toxicity for tissues, inactivation by organic matter, corrosive properties, and other factors relating to particular situations.

Use-Dilution Test

This test is sometimes used to evaluate a disinfectant. In this procedure, the test bacteria are added to broth tubes containing increasingly stronger concentrations of the test disinfectant. After incubation, the growth, or absence of such, is recorded. The result is used to rate the disinfectant.

Special tests are used to evaluate the fungicidal efficacy of disinfectants.

In-Use Test

In this procedure, various dilutions of the disinfectant are tested against a standardized preparation of bacteria on the kind of material on which the disinfectant will be normally used.

Direct-Spray Method

This is used to test chemical agents that are not water-soluble.

Tissue Toxicity Test

In this procedure, dilutions of the disinfectant are tested for toxicity through exposure to cell culture systems.

DISINFECTANTS AND ANTISEPTICS

As mentioned previously, a number of factors influence the activity of these agents.

Each class of disinfectants is represented by proprietary products.

Ethyl and Isopropyl Alcohol

MODE OF ACTION. Alcohols denature cell proteins and break down cytoplasmic membrane lipids, resulting in a loss of membrane permeability.

DILUTION. A 70% solution is most effective.

USES. Alcohols are used in thermometers (add 0.2%–1% iodine), instruments, skin preparations, hands, and spot disinfection. Their usefulness is limited in that they take about 10 minutes to kill staphylococci.

ADVANTAGES. It has a bactericidal effect on gram-positive and gram-negative organisms. It is tuberculocidal and active against enveloped and nonenveloped viruses.

LIMITATIONS. It is not sporicidal and not active against fungi. It is inactivated by organic material and corrodes metals unless a reducing agent is added (e.g., 2% sodium nitrite). It bleaches rubber tile and dehydrates skin.

Ethylene Oxide

This compound is the most widely used disinfectant gas.

MODE OF ACTION. It affects protein synthesis by alkylating proteins and consequently blocking free amino groups.

DILUTION. Gas; exposure time 4–18 hours.

USES. To disinfect blankets, pillows, mattresses, lensed instruments, polyethylene tubing, thermolabile plastics, and other items that could be damaged by heat or disinfecting solutions.

ADVANTAGES. Active against bacteria, fungi, and viruses, yet harmless to most materials.

Formaldehyde

This compound is used as a gas and also as an aqueous solution. Glutaraldehyde, used in an aqueous solution, has a similar mode of action and range of activity.

MODE OF ACTION. Same as ethylene oxide.

USES. The gas is used to disinfect rooms, cabinets, fabrics, and incubators. The solution is used for instrument disinfection.

ADVANTAGES. It is active against bacteria, fungi, viruses, and spores. The gas is not corrosive for instruments and does not lose significant antimicrobial properties in the presence of organic matter.

LIMITATIONS. A relatively long period is required for disinfection. It is odorous and toxic to skin and mucous membranes. The solution damages the cutting edges of instruments.

Halogens

These include chlorine, iodine, and iodine compounds.

MODE OF ACTION. They inactivate by oxidizing free sulfhydryl groups. They are bactericidal and active against bacteria, spore-forming bacteria, fungi, and viruses.

Chlorines

Hypochlorites or hydrochlorous acid derivates.

USES. Floors, premises, plumbing fixtures, spot disinfection; fabrics are not harmed by bleaching.

ADVANTAGES. Tuberculocidal unless highly diluted.

LIMITATIONS. Bleaches fabrics, corrodes metals, unstable in hard water, must be freshly prepared, and tarnishes silver. Chlorine is inactivated by organic material.

Iodine and Iodophores

Iodine is a tincture (ethanol) or aqueous solution (2%–5%).

Iodophores consist of iodine combined with surface-active agents. They act rapidly and have low toxicity for tissue. There are many proprietary products, including Wescodyne and Betadine.

USES. Tincture of iodine is an effective skin antiseptic. Products like Wescodyne are used for thermometers, utensils, rubber goods, and dishes or for presurgical scrub. Betadine and similar iodophors are used for presurgical scrub. Other iodophores are designed for specific purposes; for example, Iosan for milking and dairy operations.

ADVANTAGES. Iodophors are cleaning, disinfecting, and nonstaining. They leave a residual antibacterial effect and have minimal toxicity.

LIMITATIONS. Tincture of iodine stains and is irritating to tissues. Iodophors are somewhat unstable, are inactivated by hard water, and may corrode metals.

Phenolic Disinfectants

These are derivatives of phenol. They include cresol, the cresylics, and substitution products with halogen and alkyl groups. There are many proprietary products, including Amphyl, Lysol, O-Syl, Staphene, Vesphene, Tergisyl, and Armisol. Some are available as sprays as well as solutions. Some, like Lysol, are saponated.

MODE OF ACTION. They denature proteins and destroy selective permeability of cell membranes, resulting in leakage of cell constituents.

USES. Cresol, equipment, linen, excreta; Amphyl, instruments; Lysol, laundry rinse for blankets and linens; O-Syl, Staphene, and Vesphene, floors, walls, and equipment; Tergisyl and Armisol, environmental uses.

ADVANTAGES. They are effective against bacteria except for spore-formers. They are not inactivated by organic matter, soap, or hard water (except creosol). There is a residual effect if allowed to dry on surfaces.

LIMITATIONS. Phenolics are not sporicidal and are only weakly effective against nonenveloped viruses. Creosol must be used in soft water and is slow acting.

Quaternary Ammonium Compounds

Their surface-acting properties make them excellent cleaning agents.

Cationic Detergents

There are a number of proprietary products including Zephiran, Cetavolon and Roccal.

MODE OF ACTION. They injure the cell by damaging the cytoplasmic membrane and reducing cell permeability.

USES. Cleaning and disinfection of instruments, utensils, and rubber goods; also used for milking and dairy operations. Instrument soak (except for those with cemented lenses), lacquered catheters, synthetic rubber goods, and aluminum instruments.

ADVANTAGES. Low tissue toxicity.

LIMITATIONS. Although effective against many bacteria, they are not tuberculocidal or sporocidal and have limited viricidal activity. *Pseudomonas aeruginosa* is relatively resistant. They are inactivated by protein, soap, and cellulose fibers.

Anionic Detergents

These are soaps and fatty acids. Included among the proprietary products are Hexachlorophene and pHisoHex. They are incorporated in a number of hand creams and bar soaps.

MODE OF ACTION. They dissociate to yield negatively charged ions that disrupt the lipoproteins of cytoplasmic membranes.

USES. Mainly for skin cleaning and disinfection.

ADVANTAGES. Good cleansers that have prolonged antibacterial action.

LIMITATIONS. They are slow in action, have limited viricidal activity, and are not sporicidal or tuberculocidal. They are toxic if used continuously and can be absorbed into the body in increasing quantities especially through the delicate skin of infants.

ADDITIONAL DISINFECTANTS

Heavy Metals

Organic mercury compounds, such as mercurochrome and thimerosal, are less toxic than other mercuric compounds, but they have only slight bactericidal activity. Mercuric chloride and silver nitrate are used as antiseptics in a dilution of 1:1000. The former compound is currently little used because of environmental contamination, and the caustic nature of silver nitrate limits its use.

Alkalis

Lye (2% NaOH solution) is used in veterinary medicine for disinfecting stables and premises. It is bactericidal and viricidal.

Lime (calcium oxide) dissolved in water yields $Ca(OH)_2$. This solution of lime is also bactericidal and viricidal and is used to disinfect premises. Lime is added to "infected" carcasses before burial.

Acids

A 4%–5% solution of acetic acid is bactericidal and viricidal. It is mainly used to disinfect stables and premises.

A 2% HCl solution has been used to treat hides suspected of harboring anthrax spores.

Hydrogen Peroxide

This oxidizing agent, available as a 3% aqueous solution, is useful for cleaning and disinfecting wounds and as a mouthwash in humans and animals with septic gingivitis and stomatitis. The solution liberates oxygen when it contacts the catalase of tissues. There is no penetration of tissues, and its effect is of short duration.

Soaps

Soaps have only slight bactericidal activity, but they are effective in the mechanical removal of organisms. However, the act of washing appears to bring the resident flora to the surface of the skin of the hands, resulting in increased bacterial counts. For this reason, the germicides hexachlorophene (a phenolic compound) and tetrachlorosalicylanilide are added to soap.

Biguanide Compounds

Chlorhexidine (Hibitane, Nolvasan) is the most commonly used disinfectant of this group. It is bactericidal in high dilutions, but viruses (except lipophilic ones), spores, and mycobacteria are relatively resistant. It is combined with a quaternary ammonium compound to increase its germicidal spectrum and activity. This combination, called Nolvasan, is used widely by veterinarians for preoperative treatment of skin, surgical scrub, obstetric procedures, and milking and dairy operations.

Chlorhexidine is incorporated in many preparations including ointments, wound and skin cleansers, shampoos, and teat dips. It has the advantage of a low potential for local or systemic toxicity.

Dialdehydes

Glutaraldehyde (Cidex) is the most widely used compound of this group. As mentioned earlier, it is similar to formaldehyde in action and range of activity. It has one of the widest spectrums of any disinfectant, being bactericidal, viricidal, fungicidal, and sporicidal. A 2% aqueous solution buffered to pH 7.5–8.5 is useful for disinfecting surgical instruments, cystoscopes, and anesthetic equipment. However, heat sterilization is preferable. Spores are killed within 3 hours, and vegetative bacteria are killed in 10 minutes.

Miscellaneous

Merthiolate (1:10,000) is used as a preservative in serum and in biologic products. Actidione is used in Sabouraud agar to depress the growth of common saprophytic fungi. Formalin (0.3–0.5%) is used to kill bacteria in vaccines and bacterins. Gentian violet, potassium tellurate, malachite green, brilliant green, and selenite F are incorporated in a variety of media to inhibit the growth of undesirable bacteria. Thallium acetate is incorporated in mycoplasma media to inhibit growth of gram-negative bacteria. Beta-propiolactone is used to sterilize grafts, vaccines, bacterins, and sera.

Sodium nitrite (0.2%) is added to alcohol, formalin, formalin-alcohol, iodophor, and quaternary ammonium solutions to prevent corrosion. Sodium bicarbonate (0.5%) is added to phenolic solutions to prevent metallic corrosion.

DISINFECTION AND SELECTED ANIMAL DISEASES

Guidelines for disinfection relating to important animal diseases, including notifiable diseases occurring in the United States, are provided by the United States Department of Agriculture. The actual disinfection is carried out in the United States under the supervision of state, federal, and accredited veterinarians.

10 Diagnostic Veterinary Bacteriology and Mycology: An Overview

The principal procedures routinely employed in the veterinary diagnostic laboratory for the laboratory diagnosis of bacterial diseases are outlined briefly in the discussion that follows. The procedures used for the laboratory diagnosis of mycotic diseases are summarized in Table 35.1.

The term "clinical specimens" denotes those materials, such as tissues, blood, urine, skin scrapings, and body fluids, taken from animals for diagnostic purposes. In the diagnosis of microbial diseases, such materials must reach the diagnostic laboratory with as little change as possible from their original state. Suspension of microbial multiplication is usually accomplished by maintaining the specimens at refrigerator temperature until they reach the laboratory. On occasion, it may be advisable to freeze specimens.

SUBMISSION OF SPECIMENS FOR BACTERIOLOGICAL EXAMINATION

Obviously the diagnostic microbiology laboratory can function most effectively when the correct specimens are selected and properly submitted. Most diagnostic laboratories supply veterinary practitioners with detailed instructions on the selection, packing, and shipment of specimens. The submission form provides space for information on the origin and nature of the specimen, the clinical history, and the disease or diseases suspected.

Just before the death of the animal and shortly thereafter, a number of intestinal bacteria may invade the host's tissues. The significance of these organisms, including potential pathogens, is difficult to assess when tissues have been taken even a short time after death. Living, sick animals presented for necropsy are usually the best source of specimens. In all instances, the importance of fresh tissues taken as soon as possible after death cannot be overemphasized.

In the interest of protecting laboratory personnel, persons submitting specimens should inform the laboratory if they are submitting specimens from suspected zoonotic diseases. To give the reader some idea as to how clinical specimens are submitted, some instructions are provided below for the selection, preservation, and submission of some important kinds of specimens. The selection of tissues and organs for the various microbial diseases is mentioned in more detail with the discussion of the particular disease or pathogen in chapters that follow.

Veterinarians frequently submit live, sick, and recently dead animals for necropsy. This is frequently the case when small or young animals and poultry are involved.

Tissues and Organs

Place tissues in plastic bags or leakproof jars. Portions of intestines should be packed separately. If there are no apparent lesions and an infectious disease is suspected, portions of liver, lung, kidney, spleen, intestine, and lymph nodes should be submitted. Specimens taken at the margin of diseased and normal tissue are preferred.

Brains sent for examination should be halved longitudinally. One half is refrigerated or frozen over dry ice, and the other is placed in 10% buffered formalin for histopathologic examination. Tissues in formalin should not be frozen.

All specimens can be conveniently shipped in a Styrofoam box or ice chest containing a generous amount of ice. Dry ice with plenty of insulation is preferred for longer preservation. Small specimens may be shipped in an insulated container with an ice pack.

Swabs

Swabs are of value for the submission of infectious material to the laboratory. On conventional cotton swabs, many bacteria are susceptible to desiccation during shipment; therefore, the swab should be placed in a non-nutritional transport medium. The survival rate of many pathogenic bacteria is significantly increased by the use of good transport media. Special swabs are required for swabbing the cervix of cows and mares. These can be prepared by attaching absorbent cotton to the end of an 18- to 24-in-long wire with a rubber band. Several convenient swab systems using a transport medium are available commercially.

Feces

Fecal specimens should be obtained directly from the rectum. Because of contamination, "ground droppings" should be avoided.

Milk

Milk should be collected from animals aseptically in sterile screw-capped or stoppered vials. Examinations may be negative if samples are taken during treatment.

Urine

Urine should be collected aseptically by midstream, catheter, or bladder tap. In collecting urine for bacteriologic examination, the aim should be to limit to a minimum normal flora and environmental bacteria. Because urine can support the growth of bacteria, it should be refrigerated immediately and certainly not left at room temperature for longer than 1 hour. The actual number of bacteria present in the urine at the time of collection indicates whether a urinary tract infection exists.

If the urine is to be examined for leptospira by darkfield, 1.5 mL of 10% formalin should be added to 20 mL of urine. Leptospira disintegrate shortly after collection unless fixed in formalin solution.

Blood

Optimally, three to four blood samples, 5–10 mL each, should be cultured in a liquid or biphasic medium during a 24-hour period. Many convenient blood culture systems are available commercially.

Anaerobes

Some anaerobes, particularly some of the gram-negative non-spore-formers, are sensitive to oxygen. Special commercial transport systems are available for the submission of materials suspected of containing significant anaerobes. Some laboratories provide tubes with rubber stoppers containing oxygen-free gas for the submission of swabs. Liquid material can be submitted in syringes devoid of air bubbles. Unless suitable specimens are delivered to the laboratory promptly, culturing for anaerobes rarely provides useful information.

BACTERIOLOGICAL EXAMINATION OF CLINICAL SPECIMENS

The examination of clinical specimens for the purpose of isolating and identifying potentially pathogenic bacteria is referred to as diagnostic or clinical bacteriology. This part of veterinary microbiology is traditionally taught in laboratory exercises that accompany the lecture course and thus will be alluded to only briefly here.

The procedures to be followed in examining clinical specimens depend considerably on the disease(s) or pathogen(s) suspected, and thus, an adequate clinical history is extremely important.

The steps that are followed in the bacteriologic examination of most specimens are outlined briefly in Fig. 10.1. and below.

- Clinical history, suspected pathogen, and the nature of the specimen (tissue, milk, urine, tissues, feces, swabs, pus, discharges, fetal stomach contents, cervical mucus, skin scrapings, etc.) will determine the direct examination (stained smear, wet mount, dark field examination, fluorescent antibody stain, etc.) to be carried out.
- The result of the direct examination may in some submissions result in a diagnosis. On occasion, a strong presumptive diagnosis can be made on the basis of a direct examination (smear or wet mount); for example, with actinobacillosis, actinomycosis, blastomycosis, or nocardiosis. The fluorescent antibody procedure can sometimes be used to rapidly identify some organisms in clinical materials, for example, with *Clostridium chauvoei* and *Clostridium septicum*, and also in cultures, as in the case of *Listeria monocytogenes* and *Francisella tularensis*. However, in most instances, the direct examination will indicate which culture media should be inoculated. This usually includes blood agar but may also include selective media. The temperature and length of incubation of the media may also be indicated by the direct examination.
- If urgent, an antimicrobial susceptibility test may be initiated before the bacteriological examination has been completed. The direct inoculation of clinical material for antimicrobial susceptibility is not recommended because more than one type of organism may be involved and the number of organisms inoculated is not standardized.
- After incubation of the culture media, the plates are examined for growth. If colonies are present, smears are prepared and Gram-stained. Some procedures, such as the catalase and oxidase tests, are conducted on colonies. From the results, the bacteriologist will decide on the probable generic identification of the predominant colonies and will inoculate certain differential media. If gram-negative bacteria are involved, it is often, at this stage, advantageous to inoculate triple-sugar iron agar slants.
- After sufficient incubation, the differential media are read and an identification is made. In some instances, more than one isolate may be identified. Serological tests are sometimes used for final identification. Tables listing the differential characteristics of microorganisms of veterinary significance are provided in diagnostic microbiology texts.
- Following the identification of one or more organisms, antimicrobial susceptibility tests are conducted.

Special procedures are required for a number of pathogens, including mycobacteria, chlamydiae, rickettsiae, spirochetes, and mycoplasmas.

The veterinary clinician should interpret the bacteriologic findings. The microbiologist can help by indicating

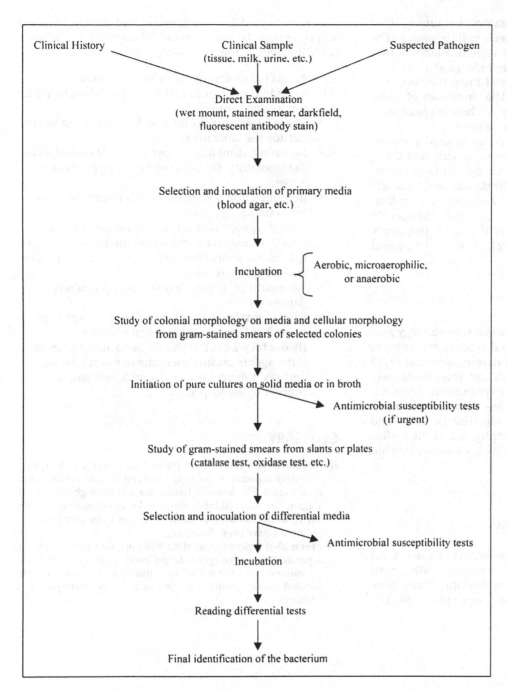

FIGURE 10.1   Routine steps in the isolation and identification of bacteria from clinical specimens.

the amount of growth of a particular organism. This may be stated as few colonies, very light growth, moderate or heavy growth of a pure culture. Interpretation may be particularly difficult if more than one species is isolated. This illustrates the importance of the veterinary practitioner having familiarity with the normal flora and pathogens of domestic animals.

Some laboratories have replaced some of procedures described above with semiautomated or automated commercial systems for identification of bacteria and yeasts. Most of these systems involve miniaturization of conventional methods. Some have a computer-generated identi-

fication database. Other automated identification systems employ fatty acid profiles, measurement of growth or metabolism, bacterial fingerprinting, and enzymatic profiling. Because of expense and an inadequate database of some systems for bacteria of veterinary significance, automated systems are not widely used in veterinary diagnostic laboratories. Many veterinary laboratories use commercial systems and kits for the identification of the Enterobacteriaciae, nonfermenters, gram-negative fermenters, staphylococci, streptococci, and other categories.

Recent years have seen the development of various molecular methods for identification of microorganisms in the clinical microbiology laboratory. Because of their expense, these procedures have been mainly used in the larger diagnostic laboratories and reference laboratories. The available newer methods include genetic probes, Southern blots, ribotyping, bacterial fingerprinting, and the polymerase chain reaction. The principles of these methods are described in Chapter 5. Their application is referred to under specific infectious agents.

Some immunological procedures can be used in the diagnosis of specific infectious diseases. Enzyme-linked immunosorbent assays (ELISAs), latex agglutination tests, and immunoblotting (**Western blot**) are used to detect antigen. ELISA, agglutination tests, and complement-fixation procedures are used to detect and measure specific antibody. The ELISA technique is the most frequently used immunological diagnostic technique in the clinical laboratory.

PRACTICE MICROBIOLOGY

Some veterinarians carry out diagnostic microbiology procedures in their clinics. Well-trained veterinary personnel using primary media and appropriate commercial rapid identification kits and systems can at least tentatively identify some of the more common pathogens. Examinations for bovine mastitis and canine urinary tract infections can be carried out effectively. The isolation and tentative identification of dermatophytes and the performance of antimicrobial susceptibility tests are well within the capacity of many clinics.

SAFETY IN THE CLINICAL MICROBIOLOGY LABORATORY

Many of the clinical specimens processed in the clinical microbiology laboratory harbor potentially dangerous pathogens. To avoid laboratory-acquired infections, laboratories should have clearly defined safety protocols. The basic rules or guidelines outlined briefly below are directed at preventing laboratory-acquired infections. Detailed guidelines will be found in clinical microbiology texts.

- Access to laboratories handling potentially hazardous specimens is restricted to laboratory and support personnel.
- Use of protective clothing and of gloves not worn outside the laboratory.
- No eating, drinking, or application of cosmetics in the laboratory. Do not insert or remove contact lenses.
- Immunization schedules for laboratory personnel; for example, against rabies.
- Effective procedures for decontamination of all infectious materials and wastes, including clinical specimens, instruments, cultures, syringes, needles, and spilled materials.
- No mouth pipetting. Aerosols are particularly dangerous.
- Use of biosafety hoods when zoonotic agents are suspected. Special containment facilities (**Biosafety Level** 3) should be used; for example, if the agents causing such diseases as tularemia, anthrax, tuberculosis, coccidioidomycosis, or brucellosis are suspected.

GLOSSARY

Biosafety Level The Centers for Disease Control and Prevention have classified etiological agents on the basis of their human hazard. The levels of hazard are one through four. Level 1 agents are the least infectious, and Level 4 (some viruses) are the most infectious. The safety measures to be employed for each level have been described.

Western blot Procedure for identifying proteins that have been separated by polyacrylamide gel electrophoresis. They are transferred from the gel to an artificial membrane. Specific antibodies are applied for identification of corresponding proteins.

PART II

Bacteria

11 Rickettsiales

In the presentation of discussions of particular bacteria, we have followed the order of the classification of the second edition of *Bergey's Manual of Determinative Bacteriology*. Thus we now begin with Volume 2, *The Proteobacteria*, Section XV, The α-Proteobacteria.

We use the term rickettsia or rickettsiae to refer to bacteria in the families Rickettsiaceae and Ehrlichiaceae, which belong in the Section α-Proteobacteria. It is of interest that these families are in the same Class, Rhodospirilli, as *Bartonella*, *Brucella*, and *Afipia*. The family Rickettsiaceae has one genus, *Rickettsia*; the family Ehrlichiaceae has seven, *Aegyptianella*, *Anaplasma*, *Cowdria*, *Ehrlichia*, *Eperythrozoon*, *Haemobartonella*, and *Neorickettsia*. The principal diseases, their causes, and their vectors are listed in Table 11.1.

Coxiella burnetii, formerly considered a rickettsia, is now placed in the Section γ-Proteobacteria, in the same Class as *Francisella* and *Legionella*.

CHARACTERISTICS OF RICKETTSIAE

The rickettsia are small, pleomorphic, coccobacillary, nonmotile, gram-negative, obligate intracellular bacteria. They multiply by binary fission and can be seen with the light microscope. They have deoxyribonucleic acid (DNA), ribonucleic acid (RNA), and cytochromes and are susceptible to many antibiotics. Most grow readily in the yolk sac of embryonated eggs and in cell cultures. Several species have been grown on artificial media. Their metabolic reactions are aerobic. The rickettsial diseases are transmitted by arthropod vectors.

They have cell walls that resemble those of gram-negative bacteria, which contain lipopolysaccharides. They stain reasonably well with Giemsa, Castaneda, Gimenez, and Macchiavello stains, but poorly with the Gram stain.

They possess many of the metabolic functions of bacteria, but require exogenous cofactors from animal cells. Rickettsiae can generate their own energy by the synthesis of adenosine triphophate (ATP) via the metabolism of glutamate. In addition, rickettsiae possess transport mechanisms that exchange ATP for adenosine diphophate (ADP) in the intracellular environment, providing a means to usurp the host cell ATP under favorable circumstances. They can lose their viability in storage because of the loss of their intracellular ATP pool and several coenzymes.

Species of the Family Ehrlichiaceae differ in some respects from the rickettsiae described above. They are referred to below under *Erhlichia*.

Table 11.1   Rickettsia of Veterinary Significance

Rickettsia	Disease	Host	Vectors
Rickettsia rickettsii	Rocky Mountain spotted fever	Humans, dogs	Ticks
Aegyptianella pullorum	Aegyptianellosis	Poultry	Ticks
Anaplasma marginale	Anaplasmosis	Ruminants	Ticks, biting diptera
Anaplasma ovis	Anaplasmosis	Sheep, goats	Ticks
Cowdria ruminantium	Heartwater, cowdriosis	Ruminants	Ticks
Ehrlichia canis	Canine monocytic ehrlichiosis	Dogs	Ticks
Ehrlichia ewingii	Canine granulocytic ehrlichiosis	Dogs	Ticks
Ehrlichia platys	Canine cyclic thrombocytopenia	Dogs	Ticks
Ehrlichia risticii	Potomac horse fever	Horses	Snail/fluke suspected
Ehrlichia equi	Equine ehrlichiosis	Horses	Ticks suspected
Ehrlichia ondiri	Bovine petechial fever	Cattle	Probably ticks
Ehrlichia phagocytophila	Tick-borne fever	Ruminants	Ticks
Eperythrozoon suis	Swine eperythrozoonosis	Swine	Lice, biting arthropods
Eperythrozoon ovis	Ovine eperythrozoonosis	Sheep, goats	Biting arthropods
Haemobartonella felis	Feline infectious anemia	Cat	Unknown
Neorickettsia helminthoeca	Salmon poisoning	Dogs, other canids	Fluke
Neorickettsia elokominica	Elokomin fluke fever	Canids, raccoon, bear	Fluke

IMMUNE RESPONSE

Immunity is both cellular and humoral. However, cell-mediated immune mechanisms and cytokines, such as gamma interferon and tumor necrosis factor alpha, are of greater significance in the immune response than are antibodies. Vaccines consisting of killed organisms are used to prevent epidemic typhus and Rocky Mountain spotted fever. Several vaccines are available to prevent rickettsial diseases of animals.

FAMILY RICKETTSIACEAE

Rickettsia

The only species of veterinary significance is *Rickettsia rickettsii*, the cause of Rocky Mountain spotted fever. Other species cause human typhus fevers. One of these, epidemic typhus fever (*Rickettsia prowazekii*; vector, lice), which is rare in the United States, has been enormously important throughout history because of its influence on the outcome of major wars. Without treatment, the case fatality rate in epidemic typhus can reach 30%.

About 50 cases of murine typhus (*Rickettsia typhi*; vector, flea) a milder disease, occurs in the United States annually.

Rickettsialpox is a mild disease, characterized by low fever and rash, which occurs infrequently in the United States. It is caused by *Rickettsia akari* and is transmitted by mouse mites.

Scrub typhus, which occurs in the Far East and Australia, is caused by *Rickettsia tsutsugamushi* and is transmitted by rodent **chiggers.**

Rickettsia felis causes a syndrome in humans that resembles murine typhus. It is characterized by chills, fever, headache, and sometimes a rash after several days. It is transmitted by the flea *Ctenocephalides felis* subsp. *felis*, which is associated with cats and the opossum. The organism is maintained in the flea by transovarian transfer. The disease has been reported in the United States, Mexico, Brazil, and France. The status of the agent in the cat has not been determined.

Rickettsia are parasites of the gut cells of arthropods; transmission usually is from arthropod to animal. Organisms proliferate in endothelial cells of capillaries, producing vasculitis. The resulting thrombi and hemorrhages are responsible for skin rashes seen in humans.

CELLULAR PRODUCTS. Noninfectious (ultraviolet irradiated) rickettsiae are toxic for mice and rats when administered intravenously. Death is caused by damage to capillary endothelial cells, producing loss of plasma, decrease in blood volume, and shock. The toxins have not been isolated and identified. Hemolysins are produced by some typhus rickettsiae. Rickettsiae contain endotoxin-like lipopolysaccharides, which are different from the true endotoxins of gram-negative bacteria in that they act strongly to stimulate production of protective antibodies.

PATHOGENESIS. Infections begin in the vascular system; organisms proliferate in endothelial and phagocytic cells and are disseminated via the bloodstream. There is obstruction of small blood vessels because of hyperplasia of infected endothelial cells and resulting small thrombi. Fever, hemorrhagic rash, stupor, shock, and patchy gangrene of subcutis and skin are among the signs and lesions noted. These clinical signs are thought to be in part caused by endotoxin-like substances of rickettsiae. Steps involved in infection include adherence, endocytosis, and phagosome destruction. The adherence is facilitated by the surface receptors of the host cell. After engulfment, rickettsiae destroy the phagosomal membrane by phospholipase and then multiply within the cytoplasm or, in certain cases (spotted fever), in the nucleus as well.

RICKETTSIA RICKETTSII. Rocky Mountain spotted fever (RMSF) is a febrile disease, mainly of humans, caused by *R. rickettsii*. Human infections (600–700 cases annually in the United States) vary from mild to quite severe and sometimes fatal. Dogs are susceptible, but the disease is usually mild; however, young dogs may sustain severe infections. The canine disease is seen most frequently in south central and southeastern United States. It is infrequent in the Rocky Mountain regions. The disease, which only occurs in the Western Hemisphere, also occurs in Canada, Mexico, and Central and South America.

The reservoir of this rickettsia is principally wild rodents, hares, and rabbits and the ticks (at least six species in the United States) that feed on them. The principal tick vectors in North America are *Dermacentor andersonii* (Rocky Mountain states) and *Dermacentor variabilis* (Eastern states). RMSF, like Lyme disease, occurs where people live near forested areas.

Most infections in humans and animals result from tick bites. The organism is maintained in ticks by transovarian transfer. Tick feces and secretions contain the organism, which can penetrate the skin and conjunctivae. Dogs may bring infected ticks into contact with humans. The organism enters the bloodstream from the tick bite and spreads hematogenously. As mentioned above it multiplies in endothelial cells, resulting in vasculitis, thrombosis, and hemorrhages.

Signs noted in dogs are malaise, fever, lymphadenopathy, polyarthritis, edema of the face and extremities, and petechial hemorrhages on mucous membranes in severe cases.

Laboratory Diagnosis. A thrombocytopenia has been a consistent finding in the canine disease.

Because the agent is highly infectious for humans, blood and tissues should be handled with great care.

Paired serum samples are required because of antibodies in endemic regions. The serologic procedures used for canine sera are the microimmunofluorescence test, ELISA, and the latex agglutination test. A fourfold increase in titer is considered significant.

Demonstration of rickettsia in fluorescent antibody-stained smears or sections of skin biopsies is significant.

Treatment and Control. Tetracyclines or chloramphenicol administered for 2 weeks is effective.

Ticks should be removed daily; prevention involves tick control where feasible.

No vaccine is currently available.

FAMILY EHRLICHIACEAE

Members of this family are generally referred to as rickettsia, although they differ from those described above in a number of respects. They propagate, depending on species, most efficiently in vacuoles in erythrocytes or mononuclear or granulocytic phagocytes. Within cytoplasmic vacuoles, microcolonies form, called morulae. Two distinct morphologic forms occur: reticulate (electron-lucent) forms and dense-core (electron-dense) forms, both of which can multiply by binary fission. Cells are lysed, releasing cell-free bacteria that are infectious for other cells.

Aegyptianella

AEGYPTIANELLA PULLORUM. Aegyptianellosis of domestic and wild fowl is caused by *Aegyptianella pullorum* and has been reported in South Africa, Indochina, and the Balkans.

This disease is spread by ticks, especially *Argas* spp., and is frequently associated with fowl spirochetosis. The acute disease is characterized by high fever, diarrhea, anorexia, and paralysis. The disease is asymptomatic to mild in endemic regions.

Giemsa-stained blood smears reveal multiple inclusions in erythrocytes, and the organisms may be present in phagocytes or free in the plasma.

Aegyptianellosis is effectively treated with tetracyclines.

Anaplasma

ANAPLASMA MARGINALE. The principal rickettsia in this genus is *A. marginale*, which occurs in spherical, coccoid, and ring forms. It causes anaplasmosis, an arthropod-borne (at least 16 species of ticks, and biting diptera) disease of cattle, water buffalos, deer, antelope, and other ruminants that occurs worldwide in tropical and subtropical countries. *Dermacentor* ticks are the principal vectors in the United States. Calves under 6 months of age are relatively resistant to the clinical disease but are infected early and become carriers. Transplacental transmission may occur.

The incubation period is usually several weeks, and the disease is seen in acute, subacute, and chronic forms. The acute disease is characterized by fever, varying degrees of anemia, and icterus with rapid loss of condition; cows may abort. Unlike babesiosis, there is no hemoglobinuria; infected erythrocytes are removed by phagocytosis. If untreated, the acute disease is frequently fatal. In endemic areas, most cattle are asymptomatic carriers. When unexposed mature animals are introduced to endemic areas, they almost invariably develop the disease if they have not been vaccinated or prophylactically protected.

Laboratory Diagnosis. Anaplasmosis is diagnosed by the demonstration of the organisms as densely stained marginal bodies (inclusions) in the erythrocytes of Giemsa-stained blood smears. It is of interest that each membrane-lined inclusion has up to 10 initial bodies that contain RNA and DNA. The initial bodies are released and infect erythrocytes.

Immunofluorescence staining is also used for demonstration of organisms. Nucleic acid probes and the polymerase chain reaction have been used in the identification of *Anaplasma*. Severe, prolonged infections with much red cell destruction may show few anaplasmas. The inclusions of *Anaplasma centrale* are more centrally located. Special staining procedures are required to demonstrate *Anaplasma caudatum* with its characteristic appendage.

Immunofluorescence assay, ELISA, card agglutination, capillary agglutination, complement fixation, and latex agglutination tests have been used to detect infected animals (Fig. 11.1).

Treatment. Tetracyclines or imidicarb dipropinate are effective if given early. They are also effective in eliminating the carrier state when administered for prolonged periods. Blood transfusion may be indicated.

Control and Prevention. Vectors should be reduced. Eradication can be accomplished by the removal of infected animals, although this is not usually feasible. In endemic areas, it is important to disinfect instruments between animals when performing procedures such as dehorning, castration, vaccination, and blood collection.

The immune response involves both humoral and cell-mediated immunity, but the latter would appear to be most important in protection. Premunition of young animals, that is, the deliberate infection with *A. marginale*, is widely practiced in tropical and subtropical countries. In adult animals, premunition should include concomitant tetracycline or imidocarb administration. Immunity after recovery is not permanent.

An adjuvant vaccine consisting of killed *A. marginale* (blood origin) is available. Other inactivated vaccines are available. They do not protect against infection, but they reduce its severity. A live *A. centrale* vaccine provides partial protection, although it cannot be used in the United States.

ANAPLASMA OVIS. This a relatively avirulent rickettsia that sometimes occurs with *A. marginale* in Central Africa

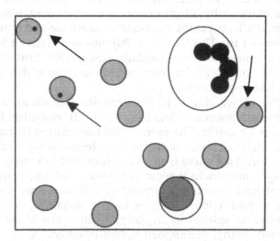

FIGURE 11.1 Illustration of a blood smear containing red blood cells infected with *Anaplasma marginale* (indicated by the arrows).

and the United States. Under some circumstances, it can cause clinical anaplasmosis in sheep and goats.

ANAPLASMA CENTRALE. This species causes a milder form of anaplasmosis. It produces central bodies in erythrocytes that are almost identical to the marginal bodies seen with *A. marginale* but that are located in the center of the cells.

ANAPLASMA CAUDATUM. This species, which has a tail-like appendage, is sometimes seen with *A. marginale*. Its significance is unclear.

Cowdria

COWDRIA RUMINANTIUM. This species is the cause of cowdriosis or heartwater, which occurs in cattle, sheep, goats, and wild ruminants mainly in Africa. In recent years, it has been reported from some Caribbean islands. It is transmitted by *Amblyoma* ticks, in which the organism is transferred transstadially (between stages).

The organism multiplies in lymph nodes, spreads to the bloodstream, and infects endothelial cells, resulting in widespread edema and hemorrhages. The disease occurs in peracute, acute, and subacute forms and is characterized by septicemia, fever, hydropericardium (heartwater), neurologic involvement, and often, a high mortality.

Laboratory Diagnosis. Squash and crush smears are made from the hippocampus and cerebral cortex and stained with Giemsa stain for rickettsiae.

An immunofluorescence assay has been used to detect antibodies.

Treatment and Control. Tetracyclines are effective if administered early.

Tick control and vaccination of young animals with virulent *C. ruminantium* is practiced in endemic areas.

Ehrlichia

EHRLICHIA CANIS. Canine ehrlichiosis (canine monocytic ehrlichiosis, tropical canine pancytopenia) is an acute to chronic rickettsial disease caused by *E. canis* and characterized by infection of monocytes and lymphocytes. It affects canids and occurs worldwide and in many regions of the United States. Puppies and German Shepherds appear to be particularly susceptible. Ehrlichiosis may be complicated by concurrent infection with babesia and haemobartonella.

The brown dog tick, *Rhipicephalus sanguineus*, is the vector and reservoir. Ticks may harbor the organism for as long as 5 months. The agent is not transmitted transovarially. All three stages of the tick can feed and transmit the infection. Tick saliva is the main source of infection.

Signs may include recurrent fever, epistaxis, mucopurulent nasal discharge, vomiting, subcutaneous hemorrhages and edema, depression, emaciation, anemia, weight loss, splenomegaly, polyarthritis, generalized lymphadenopathy, meningoencephalitis, convulsions, paralysis, and death, particularly in German Shepherds.

Laboratory Diagnosis. Unclotted blood for buffy coat and regular smears are used. In necropsied dogs, smears should be made from the lungs and other organs. Smears are stained by Giemsa and fluorescent antibody. The characteristic morulae of *E. canis* in monocytes and lymphocytes are frequently not present in stained smears. The optimum time for their demonstration is about 13 days postinfection.

Thrombocytopenia, hyperglobulinemia, nonregenerative anemia and neutropenia are supportive of a diagnosis.

A PCR procedure and a DNA probe have been used in the identification of *E. canis* in tissues.

Serum is tested for antibody by an immunofluorescence assay. The test may be negative early in the disease. Titers continue to rise as the disease progresses.

Treatment and Control. Doxycycline, tetracycline, and oxytetracycline are effective if the disease is diagnosed early; treatment should be given for at least 2 weeks. Additional treatment may be necessary, particularly in the chronic disease. Dogs cleared of infection are susceptible to reinfection. Without antibiotic therapy, dogs may remain carriers for many months.

Isolation, treatment, or elimination of seropositive animals can be effective.

Spraying and dipping to eradicate ticks also can be effective. Avoid tick-infested areas and remove ticks using gloves.

Public Health Significance. A considerable number of human infections have been reported. Infection is not thought to be acquired directly from dogs. Ticks are the probable vector.

EHRLICHIA EWINGII. This species causes canine granulocytic ehrlichiosis (CGE), a milder and much less common ehrlichiosis than canine monocytic ehrlichiosis. CGE is characterized clinically by anorexia, muscle stiffness, polyarthritis, lameness, neck pain, and weight loss. Anemia and thrombocytopenia may be present.

The disease occurs in the United States. and is transmitted by ticks, including the abundant Lone-Star tick, *Amblyomma americanum*.

Laboratory diagnosis is based on finding the characteristic morulae in neutrophils and eosinophils and serologic differentiation from *E. canis* using the immunofluorescence assay.

Treatment is the same as for canine monocytic ehrlichiosis.

EHRLICHIA PLATYS. This species causes canine infectious cyclic thrombocytopenia (ICT) that is usually subclinical but that, on occasion, can be clinical. *Ehrlichia platys* infection can potentiate *E. canis* or *Babesia* infections. Many dogs with antibodies to *E. canis* have antibodies to *E. platys*. The vector is considered to be the brown dog tick, *R. sanguineus*. ICT has been reported from the southern United States, southern Europe, and some countries of the Middle East.

Clinical disease is infrequent. Signs can include fever, dullness, anorexia, nasal discharge, anemia, petechial and ecchymotic hemorrhages, and weight loss.

Laboratory Diagnosis. Unclotted blood for buffy coat and regular smears made from lungs and other organs of necropsied dogs are used. Smears stained by Giemsa and fluorescent antibody procedures are examined for characteristic inclusions in platelets.

A finding of thrombocytopenia is supportive of a diagnosis.

Serum is tested by an immunofluorescence assay, which may be negative early in the disease.

Treatment and Control. Doxycycline or other tetracyclines should be given for at least 2 weeks.

Isolation with treatment, or elimination of seropositive animals, also can be effective.

Ticks should be eliminated.

EHRLICHIA RISTICII. This species causes Potomac horse fever (equine moncytic ehrlichiosis, equine ehrlichial colitis) a noncontagious rickettsial disease of horses characterized by fever and, frequently, a profuse diarrhea with mortality approaching 30%.

The disease was first reported in Maryland (United States) but is now known to occur widely in North America, Europe, and some countries of South America and Asia. It is seasonal in North America, occurring, often sporadically, from May to October.

The mode of infection and transmission is not known. It is suspected that a fluke/snail may be involved.

Among the clinical signs are fever, anorexia, leukopenia, listlessness, and usually, but not always, diarrhea. Upward of 30% of horses with the disease die. Laminitis may be a complication. Abortion may occur in mid- to late gestation.

Laboratory Diagnosis. Ulcerative gastroenteritis is the most visible lesion at necropsy.

Acute and convalescent sera are preferred. An immunofluorescence assay (IFA) and the ELISA are used for detection and titration of antibodies.

Unclotted blood or blood smear is needed for direct examination. Demonstration of the morulae of *Ehrlichia* in stained blood smears (in monocytes and neutrophils) is indicative of Potomac horse fever (PHF). Because of the irregular presence of the rickettsiae in smears, this procedure is not usually carried out.

There is no serologic cross-reaction between the ehrlichia of this disease and *E. equi*. Serologic procedures (IFA and ELISA) are used almost exclusively for the diagnosis of PHF. Although the IFA test does not discriminate between present and past exposure, horses that react positively and have characteristic clinical signs should be considered to have PHF.

The organism can be isolated, cultured, and identified in macrophage cultures, but these procedures are not carried out routinely.

Treatment and Control. Tetracyclines are usually effective if administered early and continued for at least 5 days.

Until the mode of transmission is known, little can be done, other than vaccination, in the way of preventing infection. Efforts directed at reducing exposure to biting insects and eliminating ticks are not thought to be helpful.

Inactivated whole-cell vaccines are available, but the duration of immunity is short. In endemic areas, it may be advisable to vaccinate twice during the period the disease occurs. A booster injection every 6 months is recommended in endemic areas.

EHRLICHIA EQUI. Equine granulocytis ehrlichiosis, caused by *E. equi*, is a sporadic, noncontagious disease that ranges in severity from unapparent to moderately severe, with acute manifestations being rare. The causal agent, *E. equi*, has a wide natural host range that includes horses, burros, llamas, dogs, and some rodents. The disease occurs in California, Florida, and a number of other states in the United States, as well as in Canada, Sweden, Great Britain, and South America.

Older horses are most severely affected; the disease is mild in young horses. The tick *Ixodes pacificus* can transmit *E. equi* to horses. There is evidence that *Ixodes dammani*, which transmits the agent of Lyme disease, may also transmit *E. equi*.

The disease is characterized by mild fever, thrombocytopenia, mild anemia, anorexia, leukopenia, edema of the limbs, and reluctance to move. Recovery is usually spontaneous in 2–3 weeks.

Laboratory Diagnosis. This involves the examination of stained smears from blood and buffy coat for the morula of *E. equi* in neutrophils and the testing of sera with an IFA. An IFA is available for the diagnosis of the other ehrlichiosis of horses, Potomac horse fever.

A PCR procedure can detect the DNA of *E. equi* in buffy coat.

Treatment. Tetracyclines daily for at least a week are effective.

Recovered horses are immune and no longer carriers.

Isolation of infected animals and arthropod control is recommended.

Vaccines are not currently available.

Public Health Significance. Whether or not humans acquire *E. equi* from horses is not clear, in that *E. equi*, *Ehrlichia phagocytophila* (tick-borne fever of cattle, etc.), and the agent that causes human granulocytotrophic ehrlichiosis (HGE) are indistinguisable. The risk of acquiring the infection from horses is not known.

EHRLICHIA ONDIRI. This species (***species uncertae sedis***) is the cause of bovine petechial fever (ondiri disease), a noncontagious disease characterized by fever, petechial hemorrhages of mucous membranes, and edema of the conjunctiva, with collapse followed by death in acute cases.

The disease occurs in the mountainous regions of East Africa. Some wild ruminants serve as a reservoir of the rickettsia, and biting arthropods are suspected as vectors.

Laboratory diagnosis is based on demonstration of rickettsiae in Giemsa-stained blood and splenic smears. The organisms are found in monocytes and granulocytes.

Tetracyclines and dithiosemicarbazone have been effective experimentally.

EHRLICHIA PHAGOCYTOPHILA. This species causes tick-borne fever, a disease of cattle, sheep, and goats that is transmitted by *Ixodes* and *Rhipicephalus* ticks. It is characterized by fever, depression, reduced milk production, respiratory distress, and occasionally, abortion. Febrile periods recur, and animals may be infected for months and years.

The disease has been reported from the United Kingdom, other European countries, India, and South Africa.

This rickettsia is indistinguishable from *E. equi* and the HGE agent referred to below.

Laboratory diagnosis is based on demonstration of rickettsiae (groups of basophilic bodies) in granulocytes and monocytes of Giemsa-stained smears in the early febrile period.

Tetracyclines are effective.

EHRLICHIA CHAFFEENSIS.
This is the cause of human monocytotrophic ehrlichiosis, a disease with a frequency in North America similar to RMSF. It occurs most often in the south central and southeastern states of the United States. The reservoir is the white-footed mouse, domestic dogs, and probably other animals; the vector is *Ixodes scapularis*.

HGE is caused by the HGE agent, which is indistinguishable from *E. equi* and *E. phagocytophila*. The disease in humans resembles the disease caused by the two aforementioned species in animals. HGE occurs in the same regions where Lyme disease is seen.

Sennetsu ehrlichiosis, which occurs in humans in Japan and Malaysia, is caused by *Ehrlichia sennetsu*. It is a rarely occurring, self-limited febrile illness.

Eperythrozoon

Species of the genera *Eperythrozoon* and *Haemobartonella* are difficult to differentiate morphologically. Unlike *Haemobartonella*, the eperythrozoa often occur as ring forms and are present on erythrocytes and free in the plasma with equal frequency. As with most other members of the family Anaplasmataceae, *Eperythrozoon* have not been cultured in cell-free media, are transmitted by arthropods or parental inoculation of infected blood, and are susceptible to tetracyclines.

EPERYTHROZOON SUIS.
This species occurs in the United States and Europe and causes a clinical disease in pigs characterized by icterus, anemia, inappetence, and weakness. The severity of the disease appears to be dose-related, and most infected pigs display no clinical signs, but carry the organism in a latent state.

Laboratory Diagnosis. This is based on the demonstration of the organism (ring-shaped bodies) on erythrocytes. Blood smears are stained by Giemsa, fluorescent antibody, and acridine orange. Complement-fixation, immunofluorescence assay, ELISA, and **indirect hemagglutination** have been employed to detect antibodies.

Another species, *Eperythrozoon parvum*, is a nonpathogenic parasite of swine and may be confused with *E. suis*.

Both organisms appear to be widespread in the United States, particularly in the Midwest.

Treatment and Control. Tetracyclines are effective in the treatment of swine eperythrozoonosis. Control of lice and other biting arthropods is important.

EPERYTHROZOON OVIS.
This species has been associated with splenomegaly, hepatomegaly, anemia, and excessive pericardial fluid in lambs. Transmission is by mosquitoes and sand flies. Affected lambs are generally unthrifty, and pastured lambs may show retarded growth.

Demonstration of the organism in blood smears and complement fixation and the immunofluorescence assay for antibodies are useful in diagnosis.

Tetracyclines in feed or water are effective in treating the disease.

Other organisms presumed to belong to the genus *Eperythrozoon* have been found in various animal species. They are thought to be of minor pathogenic significance.

Haemobartonella

HAEMOBARTONELLA FELIS.
This species causes the widespread (worldwide) disease of domestic and wild cats, feline infectious anemia. The mode of transmission is not known. An arthropod vector has not been identified, although fleas are suspected.

The disease is characterized by acute, subacute, and chronic forms, all of which lead to anemia. In the acute disease clinical signs include variable fever (103°–105°C), anorexia, jaundice, and splenomegaly. In the chronic form, the clinical signs are less severe and temperatures may be normal.

The infection may be latent in many cats and usually only becomes clinical as a result of stress or concurrent disease.

Laboratory Diagnosis. *Haemobartonella felis* is a small, coccoid, rod-like or ring-shaped organism. Diagnosis is based on the demonstration of numbers of characteristic organisms on the surfaces of erythrocytes of peripheral blood or bone marrow in Giemsa- or fluorescent antibody–stained smears (see Fig. 11.2). A number of smears may have to be examined because *H. felis* may only appear in the blood periodically (parasitemic episodes).

Treatment and Control. Blood transfusions have been helpful. Tetracyclines are administered for 2–3 weeks.

External parasites should be controlled, and blood donor cats should be screened to prevent spread of other diseases.

HAEMOBARTONELLA CANIS.
This species causes asymptomatic infections in dogs. Acute hemolytic anemia may develop when latently infected dogs are immunosuppressed by drugs, certain infections, and other means.

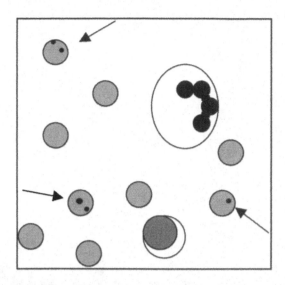

FIGURE 11.2 Illustration of a blood smear containing feline erythrocytes infected with *Haemobartonella felis* (indicated by the arrows).

Other species of the genus occur in various animals but are considered of minor pathogenic significance.

Neorickettsia

NEORICKETTSIA HELMINTHOECA. Salmon poisoning complex (SPC) is an acute, infectious, rickettsial disease of dogs and other canids, caused by *Neorickettsia helminthoeca* alone or with the Elokomin fluke fever agent, *Neorickettsia elokominica.* The latter can also, by itself, cause SPC. These rickettsial agents are present in the various stages of the liver fluke *Nanophyetus salmincola*; namely, snail (cercariae) to fish (metacercariae) to dog. The metacercaril cysts occur in the muscles of salmon and other fish. The disease is contracted from eating fluke-encysted (fluke metacercariae) raw salmon and occasionally other fish.

It is an acute, febrile disease with mortality reaching as high as 90% if untreated. The disease occurs in the western coastal United States and Canada, from northern California to Alaska. Dogs of all breeds and ages are susceptible. Dog-to-dog transmission has not been proven.

The Elokomin fluke fever agent (*N. elokominica*) resembles *N. helminthoeca*, but differs antigenically. It has a wider host range, including bear and raccoon, and sometimes occurs with *N. helminthoeca* infection.

The rickettsia from the ingested liver flukes are released into the gut of dogs or other animals. They infect the lymphatic structures of the intestine, resulting in a hemorrhagic enteritis often leading to death. Clinical signs may include diarrhea, hemorrhagic enteritis, vomiting, passage of blood, and dehydration.

Laboratory Diagnosis. The geographic region and a severe disease after eating raw fish suggest SPC.

Feces are submitted for examination for fluke eggs. Fluke ova may not be present because the prepatent period for the fluke may be longer than the incubation period of the rickettsia. The finding of the ova of *N. salmincola* in the feces supports a diagnosis of SPC.

If available, a moribund or dead animal should be submitted for necropsy examination and examination of smears from lymphoid tissue.

A definitive diagnosis can be made on the basis of demonstrating the rickettsia in smears from lymph nodes of the alimentary tract, tonsils, thymus, or spleen. Supportive of a diagnosis are the gross and microscopic lesions of SPC, including hemorrhagic enteritis, marked lymphadenopathy, lymphoid hyperplasia, and focal necrosis with organisms demonstrable by rickettsial stains.

Treatment and Control. Tetracyclines or chloramphenicol are effective. Praziquantel has been effective against flukes in dogs and coyotes.

Do not feed uncooked fish to dogs, particularly in endemic regions.

GLOSSARY

chiggers Six-legged larvae of harvest mites that suck blood from vertebrates and, thus, cause intense itching.

indirect hemagglutination In this type of hemagglutination, the antigen is adsorbed to the red cells. There is hemagglutination when specific antibody is added.

species uncertae sedis Species of uncertain affiliation.

12 *Brucella* and *Bartonella*

Brucella and *Bartonella* are placed in the Section α-Proteobacteria close to the Rickettsialles. The only genus in the family Brucellaceae of veterinary and medical significance is *Brucella*. Brucellae are small, gram-negative, nonmotile, non-spore-forming coccobacilli. They are aerobic and **carboxyphilic**, catalase- and urease-positive, and produce no acid from carbohydrates in conventional peptone media. That the species are different has been confirmed by chromosomal DNA analysis by pulsed-field gel electrophoresis, although DNA hybridization studies show that the first six species named below show a high degree of homology.

BRUCELLA

They are not found living apart from animals, and all are pathogenic, facultative, intracellular parasites with a predilection for organs rich in the sugar erythritol, such as the reticuloendothelial system and the reproductive tract. The following species with their principal animal hosts are recognized:

Brucella abortus: cattle;
Brucella melitensis: goats;
Brucella suis: swine;
Brucella ovis: sheep;
Brucella canis: dogs, coyotes, and foxes;
Brucella neotomae: recovered from rodents, not
    pathogenic for humans;
Brucella maris: marine animals, proposed new species.

Of these species, four are known to infect humans: *B. abortus*, *B. suis*, *B. melitensis*, and *B. canis*.

The common routes of infection in brucellosis of humans and animals are via the mucous membranes of the digestive tract, genital tract (cow or sow, bitch from male), and skin.

PATHOGENESIS

The invading organisms are quickly phagocytosed by polymorphonuclear leukocytes, in which some are able to survive and multiply. Their survival is attributed to inhibition of the bactericidal myeloperoxidase–peroxide–halide system by the release of 5'-guanosine and adenine. Macrophages also take up brucellae early in the infection. The organism passes from the point of entry via the lymphatics to the regional lymph nodes and, after multiplication, to the thoracic duct and then via the bloodstream to the parenchymatous organs and other tissues, where they enter fixed macrophages and parenchymal cells. There follows intracellular multiplication, with a chronic inflammatory response characterized by mononuclear infiltration resulting in giant cell and granuloma formation. Foci of the latter develop in lymphatic tissues, liver, spleen, bone marrow, and other locations. On occasion, these granulomatous foci or nodules may abscess. Hypersensitivity of tissues to elements of brucellae, including endotoxin, may play a role in pathogenesis.

The predilection that brucellae have for the **ungulate** placenta, fetal fluids, and testes of the bull, ram, and boar is attributed to erythritol. This polyhydric alcohol has been shown to stimulate the growth of *Brucella*. It is not present in the human placenta. The growth of the vaccine strain, *B. abortus* 19, is not stimulated by erythritol.

IMMUNITY

With regard to the innate immune response, the invading brucellae are most likely to encounter complement proteins, neutrophils, natural killer (NK) cells, and macrophages. The investigation into the activation of the complement alternate pathway by brucellae is mixed at best. *Brucella abortus* LPS (lipopolysaccharide) does not activate the alternate complement pathway. However, the classical complement pathway can be activated by IgM and IgG antibodies against the LPS and, effectively, the bacterial cells.

For effective phagocytosis of brucellae, opsonization is important. Neutrophils will phagocytose efficiently brucellae that have been opsonized with normal serum, most likely by serum complement protein C3b. Some of the brucellae are capable of replication inside neutrophils, and it is hypothesized that this is the route whereby they enter regional lymphatics early in the course of infection. Brucellae survive within neutrophils by preventing degranulation, possibly by interfering with myeloperoxidase. Furthermore, *B. suis* and *B. abortus* are thought to possess currently unidentified products that inhibit phagosome–lysosome fusion. Also of note is the observation that not all hosts are created equally. Bovine neutrophils are more effective at killing smooth brucellae, but they are about equal in the killing of rough strains.

Virulent strains of *B. abortus* can survive and multiply within neutrophils and macrophages better than avirulent strains. *Brucella abortus* releases 5'guanosine monophosphate and adenine that inhibit the degranulation of peroxidase-positive granules of neutrophils. This is thought to contribute to intracellular survival. The characteristic chronic granulomatous lesions found in brucella-infected tissues is the result of recruitment of neutrophils, macrophages, and lymphocytes into the region. Macrophages also secrete the cytokine, tumor necrosis factor (TNF), which is thought to enhance the formation of this lesion.

To invade macrophages, the brucellae must also be opsonized with either specific antibody or serum C3b. Within the macrophage, the intracellular brucellae inhibit, by a currently unknown mechanism, phagosome-lysosome fusion. There is much about the interaction between brucellae and macrophages that has yet to be elucidated.

As far as NK cells are concerned, there is no known indication of NK killing of brucella-infected cells.

The next step in the potential host elimination of brucellae is the specific immune response, either humoral (development of antibodies) or cell-mediated. At present, the role of antibody in the host response to brucellae is controversial at best.

The "protective" immune response appears to be the generation of a cell-mediated immune response. This response is thought to involve both CD4+ (helper) and CD8+ (cytotoxic) populations of T cells.

The immunity acquired from natural infection is not always sufficient to prevent reactivation of infection or reinfection. This low level of immunity in some humans results in chronic and relapsing brucellosis. Bactericidal serum antibodies and neutrophils can destroy organisms that are not within phagocytic cells. There is no correlation between levels of antibodies and acquired immunity. Acquired immunity is mainly cell-mediated; however, maximal immunity would seem to depend on the interrelationship of cellular and humoral responses.

ANTIGENIC NATURE

Like many other gram-negative bacteria, *Brucella* exhibit smooth (S) to rough (R) colonial dissociation. The change from S to R is associated with loss of virulence, a tendency to autoagglutination, and loss of antigens that elicit agglutinins specific for smooth strains. The S and R colonial variants are detected by examining colonies in oblique light. The vaccine strain *B. abortus* 19 is an intermediate mutant that, although low in virulence, is antigenic (elicits agglutinins). The vaccine strain RB51 is rough and has the advantage of not eliciting antibodies of the kind detected by commonly used serological tests. This is because most of the antibody detection methods test for antibodies against the O-polysaccharide of the LPS, which is a sign of infection. However, RB51 is thought to possess very little of the O-polysaccharide on its LPS. Therefore, these characteristic antibodies are not generated.

All *Brucella* spp. are closely related, and some share a number of antigens. *Brucella abortus*, *B. melitensis*, and *B. suis* possess two important surface antigens, designated A and M, which are present on the LPS protein complex. *Brucella abortus* contains more A antigen than M, *B. melitensis* has more M than A, and *B. suis* has an intermediate pattern but, like *B. abortus*, has more A than M. *Brucella canis* and *B. ovis* are antigenically rough and do not possess the A and M antigens. Both possess an R surface antigen.

It is of interest that some strains of *Yersinia enterocolitica* share an antigen with *B. abortus* and that a cross-reaction results in serological procedures.

BRUCELLA ABORTUS, *BRUCELLA MELITENSIS*, *BRUCELLA SUIS*, AND *BRUCELLA CANIS*

Cattle

Brucellosis is one of the most important diseases of cattle. It has great public health and economic significance. The disease in cattle is almost always caused by *B. abortus*. The organism is highly infectious and usually gains entrance to the body as a result of ingestion of food, water, and milk contaminated with uterine discharges, urine, or feces of an infected animal; penetration of the skin; or service by an infected bull.

The incubation period is usually from 30 to 60 days. In the cow, the infection localizes, usually after a bacteremia, in the placenta of the gravid uterus (placentitis). If the animal is not pregnant, there is usually localization in the udder (interstitial mastitis) and adjacent lymph nodes. Organisms are shed in the milk. It may also localize in the liver, lungs, lymph nodes, or spleen, where it produces granulomatous foci. Cows may remain infected for years.

In the bull, infection may localize in the testicle (epididymis) and seminal vesicle; abscessation is a common sequela; and brucellae may be discharged in the semen. Noninfected bulls usually do not become infected as a result of serving an infected cow, but infected bulls may infect cows.

The consequences of the bovine disease are loss of calves as a result of abortion at 6 months or later (about one-third of infected animals usually abort) and sterility or infertility of either the male or female.

CONTROL. Bovine brucellosis has been eliminated from several countries and from many states in the United States. The procedure that has been followed involves blood testing (agglutination test) of all cattle and the removal of reactors (titer 1:100 or higher). So that cattle will be less susceptible to reinfection, calfhood vaccination is recommended, and in some circumstances, is mandatory. The attenuated live vaccine (Strain 19 *B. abortus*, biotype 1) is used in female calves 4–12 months of age. They develop an agglutination reaction, which usually decreases or disappears soon. If the reaction at 1:200 or higher persists past 30 months of age, the animal is considered a reactor. Because strain 19 may cause infertility in some male calves, its use is restricted to females. The rough, attenuated vaccine strain RB51 is replacing Strain 19, as it does not produce antibodies detected by the commonly used serological tests. It has been approved for use in the United States, Mexico, and Chile.

The card test, which uses only one serum dilution and stained antigen, is rapid, sensitive, and useful as a field screening test. The agglutination test, enzyme-linked immunosorbent assay (ELISA), and complement-fixation test have been adapted to the rapid microtiter system. A number of other tests are performed either when the specificity of the reaction is in doubt or in the case of persisting vaccinal reactions (Strain 19). Complement fixation, rivanol precipitation, and mercaptoethanol agglutination detect primarily IgG antibodies. Rivanol and mercaptoethanol break down IgM. A drop in titer with the rivanol and mercaptoethanol tests may indicate a vaccinal titer (Strain 19) as opposed to one caused by chronic natural infection. The particle concentration fluorescence immunoassay (PCFIA) is another sensitive test that uses submicron polystyrene beads to which soluble antigens and a fluorescence marker are attached.

The **brucellosis ring test (BRT)** for agglutinins shed from the udder in the milk is performed at dairies three times each year on milk from herds whose milk is sold. If there are reactors to this very sensitive test, or if there is any evidence of brucellosis in a herd, a blood test is carried out. Serum is taken from market cattle, dairy and nondairy, before slaughter, for serologic screening. Herds with positive reactors are then blood tested.

Readers are referred to publications of the U.S. Department of Agriculture for further details on regulations and procedures relating to the brucellosis eradication programs.

LABORATORY DIAGNOSIS. The culture and identification of *B. abortus* and other species are discussed in general below.

Swine

Although considered low in the United States, the incidence of swine brucellosis (*B. suis*) is difficult to estimate, because testing is not compulsory. *Brucella abortus* and *B. melitensis* rarely infect swine. Swine of all ages are susceptible; feral swine are sometimes infected. Nursing pigs may become infected as a result of ingesting milk from infected sows. Older animals usually become infected by ingesting contaminated food, water, or soil. Infected boars transmit the disease by coitus.

Swine brucellosis is characterized by abortion, sterility, birth of stillborn or weak pigs, focal abscessation in various organs, spondylitis, and lameness. If given sufficient time, many animals will fully recover and free their tissues of the organism. Abortion may occur at any time during gestation; gilts and sows usually abort only once. Unlike cattle, infected sows may eliminate the infection but remain susceptible to reinfection.

Brucellosis is a more generalized infection in pigs than in cattle. Following bacteremia, the organism may localize in lymph nodes, spleen, liver, kidneys, uterus, mammary glands, urinary bladder, seminal vesicles, testicles, accessory sex glands, and bones. Unlike *B. abortus* in the cow, *B. suis* may persist for some time in the sow's uterus, causing metritis and sterility. In some instances, it has been isolated from uterine discharges after 30 months.

CONTROL. Three plans are used to eradicate swine brucellosis:

1. Elimination of the infected herd and restocking with brucellosis-free swine is the most severe.
2. Infected animals are separated from the noninfected ones and eventually slaughtered. The noninfected gilts, boars, and weanling pigs serve as the nucleus for a clean herd. Testing is carried out frequently and all infected animals are removed.
3. If the incidence of infection is low, reactors are removed and the herd is retested at 30-day intervals. Reactors are removed until the entire herd is negative on retest.

Swine do not react immunologically (humoral) to the same degree that cattle do, and as a consequence, the agglutination test is less reliable. The card test is considered more accurate than the agglutination test. The other serological tests used for cattle may also be used for swine.

Following two consecutive negative herd tests not less than 90 days apart, the herd is eligible for Validated Brucellosis-Free Herd status in the United States. Vaccination is not employed.

LABORATORY DIAGNOSIS. The culture and identification of *B. suis* and other species are discussed in general below.

Dog

Brucella abortus and *B. suis* have been isolated occasionally from sporadic infections in dogs. Canine brucellosis caused by *B. canis* was first recognized as a problem in beagle breeding kennels. The disease is known to be widely distributed throughout the general dog population, although the incidence is low.

The mode of infection, transmission, and pathogenesis of the canine disease is similar to that of brucellosis in cattle, swine, and goats. Expelled tissues and vaginal discharges of aborted bitches and the urine of infected males are primary sources of the infectious agent. Other means of transmission are copulation and nursing.

The incubation period after oral infection is 6–21 days. The bacteremic phase of the disease may last as long as 2 years, and other than a lymphadenopathy, dogs show little evidence of infection. Infected bitches usually abort in the last trimester. Those puppies that are not dead when aborted soon die. Following abortion, there is a yellow-brown to dark brown discharge that persists for 1–6 weeks. Another possible result of infection of the bitch is resorption of the fetuses. Females may subsequently fail to conceive. Infections of bones may give rise to chronic osteomyelitis and **diskospondylitis**.

Prostatitis, epididymitis, and testicular atrophy with decreased or no spermatogenesis are common in the male and may result in irreversible sterility. Infected males may harbor the organism in their genital tract for several months.

DIAGNOSIS.   This is best accomplished by culture of the organism from blood (blood culture), urine (male), fetal organs, and vaginal swabs. Positive blood cultures are the most reliable evidence of *B. canis* infection.

The following serological procedures are employed, but they are not as reliable as culture:

- **Rapid slide agglutination test (RSAT).** The original form of this office screening test used stained *B. ovis* as antigen. Serum was treated with 2-mercaptoethanol. This test was reliable when negative, but about 40% of positive samples were false.
- **M-RSAT.** An improved test uses a *B. canis* strain (mucoid negative) and has greater specificity.
- **Agar gel immunodiffusion test.** This test, using cell wall antigens, is subject to false positives. When highly specific protein antigens are used, the procedure has been found to be sensitive and accurate in detecting infection.
- **Tube agglutination test.** This procedure is also prone to false positives.
- **ELISA.** This procedure, using "specific antigens," has been reliable and may be adapted to commercial kits.
- **Indirect fluorescent antibody test.** This procedure has also been found to have a high rate of false-positive reactions.

The culture and identification of *B. canis* is discussed later.

CONTROL.   Treatment is not practiced. The disease is eliminated from kennels by blood testing, followed by elimination of reacting dogs. Only dogs free of brucellosis, specifically those that are negative to at least two tests, are added to brucellosis-free breeding kennels. A satisfactory vaccine has not yet been developed.

Goats

Although accurate data are not available, tests indicate that the incidence of brucellosis in goats in the United States is approximately 1%. The majority of infections in goats are caused by *B. melitensis*.

Laboratory diagnosis and control are essentially the same as for cattle.

Horse

Brucella abortus and *B. suis* have been recovered, along with other organisms, from cases of suppurative bursitis (fistulous withers and poll evil). Brucellae have also been recovered from muscles, tendons, and osteoarthritic lesions in various locations in the horse. There is little information on the relationship between serological titers and infection.

Sheep

Brucella abortus and *B. melitensis* cause occasional infections similar to that seen in goats. Abortions may occur. *Brucella ovis* infection is discussed below.

GENERAL

Direct Examination

The Modified Ziehl-Neelsen (MZL) is useful in demonstrating brucellae in smears from the placenta (cotyledons) in bovine abortion. Cells of the chorion are packed with organisms that stain red against a blue background. Organisms can also be demonstrated directly in smears from vaginal mucus, semen, and various tissues. Direct and indirect fluorescent antibody staining can also be used.

Laboratory Diagnosis

Good growth is obtained on tryptose, potato, liver infusion, and blood agar. Colonies are round, entire, smooth, glistening, and translucent. Young colonies are 1–2 mm in diameter; they may become 5–8 mm on continued incubation. *Brucella abortus* requires 10% CO_2 for initial isolation. Plates should be incubated for as long as 30 days. Small rods, single or in pairs or short chains, are seen in smears from colonies. CO_2 is inhibitory to *B. canis*.

The different species can be identified by the characteristics listed in Table 12.1. With additional tests, a number of biotypes (biovars) of each of the classic species can be identified. For growth in the presence of dyes, the latter are incorporated in tryptose agar. A number of bacteriophages are available to aid in the identification of *Brucella* spp.

Monospecific sera prepared to react with A, M, and R antigens are used to aid identification (see Table 12.1). They are prepared by adsorption of the sera with the appropriate *Brucella* species (see Antigenic Nature). Fluorescent antibody staining is used for generic identification. Organisms from colonies can be presumptively identified as brucellae by a slide agglutination test using *B. abortus* antiserum.

Experimental Animals

Guinea pigs can be readily infected with infectious material. They are useful if material is badly contaminated or the numbers of organisms are very small. Infected guinea pigs will yield pure cultures and develop a significant agglutination titer.

Resistance

All species are readily killed by commonly used chemical disinfectants and pasteurization. Organisms are fairly resistant to some environmental conditions; for example, *B. abortus* will survive for 4–5 hours when exposed to direct

Table 12.1   Differentiation of *Brucella* Species and Their Biotypes (Biovars)

Species	Biotype	Urease	CO_2 requirement	H_2S production	Growth on Dyes		Agglutination in Sera		
					Thionin (20 μg/mL)	Basic Fuchsin (20 μg/mL)	A	M	R
B. melitensis	1	V	−	−	+	+	−	+	−
	2	V	−	−	+	+	+	−	−
	3	V	−	−	+	+	+	+	−
B. abortus	1	+	(+)	+	−	+	+	−	−
	2	+	(+)	+	−	−	+	−	−
	3*	+	(+)	+	+	+	+	−	−
	4	+	(+)	+	−	(+)	−	+	−
	5	+	−	−	+	+	−	+	−
	6*	+	−	(−)	+	+	+	−	−
	9	+	+	+	+	+	−	+	−
B. suis	1	+	−	+	+	−	+	−	−
	2	+	−	−	+	−	+	−	−
	3	+	−	−	+	+	+	−	−
	4	+	−	−	+	(−)	+	+	−
	5	+	−	−	+	−	−	+	−
B. canis		+	−	−	+	−	−	−	+
B. ovis		−	+	−	+	(+)	−	−	+
B. neotomae		+	−	+	−	−	+	−	−

Note: V, variable; (+), most are positive; (−) most are negative.
*To differentiate between biotypes 3 and 6, examine growth at 40 μg/mL thionin. Biotype 3 = (+), biotype 6 = (−).

sunlight; 4 days in urine; 5 days on cloth at room temperature; and 75 days in an aborted fetus during cool weather.

Immunization

Strain 19 vaccine, a live attenuated (*B. abortus* biotype 1) strain, was developed by Buck in 1930. It is not considered transmissible. In vaccinated calves, agglutination titers usually fall to negative levels in 4–6 weeks. As mentioned above, there is the problem of persisting reactors. If an animal is positive (1:200) after 30 months, it is considered a reactor.

Adjuvant bacterins, such as those prepared from vaccine strain 45/20, are used in some countries; 45/20 has been used live or dead to reduce losses in adult cattle. Strain 19 has also been used in adult cattle. Because 45/20 is a rough strain, the immune response to it can be distinguished from that caused by infection. When used as a killed vaccine, two doses provide protection for about a year. The use of strain 45/20 has been discontinued in many countries as the strain readily reverts to smooth and is capable of causing disease.

The recently developed, live attenuated strain RB51 (*B. abortus*) is replacing Strain 19. It is a stable rough strain that elicits good protection but does not induce the serological responses that cause difficulty in the use of serological tests for detecting infected animals.

As mentioned above, protective immunity in brucellosis is predominantly cell-mediated. Several protein candidates of *Brucella* have been implicated as "protective antigens" in the generation of a cell-mediated immune response. These include the Cu/Zn superoxide dismutase, the L7/L12 ribosomal protein, and the O-polysaccharide of the LPS. The efficacy of any of these antigens in vaccine development has yet to be established.

BRUCELLA OVIS

This organism causes a widespread, sexually transmitted disease of sheep characterized in the ram by orchitis, epididymitis, and impaired fertility and in some ewes by placentitis and abortion. The ram is more susceptible than the ewe, and more rams develop lesions than ewes. Infection of ewes originates almost exclusively from infected rams, and the disease is effectively controlled by the elimination of the infected rams.

Various vaccination procedures have been used successfully to prevent rams from becoming infected. *Brucella melitensis* Rev.1 live attenuated vaccine has been used with success to immunize rams against *B. ovis* infection. This vaccine and the *B. melitensis* H 38 killed vaccine result in rams being positive in *B. melitensis* serologic tests.

Brucella melitensis occasionally causes disease in sheep that resembles *brucellosis* in goats.

Brucella ovis, like *B. canis*, is in a rough form, and colonies are dull, opaque and yellowish. CO_2 is required for isolation, and identification is based on the criteria given in Table 12.1.

Control and elimination of the disease are accomplished by complement fixation testing, semen examination (staining, including fluorescent antibody (FA) and

MZN method, and culture), and culling of rams with palpable lesions. ELISA, hemagglutination, and immunodiffusion tests have also been used successfully to detect infections. Two consecutive negative tests of flocks indicate absence of the infection.

Public Health Significance

Human infections are caused by the three classic species and *B. canis*. In heavy swine-raising areas, *B. suis* infections are more prevalent; *B. melitensis* infections are seen in goat-raising areas, and *B. abortus* infections occur in areas with infected cattle. Pasteurization has greatly reduced the incidence of brucellosis in humans. In recent years, there have been ~100 human cases in the United States annually. The three principal species of brucellae are highly infectious for humans.

Organisms are thought to penetrate the unbroken skin and mucous membranes. Important sources are microbiology laboratories, infected cows (obstetrical procedures), and unpasteurized milk and other dairy products. Multiple infections in laboratory workers caused by *B. abortus* and *B. melitensis* have been reported. Slaughterhouse workers and veterinarians frequently contract the disease in endemic regions.

The disease can vary from quite mild to very severe. The incubation period ranges from 8 to 90 days. Those under 14 years of age are less susceptible. There is usually a bacteremia, resulting in a variety of symptoms, including undulating fever, profuse perspiration, and rheumatic and neuralgic pains. The course is variable and relapses are frequent. Most patients totally recover within a year or two, even without treatment.

The organism may localize in the liver, lymph nodes, or bones, resulting infrequently in the chronic disease, which may last as long as 20 years with intermittent relapses of varying intensity. Abortion is rare in women, perhaps resulting from the absence of erythritol in the human placenta. Symptoms in the chronic form are thought to be mainly caused by hypersensitivity to *Brucella* protein.

Infections caused by *B. suis* and *B. melitensis* may be more serious than those caused by *B. abortus*. Brucellosis caused by *B. canis* is relatively mild. Infections caused by strain 19 have been reported. There do not appear, as yet, to be unequivocally documented human infections caused by RB51. A large dose of vaccinal organisms or impaired immunity could conceivably contribute to human infections.

Diagnosis

The agglutination test, although useful in the early and acute disease, may be negative in chronic infections. The anti-*Brucella* **Coombs test**, which detects incomplete antibody, is usually positive in the chronic disease. The complement-fixation test is superior to the agglutination test for chronic infections. Reagents for ELISAs are available commercially. These procedures measure total IgG and IgM anti-*Brucella* antibodies. They are highly sensitive and

eliminate the troublesome **prozones** of agglutination procedures. The *B. canis* agglutination test must be used for the diagnosis of human infections caused by that species.

Multiple blood cultures have been useful in the diagnosis of human brucellosis.

Treatment

Treatment is effective in humans if begun early. Oral doxycycline with rifampin administered for 30 days is preferred to prolonged treatment with a tetracycline and streptomycin. With the former two drugs, there are fewer side effects and infrequent relapses. Treatment of the chronic disease is not always satisfactory because organisms are intracellular and there are inaccessible foci (or focus), often in bone.

BARTONELLA

The genus *Bartonella* is closely related to the genus *Brucella*. The genus *Afipia* is closely related to *Brucella* and has only one species, *Afipia felis*, which is of minor veterinary significance.

Bartonellae are small, gram-negative, oxidase-negative, aerobic, fastidious rods. The following species are of veterinary interest:

- ***Bartonella henselae.*** Habitat, cat; cause of cat-scratch disease (CSD), **bacillary angiomatosis**, and **peliosis hepatitis** in humans.
- ***Bartonella clarridgeiae.*** Habitat, cat; thought to be an infrequent cause of CSD.
- ***Afipia felis.*** Habitat, cat, but uncommon; considered an infrequent cause of CSD.

Several *Bartonella* species are found parasitizing erythrocytes of birds, fish, small rodents, and other animals.

BARTONELLA HENSELAE

This small, gram-negative rod, a facultative intracellular parasite, is the cause of CSD, a frequently occurring noncontagious human disease acquired from cats. The cause was unknown for many years, but recently it has been determined that most cases of CSD are caused by *B. henselae*. This organism can infect cats for long periods without causing any apparent disease.

Transmission and Pathogenesis

CSD affects children predominantly, and there is almost always a history of contact with a cat. Most cases occur in the late summer and autumn. The cats involved are normal and usually less than a year of age. The causal bacterium is a commensal of the mouth and skin of at least 30% of cats.

Infection may result from a cat scratch, a puncture wound, or entrance via the conjunctiva (Parinaud's oculoglandular syndrome). It is thought that claws acquire the organism from saliva during grooming. There is strong evidence that fleas and ixodid ticks including *Amblyoma americanum* (Lone-Star tick) can transmit the infection.

Little is known of factors leading to the pathogenicity. *Bartonella henselae* have pili that facilitate adherence and contribute to intracellular location in erythrocytes and endothelial cells. A 43-kDa adhesin, omp43, has yet to be characterized. The current understanding of the mechanism is that pili of *B. henselae* are involved with the stimulation of the production of growth factors of its target cells, causing the target cells to proliferate. In addition, *B. henselae*, by an unknown mechanism, stimulates the expression of ICAM-1 (intercellular adhesion molecule) by the target cells. Contact with the target cell allows for aggregation of the *B. henselae* cells. These aggregates are then engulfed into the target cells by novel structures known as invasomes. Invasomes can be distinguished from phagosomes in the target cells and are, thus, unique. Cortical F-actin, ICAM-1, and phosphotyrosine are thought to be associated with the process of creating and engulfing the invasome. Beyond this, much of the pathogenesis of *B. henselae* has yet to be determined.

The incubation period ranges from 3 to 90 days. The course may be as long as 4 months. A red or pink macule develops at the site of entrance, followed by a vesicle that ruptures and encrusts. A papule less than 1 cm in diameter persists for a number of weeks. Unilateral regional lymphadenopathy (axillary, cervical or trochlear) develops with enlargement and occasional suppuration. This regional lymphadenopathy is the predominant sign of CSD. It may be accompanied by low-grade fever and mild, systemic symptoms. The lymph nodes involved depend on the site of the entrance of the agent.

Serious illness with bacillary angiomatosis, peliosis hepatitis, or other disseminated infection is seen in immunocompromised patients, such as those with HIV infection.

As mentioned above, *B. clarridgeiae* and *A. felis* are infrequent causes of CSD.

Laboratory Diagnosis

This is usually accomplished by staining smears of material, usually biopsies, collected from the early lesion. When stained by the Warthin–Starry silver stain, the bacteria are pleomorphic, coccoid, and small (less than 1 μm in diameter). They are usually extracellular and may appear as microcolonies.

Although isolation and identification are not necessary for diagnosis, cultivation can be accomplished on blood agar. Five weeks' incubation may be required for the appearance of colonies. The latter are whitish, invaginated, and tenacious and may be imbedded in the medium.

A highly specific skin test using an "antigen" consisting of heat-treated pus from lymph nodes has been used effectively in diagnosis. Serologic test systems (including indirect immunofluorescence assay and ELISA) for antibodies to *B. henselae* in humans and cats are available commercially. A PCR procedure has been used to amplify the causal agent in tissues.

Treatment and Prevention

The disease is usually self-limiting, with most infections resolving spontaneously without treatment. Inflamed, fluctuant abscesses may be aspirated for relief of pain. Tetracyclines, erythromycin, rifampin and ciprofloxacin for 1–3 months have been effective in disseminated forms of the disease as in acquired immune deficiency syndrome. Disposal of cats thought to be involved is not indicated. Transmission to humans is prevented by avoiding intimate contact with cats, cat bites, and scratches. Removal of cats from the household may be recommended for individuals at particular risk.

A vaccine is now available to prevent CSD.

GLOSSARY

bacillary angiomatosis Disorder characterized by proliferation of neovascular tissues (angiomas). The lesions may be single or many and involve many organs. They are red (cranberry-like) initially, then enlarge to several centimeters in diameter and may ulcerate.

brucellosis ring test Test for agglutinins in cow's milk. A stained *B. abortus* antigen is added to several milliliters of milk. If agglutinins are present, they combine with the antigen and rise to the top of the milk sample, producing a discernable ring.

carboxyphilic Growth requires CO_2.

Coombs test Test that employs an antibody directed against immunoglobulins to agglutinate particles (e.g., erythrocytes) carrying nonagglutinating ("incomplete") antibody on their surface.

diskospondylitis Inflammation of the vertebrae and vertebral disk.

peliosis hepatitis Liver disorder characterized by the presence of small, blood-filled cystic lesions containing the causal bacteria. It is accompanied by weight loss, fever, and abdominal pain.

prozone Absence of serological reaction, for example, agglutination, at low dilutions of potent antisera.

ungulate Hoofed mammals, many of which are herbiverous and horned.

13 *Burkholderia, Bordetella, and Taylorella*

The genus *Pseudomonas* had originally included many species. On the basis of ribonucleic acid (RNA) homology, the genus was divided into five groups that were later, based on nucleic acid analyses, reclassified to several new genera in addition to a reduced *Pseudomonas* genus. One of these genera, *Burklolderia*, includes two species of veterinary importance, *Burklolderia mallei* (formerly *Pseudomonas mallei*) and *Burklolderia pseudomallei* (formerly *Pseudomonas pseudomallei*).

The genera *Bordetella* and *Taylorella* belong in the family Alcaligenaciae, which is closely related to the family Burkholderiaceae. The widespread free-living organism *Alcaligenes faecalis* is in the same family as *Bordetella* and *Taylorella*.

BURKHOLDERIA PSEUDOMALLEI

This organism is found in tropical and subtropical soils and water in Southeast Asia, Central Africa, and Australia, where the disease melioidosis most frequently occurs.

The modes of infection are by ingestion, inhalation (dust), and via wounds and abrasions. Outbreaks occur most frequently during or after heavy rainfall and flooding.

Pathogenesis and Pathogenicity

Burkholderia pseudomallei is a facultative intracellular parasite, and thus, the immune response is mainly cell-mediated.

Endotoxin, exotoxin, proteases, and hemolysin are thought to be some of the biologically active substances associated with *B. pseudomallei*. However, their precise role in the pathogenesis of melioidosis is not known.

The disease in humans and animals varies from a benign pulmonary form to a systemic form with visceral nodules (little pus unless secondary bacteria) and a terminal septicemia. The disease is called melioidosis or pseudoglanders. Although melioidosis is frequently seen in immunodeficient subjects, it can occur as a single independent disease without any apparent predisposing condition.

Although the disease in animals can be septicemic, often it is chronic and characterized by purulent granulomatous nodules in the lungs, liver, spleen, lymph nodes, and subcutis. The acute disease occurs more often in young animals, and those with impaired immune systems are particularly susceptible. In spite of extensive lesions, animals may appear normal. Lesions of melioidosis are frequently seen in slaughterhouses in endemic regions.

Among the animals infected are cattle, sheep, goats, pigs, horses, dogs, cats, primates, wild animals, rodents, dolphins, and tropical fish. Infected primates and dogs have occasionally been brought into the United States from endemic regions.

Laboratory Diagnosis

Mainly pus and material from nodular lesions are submitted.

Burkholderia pseudomallei grows well on standard laboratory media, including blood and MacConkey agar. Selective media are used to eliminate contaminating organisms such as *Pseudomonas aeruginosa* and other pseudomonads. Colonies are smooth and mucoid to dry and wrinkled. The growth has a pungent, earthy odor. Strains are nonhemolytic, motile, and oxidase positive. Final identification is based on biochemical tests.

Enzyme-linked immunosorbent assay (ELISA) and immunofluorescence assay are used as diagnostic aids.

Treatment and Control

Treatment of animals has not been satisfactory because of relapses when treatment is stopped. Susceptibility testing should be carried out, in that resistance to some agents has been encountered. Tetracyclines, chloramphenicol, trimethoprim-sulfamethoxazole, imipenem and related drugs, and ceftazidime have been effective. The response largely depends on the extent of the lesions.

Control involves keeping animals, as much as is feasible, on dry pastures and premises, detection and treatment of infected individuals, and vaccination.

Public Health Significance

Infected animals are not considered the source of human infections, nor are other humans.

BURKHOLDERIA MALLEI

Burkholderia mallei is an obligate pathogen of horses, other solipeds, humans, and carnivores. Glanders, the disease it causes, has been eradicated from North America and Central and Western Europe. It still occurs, however, in parts of Asia, the Middle East, and Africa.

Burkholderia mallei is a facultative intracellular pathogen that does not occur in nature.

Infection is usually via the respiratory tract. The disease is spread directly from animal to animal and indirectly by fomites. Human infections are acquired from infected animals directly or indirectly.

Pathogenicity

No exotoxin has been described; endotoxin is probably significant. Presence of a capsule has been determined to be a virulence factor, but other factors have yet to be elucidated.

Glanders is a contagious, usually chronic disease particularly of horses, mules, and donkeys, and it is characterized by the formation of tubercle-like nodules (granulomas) that frequently break down to form ulcers. Three forms of the disease are seen, depending on the principal location of the lesions: nasal, pulmonary, or skin (farcy).

Cattle, swine, rats, birds, and probably some other animals are resistant to infection. Humans, members of the cat family, and other carnivores are susceptible. All infections usually terminate fatally if not treated.

Laboratory Diagnosis

Tissue containing early nodules or pus from ulcers are submitted.

Burkholderia mallei grows well on standard laboratory media, including blood agar. Colonies are shallow, round, convex, and opaque and become yellowish green or brown on aging. On blood agar, colonies tend to be slimy. *Burkholderia mallei* differs from *B. pseudomallei* and *Pseudomonas* spp. in being nonmotile. Definitive identification is based on a number of biochemical tests.

Treatment and Control

Trimethoprim-sulfamethoxazole has been effective. No vaccines or bacterins are used.

Control is by mallein testing (analogous to tuberculin testing) and the complement-fixation test on horses and horse-kind, with the elimination of animals that react positively. Mallein (an extract of *B. mallei* cultures) is injected **intrapalpebrally.** Immunity is predominantly cell-mediated.

Public Health Significance

Human glanders, which is rare, is seen almost exclusively in those whose occupation brings them in contact with infected animals and infectious materials; for example, veterinarians, butchers, slaughterhouse workers, farmers, and laboratory workers. The disease does not occur in the Western Hemisphere.

BORDETELLA

Species of the genus *Bordetella* are small, gram-negative rods and coccobacilli. They are aerobic, catalase, and oxidase-positive and do not ferment carbohydrates (metabolism respiratory). There are both motile and nonmotile species.

Seven species have now been recognized:

- ***Bordetella bronchiseptica.*** Natural hosts are animals; causes respiratory disease including infectious atrophic rhinitis (IAR) of pigs.
- ***Bordetella avium.*** Causes turkey coryza or avian bordetellosis.
- ***Bordetella pertussis.*** Causes whooping cough (pertussis) in humans.
- ***Bordetella parapertussis.*** Causes parapertussis, a mild form of whooping cough.
- ***Bordetella hinzii.*** Has been recovered from poultry and humans. It is an opportunist causing infections in immunocompromised humans.
- ***Bordetella holmesii.*** A human opportunist causing various infections, including pertussis-like disease, endocarditis, and septicemia.
- ***Bordetella petrii.*** Recovered from an anaerobic bioreactor and of no pathogenic significance.
- ***Bordetella trematum.*** A proposed new species, recovered from wounds and ear infections in humans.

BORDETELLA BRONCHISEPTICA

Bordetella bronchiseptica is a commensal in the upper respiratory tract of dogs, cats, swine, rabbits, horses, guinea pigs, rats, and possibly other animals.

Infections may be endogenous or exogenous. Inhalation is the principal mode of infection. Spread is by direct and indirect contact and fomites.

Pathogenesis

Considerable variation exists in the ability of *B. bronchiseptica* strains to colonize and produce disease in pigs and other animals. Among the products and factors contributing to pathogenesis are

- Most *B. bronchiseptica* strains possess pili and flagella. These structures appear to correlate with growth phase and colonial morphology. Adherence of *B. bronchiseptica* to epithelial cells of the respiratory tract is facilitated by the presence of pili. *Bordetella bronchiseptica* seems to have a strong affinity for respiratory mucin. This affinity for mucin receptors appears to help the organism to adhere and colonize the nasal mucosa of young pigs.
- Virulent strains of *B. bronchiseptica* produce an extracellular enzyme, adenylate cyclase toxin, which is capable of altering cellular functions of

the host including phagocytosis and intracellular killing. In addition, the enzyme has the ability to immobilize the respiratory tract cilia (ciliostasis).

- *Bordetella bronchiseptica* possesses an intracellular, heat-labile toxin with a molecular weight of approximately 145 kDa. The toxin, a single-chain polypeptide, is inactivated by trypsin, formalin, and glutaraldehyde. It is lethal when injected intraperitoneally into mice and produces necrosis when injected intradermally into the guinea pig. The toxin, also known as dermonecrotic toxin, is at least partially responsible for the production of nasal turbinate atrophy (atrophic rhinitis) in piglets and experimentally in rabbits, rats, and mice. The toxin impairs the ability of osteoblasts to differentiate, which leads to turbinate atrophy. It appears that the severe turbinate atrophy sometimes seen in pigs is caused by mixed infection with *B. bronchiseptica* and toxigenic *Pasteurella multocida*.
- Other factors that may have a role in the pathogenesis of the disease are production of endotoxin, hemolysin, hemagglutinin, and tracheal cytotoxin. The tracheal cytotoxin is partially responsible for ciliostasis and the extrusion of the ciliated epithelium. The filamentous hemagglutinin is associated with the attachment of the bordetellae to the respiratory epithelial cells. The exact role of these enzymes and toxic products is not clearly understood.

Pathogenicity

Infection results in respiratory disease that is usually subacute to chronic in nature. Diseases or conditions with which *B. bronchiseptica* has been associated are

- **Swine.** It has a role along with *P. multocida* in the etiology of infectious atrophic rhinitis of swine (see Chapter 19). *Bordetella bronchiseptica* by itself causes a relatively mild form of IAR. The severe, progressive form of IAR leading often to atrophy of the turbinate bones and distortion of the nasal septum is caused by infection with both *B. bronchiseptica* and toxigenic strains of *P. multocida*. *Bordetella bronchiseptica* also causes a severe bronchopneumonia of young pigs.
- **Dogs.** Canine infectious tracheobronchitis (CIT; kennel cough) may be primarily caused by viruses or *B. bronchiseptica*. It is a widespread, highly contagious disease usually associated with bringing dogs from various sources together, as in clinics, hospitals, dog shows, and boarding kennels. The course is 7–10 days, and signs include a harsh dry cough, nasal discharge, anorexia, and fever. Bronchopneumonia may develop. The disease may be fatal in puppies and may leave older dogs with chronic bronchitis.
- **Horses.** *Bordetella bronchiseptica* is occasionally the cause of primary respiratory infections and also

may have a secondary role in a primary respiratory virus infection.
- **Cats.** *Bordetella bronchiseptica* is recognized as an important cause, either primary or secondary (to respiratory viruses), of upper respiratory infections. Serious outbreaks of bronchopneumonia, resulting sometimes in death, have been reported in breeding colonies and laboratory cats.
- **Rabbits, guinea pigs, and rats.** Bronchopneumonia, upper respiratory infections, and septicemia occur most commonly in breeding colonies and laboratory animals.

Respiratory infections of varying severity are seen infrequently in other animals.

Laboratory Diagnosis

The organism is aerobic, can be cultured on blood or serum agar, and may be beta-hemolytic. MacConkey agar is useful if specimens are heavily contaminated. Small, circular, dewdrop colonies appear in 48 hours. On further incubation, colonies enlarge, becoming flat and glistening. Stained smears disclose small gram-negative rods or coccobacilli.

Special media are available for culturing material from nasal swabs in the testing of swine herds for *B. bronchiseptica* and, thus, for infectious atrophic rhinitis. Because of the great difficulty of eliminating IAR from herds, this approach has been largely abandoned. *Bordetella bronchiseptica* forms distinctive colonies on Bordet-Gengou agar, a blood-based medium used routinely for isolation of *B. pertussis*. The colonies of *B. bronchiseptica* on this medium are smooth and dome-shaped and have a "mercury droplet" appearance.

Bordetella bronchiseptica is motile and indole-negative and does not produce H_2S. Urease is produced, and the tests for oxidase and catalase are positive. The reaction in litmus milk is alkaline, turning from blue to black in 5–10 days. Carbohydrates are not fermented. Additional biochemical criteria are required for definitive identification.

Antigenic Nature and Immunity

Bordetella bronchiseptica have flagellar H antigens, heat-labile surface K antigens, heat-stable surface O antigens, and fimbrial antigens. Based primarily on heat-stable surface antigens, *B. bronchiseptica* cell types have been divided into three smooth phases and one rough phase. These phases are reflected in differences in colonial characteristics, toxigenicity, hemolysis, and capacity for colonization. A 68-kDa outer membrane protein has been shown to be an important antigen in eliciting protection in piglets.

Both humoral and cell-mediated immunity would appear to be important. *Bordetella bronchiseptica* is included with *P. multocida* in bacterins to prevent IAR and respiratory disease in swine. Bacterin–toxoid preparations are given to sows before farrowing so that the colostrum contributes to protection against IAR. Piglets up to 4 weeks of age may also be vaccinated. Modified live, intranasal vaccines prepared from the agents of IAR are administered to young pigs.

In addition to viral vaccines, both live, intranasal vaccines and bacterins containing *B. bronchiseptica* are used to prevent canine infectious tracheobronchitis.

Bordetella bronchiseptica is combined with *Pasteurella multocida* in bacterins to prevent snuffles in rabbits.

Treatment and Control

The treatment and control of IAR of pigs is discussed under *P. multocida* (Chapter 19). The drugs tylosin, tetracyclines, ceftiofur, and sulfonamides, which are usually effective against both *P. multocida* and *B. bronchiseptica*, are administered in feed or water to pigs at various ages to aid in the control of IAR.

Bordetella bronchiseptica is ordinarily susceptible to many antimicrobial drugs; a notable exception is penicillin.

Antimicrobial therapy is usually reserved for severe cases of canine infectious tracheobronchitis. Tetracyclines or chloramphenicol are given parenterally. Kanamycin is administered by aerosol to unresponsive dogs. Sanitary and management practices are employed to prevent spread.

Public Health Significance

Bordetella bronchiseptica from animals rarely infects humans. It has been implicated as the cause of bronchitis, pneumonia, septicemia, bacteremia, sinusitis, endocarditis, peritonitis, meningitis, wound infections, and terminal sepsis in humans.

BORDETELLA AVIUM

This organism is the cause of the widespread, economically important disease of young turkeys and quail, avian bordetellosis, or turkey coryza. The disease is spread by direct and indirect contact and is highly contagious. The organism is harbored in the upper respiratory tract of turkeys.

Pathogenesis

The organism colonizes ciliated tracheal epithelium, leading to inflammation and destruction of the epithelium and damage to the tracheal rings.

Adherence of *B. avium* is associated with pili and hemagglutinin. Organisms agglutinate guinea pig red cells.

Some strains adhere to epithelial cells and produce toxins that are similar to those produced by other bordetellae and that include tracheal cytotoxin, and dermonecrotic toxin. Those strains producing the tracheal cytotoxin can cause deciliation and loss of mucous gland function of respiratory epithelium. In contrast with *B. broncheseptica* and *B. pertussis*, *B. avium* does not produce an adenylate cyclase toxin.

Bordetella avium produces a dermonecrotic toxin, which is a heat-labile protein, with a molecular weight of approximately 155 kDa. It is lethal to mice, guinea pigs, young chickens, and turkey poults and produces dermonecrosis when injected intradermally into guinea pigs, chickens, and turkey poults. Other virulence factors include pili, tracheal cytotoxin, and hemagglutinin.

Bordetella avium has also been isolated from the respiratory tracts of other avian species. The organism appears to have a primary or secondary role in respiratory disease in chickens.

Pathogenicity

The disease affects young turkeys and quail; young chickens are not naturally affected. It is an acute rhinotracheitis with a high morbidity and usually a low mortality. Contributing to more severe infections are various stresses and secondary viruses and bacteria, such as Newcastle disease virus and *Escherichia coli*. Turkeys usually suffer no adverse consequences in the absence of secondary agents. There may be deciliation and loss of mucous gland function of the respiratory epithelium

Signs include oculonasal discharge, a characteristic cough, sneezing, and dyspnea, with decreased weight gain. In severe cases, the tracheal cartridge is distorted and discolored. Collapse of the trachea may result in suffocation.

Laboratory Diagnosis

Bordetella avium resembles *B. bronchiseptica* in its growth and cultural characteristics, but it differs from it in that it does not produce urease. *Bordetella avium* has two colony types: a large, dry colony and a small, smooth, round colony.

The best cultural source of the organism is the anterior trachea. It grows slowly, producing small colonies on blood and MacConkey agars. The latter medium is particularly useful if there are contaminating organisms. Colonial growth agglutinates guinea pig red cells. *B. avium* resembles closely *Alcaligenes faecalis,* which is found in soil, water, and feces and that occurs occasionally in clinical specimens. The latter organism can be differentiated from *B. avium* by its failure to agglutinate guinea pig red cells.

Prevention and Treatment

Live attenuated vaccines of *B. avium* appear to offer considerable protection against the disease. A live vaccine consisting of a temperature-sensitive mutant is administered by spray to day-old poults in the hatchery. Killed vaccines are used in breeders.

Most antibiotics to which the organism is sensitive do not reach therapeutic levels at the tracheal surface. Antibiotics such as tetracyclines are used to prevent or treat secondary colibacillosis.

TAYLORELLA: TAYLORELLA EQUIGENITALIS

This small, nonmotile, microaerophilic, encapsulated, gram-negative coccobacillus causes contagious equine metritis (CEM), an acute, highly contagious venereal disease of mares, female ponies, and donkeys characterized by a metritis, cervicitis, and copious, purulent, vaginal discharge. Abortions are rare. Stallions are infected and spread the disease during coitus but show no clinical signs. Spread may also be by contaminated equipment and attendants.

The disease has been reported from the United Kingdom, France, many other European countries, Australia, and Japan. It is most prevalent in Europe and is rare in North America.

Pathogenesis and Pathogenicity

Cilia may contribute to adherence to epithelial cells, and the capsule may aid in the survival of the organism in tissues.

The infection is mainly transmitted to the mare at coitus from infected stallions. The organism is found on the surface of the penis, in the preputial smegma, and in the urethral fossa. The infection can also be spread between mares and stallions by attendants, fomites, and, especially, by instruments.

The infectious process appears to be confined to the mucous membrane of the uterus, cervix, and vagina, with accompanying endometritis, cervicitis, and vaginitis. The damage mainly involves the uterine mucosa, which spontaneously heals after several weeks, after which, breeding capability is restored. There has been no evidence of spread to other tissues and organs. The organism may reside for long periods in the clitoral sinuses and fossa of mares. The mare does not usually conceive when infected during mating. If she does, the foal may be infected and become a carrier.

The discharge from the vulva contains large numbers of neutrophils, many of which harbor *T. equigenitalis*. The edematous uterine mucosa initially contains many neutrophils and mononuclear cells. No lesions are seen in the stallion.

Laboratory Diagnosis

The disease should be suspected when there is a copious mucopurulent vaginal discharge occurring after breeding or during the breeding season.

The disease can only be diagnosed definitively by the isolation and identification of the causal agent.

Swabs from the cervix, urethra, and clitoral fossa, including the clitoral sinuses of the mare and the prepuce, urethral fossa, and penile sheath of the stallion, should be refrigerated and sent to the laboratory in a transport medium (preferably Amies) as soon after being collected as possible.

The organism can be isolated on chocolate agar with a base of Eugon or Columbia agar that has been incubated for several days in an atmosphere containing 5%–10% CO_2. Small colonies, similar in appearance to those of *Haemophilus* spp., appear after 24 hours of incubation. Although fastidious and rather unreactive biochemically, *T. equigenitalis* can be shown to be oxidase- and catalase-negative, phosphatase-positive, nonfermentative, non-

hemolytic, and strictly microaerophilic. *Taylorella equigenitalis* is agglutinated in a slide test by specific antiserum. Strains both susceptible and resistant to streptomycin occur.

A PCR procedure has been used to identify organisms in clinical materials and, in particular, in those that are culturally negative.

Complement fixation, agglutination (plate and tube), ELISA, and passive hemagglutination tests have been used, but none is reliable for the detection of carriers.

A new species, *Taylorella asinigenitalis*, has been proposed for isolates from male donkeys based on sequence analysis of DNA encoding 16S rRNA. This new species, which was phenotypically identical to *T. equigenitalis*, did not produce CEM experimentally.

Taylorella equigenitalis–like organisms are encountered that do not produce disease. They have been distinguished from pathogenic *T. equigenitalis* strains by a **multiplex PCR**.

Treatment

Intrauterine irrigation with nitrofurazone, ampicillin, or penicillin daily for 5–10 days is effective. Ampicillin or penicillin is given parenterally for the same period. The penis should be cleaned and the prepuce irrigated on at least five occasions with chlorhexidine, followed by application of nitrofurazone ointment. One week after treatment, mares and stallions must be checked to determine whether they are negative for the organism. Three successive cultures at weekly intervals should be negative.

Conception rates for mares and breeding rates for stallions return to normal the following breeding season.

Immunity

Immunity would seem to be of a low order and mainly antibody-mediated. There is evidence that previously infected mares can be reinfected several weeks after being culturally negative. Both local and systemic antibodies can be demonstrated by various procedures in mares, but not in stallions. Effective vaccines or bacterins are not available.

Control

CEM is a reportable disease. The suspected infected stallion should not be used for further breeding until shown to be culturally negative. All animals suspected or known to be infected should be kept under strict isolation until shown to be negative by culture.

The organism is fragile, and evidence indicates that it will not survive in discharge material outside the host for more than several days.

GLOSSARY

intrapalpebral Within an area near the eyelid.
multiplex PCR Polymerase chain reaction designed for the amplification of more than one DNA fragment per reaction.

14

Francisella and Coxiella

The Family Francisellaceae is in a different Section, the γ-Proteobacteria, than *Bartonella* and *Brucella*, and it comprises only one genus, *Francisella*. *Francisella tularensis* is the principal species.

Coxiella was previously considered a rickettsia. It has recently been placed in the γ-Proteobacteria, close to *Francisella* and *Legionella*, based upon comparisons of the 16S rRNA-encoding gene sequences.

FRANCISELLA TULARENSIS

Francisella tularensis is a small, pleomorphic, nonmotile, noncapsulated, aerobic, gram-negative rod or coccobacillus. It is a facultative intracellular parasite that is oxidase-negative and nonfermentative and requires cystine for isolation.

The following species and biovars are recognized:

- *Francisella tularensis*, biovar *tularensis*, type A. Occurs in North America; reservoir is the cottontail rabbit; highly virulent and infectious for most mammals including humans; has an LD_{50} in rabbits of fewer than 10 organisms.
- *Francisella tularensis*, biovar *palaeartica*, type B. Occurs in Asia, Europe, and North America; less virulent than type A; the cause of epizootics in beavers, muskrats, and voles; has an LD_{50} in rabbits of greater than 10^7 organisms.
- *Francisella tularensis*, biovar *novicida*, type C. Recovered from water; not considered a significant pathogen.
- *Francisella philomiragia* (formerly *Yersinia philomiragia*). Associated with salty or brackish water; cause of infrequent illness in humans with underlying disease, including chronic granulomatous disease or myeloproliferative disorders.

Transmission

Tularemia is principally a disease of wild animals; however, humans, as well as some domestic animals and fowl, are susceptible. In nature, the disease is frequently transmitted from infected to susceptible hosts by insect vectors. These include wood ticks, dog and rabbit ticks, deer flies, fleas, black flies, mites, mosquitoes, and lice.

Resistance

The organism will live for months at subfreezing temperatures and in frozen meat for years. Flies are infective for up to 2 weeks and ticks for their lifetime (about 2 years).

Pathogenesis

Type A biovar exhibits **citrulline ureidase** activity, but type B biovars do not. About 80% of human cases of tularemia in the United States are caused by type A serovar.

The manner in which *F. tularensis* causes disease is not understood. It possesses a thin, mainly lipid, capsule. The capsule is thought to help the organism resist phagocytosis by neutrophils and macrophages. Another virulence factor is the production of a unique acid, phosphatase, which suppresses the destructive respiratory burst associated with phagocytes. The organism is highly toxic for macrophages and has been observed to stimulate **apoptosis** in macrophage cell lines in vitro. Endotoxin is probably an important factor; an exotoxin has not been found. Immunity is primarily cell-mediated, and delayed hypersensitivity may contribute to tissue damage.

Pathogenicity

The prevalence of tularemia in wild rabbits in the United States has been estimated to be approximately 1%. In North America, the cottontail rabbit is the reservoir of infection for nearly 70% of the human cases. Other naturally susceptible animals are squirrel, opossum, beaver, woodchuck, muskrat, skunk, coyote, fox, cat, sheep, deer, bullsnake, game birds, and domestic fowl.

The most characteristic feature of the disease is focal, granulomatous lesions in a variety of organs and lymph nodes. After spread from the point of entry to dependent lymph nodes, a bacteremia results in small abscessing granulomas in visceral organs and lymph nodes. Small, necrotic, granulomatous foci in the liver, spleen, and lymph nodes are the characteristic gross lesions observed in wild rabbits. Different forms of the disease are seen in humans (see below), but systemic disease is seen most often in animals near death or at necropsy.

Tularemia is rarely seen in dogs, but there have been a number of reports of the disease in cats with, on occasion, transmission to humans by bites. Cats are thought to be infected by ticks, by eating infected rabbits, or by consuming contaminated food or water. Fever, weakness, inappetance, sometimes diarrhea, and dyspnea are followed by prostration and frequently death if untreated.

Human Disease

Humans may become infected by the bites of ticks, black flies, lice, mosquitoes, and deer flies; contact with infected animals (handling carcasses, skinning, and dressing) or their discharges; animal bites (cat most frequently, dog, and other animals); and ingestion of contaminated water and partially cooked meat. All ages are susceptible. Domestic rabbits are not a source of infection.

The human disease may assume several forms, but the most common is the ulceroglandular form, with the development of papule, ulcer, and lymph node enlargement, in that order. Depending on the portal of entry, the other forms are the oculoglandular (via conjunctiva), glandular, gastrointestinal, pneumonic, and typhoidal. All forms may give rise to the systemic form; the pneumonic and typhoidal forms are considered the most serious. The number of human cases reported annually in the United States is 100 to 200.

Laboratory Diagnosis

The organism is highly infectious for humans, and isolation should not be attempted without adequate biocontainment facilities. Depending on portal of entry, as few as 10 organisms are enough to establish disease.

Francisella tularensis grows well on cystine-blood agar; cystine is considered essential for growth although there are reports that some strains will grow on blood agar without added cystine. Plates should be incubated for at least 3 weeks. Minute, dewdrop-like colonies yield small, gram-negative rods and coccobacilli. There is a characteristic greenish discoloration (alpha hemolysis) surrounding the colonies.

Guinea pig inoculation is sometimes used to overcome contaminants. The organism can be recovered without difficulty from the organs of terminally ill guinea pigs.

Biochemical tests are difficult to perform and are not usually carried out. The fluorescent antibody (FA) procedure is widely used to identify the organism. A slide agglutination procedure using organisms from colonies and a specific *F. tularensis* antiserum is used. Biovar identification is carried out in reference laboratories.

Identification of specific antibodies by an ELISA or agglutination in the sera of guinea pigs inoculated with infectious material is confirmatory. A substantial rise in titer in the agglutination test or ELISA with paired sera is supportive of a diagnosis in humans and cats. The agglutination test is usually positive late in the disease.

Immune Response

This is primarily cell-mediated. Recovery from tularemia confers long-lasting, highly protective immunity. A live attenuated vaccine has been used in people whose risk of infection is high; however, it is no longer available in the United States.

Treatment

Streptomycin or gentamycin, given for 7–14 days, is the drug of choice. Tetracycline and chloramphenicol are also used but must be given for at least 14 days. Early treatment is important.

COXIELLA BURNETTII

This is the only species in the genus and is a small, pleomorphic coccobacillus with a gram-negative type cell wall. It stains poorly with the Gram stain; Gimenez stain is recommended. It is an obligate intracellular parasite with a developmental cycle that includes large- and small-cell variants. The small-cell variant attaches to macrophages, is ingested, and develops within the phagosome. After maturation to the large-cell variant, sporogenesis begins and spores are produced, which account for the remarkable resistance of the species, including the ability to survive at 15° to 25°C for nearly a year. High-temperature pasteurization kills the organism. After multiple passages in cell culture, the organism also undergoes an antigenic phase variation in which its lipopolysaccharide is reduced.

The organism occurs worldwide and exists in two patterns. One involves infection of wild animals and arthropod vectors, mainly ticks. The other involves domestic ruminants and is spread among these mainly by ticks, inhaled infectious aerosols, and also ingestion. Ticks infrequently infect humans. It is said that the organism has more nonhuman reservoirs than any other human malady. In addition to ticks, lice, chiggers, and flies may also carry the organism.

Transmission can be via direct or indirect contact, in that the organism may be present in placentas, reproductive discharges, milk, contaminated dust, and fomites.

Pathogenicity

The disease caused by *C. burnettii* is Q fever, which occurs worldwide, most often in a subclinical form. Abortions occur in sheep and goats. The organism can localize in the mammary gland, supramammary lymph nodes, uterus, and placenta of cows, resulting sometimes in infertility and abortion. Organisms can be discharged during lactation and at parturition.

Laboratory Diagnosis

Paired serum samples are preferred for complement fixation, microagglutination tests, and immunofluorescence assay. Smears from infectious materials are stained by the Giminez method. Isolation and cultivation of the organism in embryonated chicken eggs and cell cultures is rarely attempted.

Treatment

Tetracycline and chloramphenicol are the drugs of choice, although treatment may not be feasible. A vaccine has been used in some countries in endemic areas but is not available in the United States. If there are multiple abortions, pregnant animals should be segregated. Infectious materials such as placentas and aborted fetuses should be burned or buried, as the organisms are resistant to heat, drying, and many common disinfectants.

Public Health Significance

The human disease is uncommon but occurs occasionally, particularly in ranchers, farmers, veterinarians, and laboratory workers. Although cases are ordinarily sporadic, small outbreaks have been reported. Humans are infected in the same way that animals are infected and by consumption of unpasteurized milk. The signs are influenza-like with varying degrees of pneumonitis, cough, chest pains, weakness, and anorexia. The course is usually 1–4 weeks with resolution; however, the infection can infrequently persist for weeks. The mortality in untreated cases is 3%–4%.

GLOSSARY

apoptosis Programmed cell death; that is, a regulated set of events that result in cell death.

citrulline ureidase Enzyme, also known as citrullinase, that converts citrulline + H_2O to ornithine + CO_2 + NH_3 in amino acid metabolism.

LD$_{50}$ Least number of microorganisms or toxic substance required to kill 50% of the test animals.

15

Pseudomonas and Moraxella

As was pointed out earlier, the genus *Pseudomonas* was reduced in size and the important species *Pseudomonas pseudomallei* and *Pseudomonas mallei* were reclassified as *Burkholderia* species. The genus *Moraxella* is placed, taxonomically, close to *Pseudomonas* and also contains a number of species.

The pseudomonads are gram-negative, aerobic or facultatively anaerobic, nutritionally versatile, medium-size rods. They are motile by one or several polar flagella, catalase and oxidase-positive, and some species produce water-soluble pigments. They are free-living, being found widely in soil and water.

There are numerous pseudomonads, but only one species, *Pseudomonas aeruginosa*, is of considerable pathogenic significance in animals. Its natural habitat is water, soil, and decaying vegetation, and it causes a wide variety of infections. *P. aeruginosa* also may be found on the skin and mucous membranes and in feces.

The following species, *Stenotrophomonas maltophilia* (formerly *Pseudomonas maltophilia*), *Pseudomonas stutzeri*, *Pseudomonas fluorescens*, *Burkolderia cepacia* (formerly *Pseudomonas cepacia*), *Pseudomonas putida*, and other pseudomonads are occasionally recovered from clinical specimens, but they are rarely pathogenic in animals. Humans with cystic fibrosis are particularly susceptible to *B. cepacia* infections.

PSEUDOMONAS AERUGINOSA

Pathogenesis

Pseudomonas aeruginosa possess pili and flagella, which facilitate adherence to injured epithelial cells with subsequent colonization. As with other gram-negative bacteria, the capsule and lipopolysaccharide of *P. aeruginosa* offer considerable protection against phagocytic destruction.

Among the extracellular products produced by some strains and associated with pathogenicity are

- Proteases, including elastase, are involved in the invasiveness of the organism and destruction of tissue. They are produced by many clinical isolates.
- Some strains produce an alginate-containing polysaccharide slime layer that contributes to adherence and is antiphagocytic.

- Lecithinases and lipases enhance invasiveness, destroy tissue, and contribute to the inflammatory response.
- Exotoxin A inhibits protein synthesis, causes tissue necrosis, and contributes to lethality in severe infections.
- Exoenzyme S catalyzes the transfer of adenosine diphosphate–ribose to various guanosine triphosphate–binding proteins, including the product of the proto-oncogene *c-H-ras* (*p2lC-H-ras*). Its role in pathogenesis is unclear, but strains lacking exoenzyme S are less virulent than the parent strain.
- Leukocidin, a cytotoxin, acts on cell membranes, inhibiting and ultimately destroying neutrophils and damaging endothelial cells.
- The heat-labile hemolysin, phospholipase C, destroys a lecithin-containing lipoprotein of the alveolus (pulmonary surfactant) and thus contributes to tissue destruction and **atelectasis**.
- Pyocins prevent or reduce colonization of infected sites by other bacteria.

In addition, *P. aeruginosa* produces a deep-blue, chloroform-soluble pigment, pyocyanin, and a yellow-green, water-soluble pigment, fluorescein. These pigments exhibit antimicrobial activities against a wide range of bacteria and some fungi.

Pathogenicity

This species is a frequent contaminant in disease processes, and isolation alone is not necessarily significant. Its significance in mixed infections, particularly with streptococci and staphylococci, may be questionable. Repeated isolation in pure culture strongly indicates pathogenicity. *Pseudomonas aeruginosa* is an opportunist in weakened tissues (burns), wounds, debilitated patients, individuals with malignancies and immunodeficiencies, and young animals. It may replace bacteria that have been eliminated from infectious processes by antimicrobial treatment, and it sometimes causes a fatal septicemia. Infections are rare in healthy, normal individuals.

Only some of the many infections with which *P. aeruginosa* has been associated are listed below:

- **All animals.** Wound infections; abscess formation; diarrhea; and ear, urinary, and genital infections; nosocomial infections.
- **Horse.** Abortion, corneal, and guttural pouch infections.
- **Cattle.** Mastitis, abortion, and genital infections.
- **Dogs and cats.** Prostatitis, cystitis, dermatitis, postoperative septicemia, ear infection, and endocarditis.
- **Fowl.** Septicemia and respiratory infections.
- **Mink.** Hemorrhagic pneumonia.
- **Sheep.** "Green wool" and dermatitis.
- **Humans.** Wound, urinary, corneal, and inner-ear infections and fatal infections involving trachea, lungs, heart valves, meninges, and brain; septicemia, osteomyelitis, arthritis, cellulitis, and phlebitis; diarrhea caused by intestinal infection; infection complicating cystic fibrosis and nosocomial infections.

Laboratory Diagnosis

Specimen includes urine, pus, affected tissues, and swabs from infected tissue surfaces.

All strains grow well on ordinary nutrient media. Colonies are irregular, spreading, translucent, and 3–5 mm in diameter and may show a bluish-metallic sheen. Beta-hemolysis is usually observed around colonies growing on blood agar. A distinctive grapelike odor is usually apparent, regardless of the medium used. *Pseudomonas aeruginosa* does not grow anaerobically. Medium-sized, gram-negative rods are seen in smears. They cannot be distinguished morphologically from the enterobacteria.

Two pigments are commonly produced by *P. aeruginosa*, both of which are water-soluble: pyocyanin (bluish-green), which is chloroform-soluble ("blue pus bacillus"), and fluorescein or pyoverdin (yellowish-green), which is not chloroform-soluble. Both pigments may be found in media, but not always. Occasionally, a strain produces a dark-red pigment (pyorubin) or a brown-black pigment (pyomelanin). Pyocyanin can be extracted from the brown-black pigment of a slant culture by pouring chloroform over the growth. All strains are oxidase-positive.

Fluorescein fluoresces under ultraviolet light, but *P. fluorescens*, an occasional contaminant, also produces fluorescein. *Pseudomonas fluorescens* does not grow well at 37°C, however.

Other features of *P. aeruginosa* are motility by polar flagella and gelatin liquefaction. It is oxidase-positive, peptonizes litmus milk, uses citrate, is indole negative, and reduces nitrate. The oxidation/fermentation (O/F) test is positive for oxidation. Definitive identification is based on biochemical tests. The characteristic colonial appearance and odor of primary cultures can be highly suggestive of *P. aeruginosa*.

Antigenic Nature and Immunity

The species is antigenically heterogeneous, with a number of serotypes based on differences in O antigens. Strains can also be typed by bacteriophages and pyocins (**bacteriocins**); however, **nucleic acid fingerprinting** has largely replaced the other typing schemes in epidemiological studies.

Killed vaccines have been used in human burn patients. Autogenous bacterins have been used in mink and chinchillas. Immunity is short-lived, and there is no specific immunity to reinfection.

Resistance

Pseudomonas aeruginosa is resistant to some disinfectants including quaternary ammonium compounds; chlorine-containing disinfectants are effective. With minimal moisture *P. aeruginosa* can survive for long periods on water faucets, utensils, floors, instruments, baths, humidifiers, and medical equipment. Pseudomonads are susceptible to ethylene oxide or heat (boiling for 20 minutes).

Treatment and Control

Where applicable, surgical debridement and drainage should be provided.

Susceptibility testing should be performed although the clinical efficacy of antimicrobial drugs against pseudomonads does not always correlate well with in vitro data. Drugs that have been effective are tobramycin, gentamycin, amikacin, ciprofloxicin, colistin (polymyxin E), and carbenicillin. Resistance may develop to a single drug; thus, a combination of a β-lactam agent such as ticarcillin with an aminoglycoside may be preferred for serious infections. Because of the high concentration of polymyxin in the urine, this drug is especially effective in urinary tract infections.

Where feasible, exposure to pseudomonads should be kept to a minimum by effective sanitary measures. Multiple *P. aeruginosa* infections are uncommon in veterinary practice. When encountered, proper isolation procedures, strict sanitary measures, and effective disinfection should be applied.

MORAXELLA

Moraxella are small, gram-negative, aerobic, nonmotile rods or coccobacilli. They are catalase- and oxidase-positive, do not use carbohydrates, and do not require X or V factors.

There are at least 10 species, but only *Moraxella bovis* causes a significant disease in animals, namely, infectious bovine keratoconjunctivitis.

Moraxella spp., including *M. bovis*, occur as commensals frequently on the skin and mucous membranes of the upper respiratory tract. Some species and the animals from which they are recovered are as follows:

- **M. bovis.** Cattle and horses.
- **Moraxella canis.** Dogs and cats; human bite wounds.
- **Moraxella caprae.** Goats.
- **Moraxella cuniculi.** Rabbits.

- *Moraxella caviae.* Guinea pigs.
- *Moraxella ovis.* Sheep and goats; keratoconjunctivitis in mule deer and moose.
- *Moraxella boevrei.* Goats.
- *Moraxella lacunata.* Many animal species and humans; isolated from aborted equine fetuses, septicemia in a goat, and goats with viral pneumonia and encephalitis.
- *Moraxella phenolpyruvica.* Cattle, sheep, swine, goats.

With the exception of *M. bovis* and *M. lacunata*, organisms of this genus rarely cause disease; however, they are encountered in clinical specimens. The infections are infrequent and mainly opportunistic.

MORAXELLA BOVIS

The organism occurs as a commensal on the conjunctiva and in the nasopharynx of cattle.

Moraxella bovis is spread most commonly by flies (*Musca autumnalis*, *Musca domestica*, and *Stomoxys calcitrans*), but it can also be spread by direct contact.

Pathogenesis and Pathogenicity

Moraxella bovis is the cause of infectious bovine keratoconjunctivitis (pinkeye) (IBK), a worldwide disease of considerable economic importance. It is most prevalent during the summer, and both young and adult cattle are susceptible, although the young are more susceptible. It is seen more commonly in beef breeds and is aggravated by grazing in tall grass, by a dry dusty environment, and by insects. Other predisposing factors include prolonged exposure to sunlight (ultraviolet light), breed susceptibility, and concurrent viral (particularly infectious bovine rhinotracheitis), mycoplasmal, or ureaplasmal infections. Vitamin A deficiency is known to be a contributing factor in some outbreaks. Virulent strains produce hemolysin and have different plasmid profiles than nonpathogenic strains. Carrier animals are an important source of infection.

The disease spreads rapidly, and one or both eyes are affected. Signs accompanying the keratoconjunctivitis are photophobia, **blepharospasm**, and profuse lacrimation followed by a discharge that may become mucopurulent. There may be corneal ulcers, and within 72 hours, in severe cases, the cornea may perforate and become opaque, followed by blindness. In some cattle there is early regression of lesions.

Virulent strains produce hemolysin, are piliated, and have different plasmid profiles than nonpathogenic strains. **Pili (type IV)** aid in adherence and corneal colonization. Virulent strains are piliated and produce rough colonies that are beta-hemolytic. In addition, certain strains of *M. bovis* produce a cytotoxin that is toxic to bovine neutrophils. It is produced only by hemolytic strains and is thought to play an important role in the pathogenesis of the disease. Interestingly, the *M. bovis* hemolysin acts as a pore-forming cytolysin. Additional virulence factors include the production of proteases, fibrolysins, and phospholipases. However, these have not been well characterized in the pathogenesis of disease at this time.

Laboratory Diagnosis

Good growth is obtained on standard media; it is enhanced by the addition of blood or serum. Colonies are usually round, translucent, grayish-white, 1–2 mm in diameter, and surrounded by a narrow zone of beta hemolysis. After 48–72 hours, colonies enlarge and become somewhat flattened, with raised centers.

Stained smears reveal gram-negative or gram-variable coccobacilli, usually occurring in pairs (diplobacilli) and less frequently in short chains. *Moraxella bovis* is nonmotile, non-spore-forming, and encapsulated.

Moraxella bovis, like other species of the genus, does not ferment carbohydrates. Litmus milk becomes alkaline, nitrates are not reduced, and indole is not formed. It liquefies gelatin slowly and does not grow on MacConkey agar, and catalase production is variable. Definitive identification is based on biochemical characteristics. A fluorescent antibody test is also used frequently for rapid identification of *M. bovis* in tears and ocular discharges and from cultures.

Immunity

Immunity to the disease is of short duration and relapses are common.

Although a number of vaccines and bacterins have been developed and used in recent years, their efficacy in field trials has been variable, ranging from no effect to a reduced morbidity.

Treatment and Control

IBK is not yet considered a preventable disease. When feasible, affected animals should be separated from the nonaffected animals. Isolation and preventive treatment of newly introduced animals is recommended. Measures to reduce face flies and other insects, such as the use of insecticide tags, are helpful. Cattle should be confined to shady areas, and adequate vitamin A should be provided.

Gentamicin, ampicillin, kanamycin, and penicillin can be injected subconjunctivally. The aim of systemic treatment is to achieve an effective concentration in tears. Oxytetracycline has been useful in this regard. Other drugs to which *M. bovis* is susceptible are sulfonamides, erythromycin, ceftiofur, tilmicosin, and tylosin. Repeated treatment is required. Reduction in the number of carrier animals may be accomplished by the use of systemic antibiotics.

Public Health Significance

A number of species of *Moraxella* of animal origin have been responsible for a wide variety of infrequent infections in humans. *Moraxella canis* has been implicated in bite and wound infections.

GLOSSARY

atelectasis Collapse of the lung.

bacteriocins Agents produced by some bacteria that kill or inhibit the growth of closely related bacteria.

blepharospasm Involuntary spasmodic winking caused by contraction of the orbital muscle of the eyelids.

nucleic acid fingerprinting Refers to PCR-RFLP (polymerase chain reaction–restriction fragment length polymorphism) used first for the detection of *P. aeruginosa* species. The method amplifies the *OprI* lipoprotein gene by PCR and the resulting genes are digested with different restriction enzymes and separated by gel electrophoresis. This fingerprint is used in the molecular taxonomy of this genus.

Deoxyribonucleic acid (DNA) fingerprinting is discussed at further length in Chapter 23 under *"Bacillus anthracis* Genetics." The form of electrophoresis called pulsed field-gel electrophoresis (PFGE) is used in DNA fingerprinting for strain identification in clinical microbiology. PFGE allows the separation of extremely large (several thousand kilobases in length) DNA fragments.

pili (type IV) Generally classified as glycolipid binding proteins. Many gram-negative bacteria posses type IV pili. As a result, they are grouped based on amino acid similarities of the major pili component. In pseudomonads, type IV pili mediate adhesion to host cells.

16   Enterobacteriaceae I

The family Enterobacteriaceae, enterobacteria, or enteric bacteria are a large group of heterogeneous, gram-negative, facultatively anaerobic, medium-sized rods. The habitat of many of the species is the intestinal tract of animals and humans. Some species are free-living, occurring in soil and water. The family includes more than a dozen genera. The important genera, *Escherichia, Klebsiella, Proteus, Shigella,* and *Serratia,* are discussed in this chapter. The genera *Salmonella* and *Yersinia,* of considerable veterinary significance, are discussed separately in Chapter 17.

The enteric bacteria are oxidase-negative, catalase-positive (some exceptions), non-spore-forming, fermentative (often with gas), and usually motile. They are worldwide in distribution, and there are many nonpathogenic species and a relatively small number of potentially pathogenic species. Many enterobacteria are part of the normal flora of the intestinal tract. Fecal contamination of water is indicated by the presence of *Escherichia coli,* whose habitat is the intestine. *Klebsiella* (including *Klebsiella pneumoniae*), *Enterobacter,* and *Citrobacter* species have been recovered from vegetables and wood products of the kind used for stable bedding.

The mode of infection is almost always by ingestion. Fomites are especially important. Some infections are endogenous. Urinary tract infections are an exception.

Some strains of *E. coli* cause important diseases of domestic animals. Salmonellae, shigellae, and *Yersinia pestis* (the cause of plague) are frankly pathogenic. Some species of such genera as *Proteus, Serratia, Klebsiella,* and *Enterobacter* are mostly opportunists that produce disease under certain circumstances, such as impaired immunity, trauma to tissues, debilitation, wounds, malnutrition, and exposure to heavy doses of bacteria (bovine mastitis).

ESCHERICHIA

Escherichia coli

Although there are six species in the genus, only *E. coli* is of veterinary significance. It is recovered from a wide variety of infections in many animal species. It may be a primary or secondary agent. Nursing and young animals are particularly susceptible, and urinary tract infections are not uncommon. Colibacillosis is a general term that denotes an *E. coli* infection characterized by one or more of the following: diarrhea, enteritis, bacteremia, or septicemia. Rota- and coronaviruses, bovine viral diarrhea virus, coccidia, and cryptosporidia may sometimes be involved as well.

PATHOGENESIS AND PATHOGENICITY

From the standpoint of pathogenic mechanisms and diseases, five major categories of *E. coli* are recognized:

- Enterotoxigenic (ETEC)
- Enteropathogenic (EPEC)
- Enteroinvasive (EIEC)
- Enterohemorrhagic (EHEC)
- cytotoxin necrotizing factor–producing *E. coli.*

These categories are represented by different serotypes. Certain serotypes show a host preference and are encountered more frequently in some disease syndromes. Of the four major categories, ETEC is the most common cause of diarrhea in calves, lambs, and pigs. Strains in the other categories cause the less common disease syndromes.

Enterotoxigenic Diarrhea

ETEC is recognized as the cause of enterotoxigenic diarrhea, which is seen in nursing calves, pigs, and lambs; weanling pigs; and less frequently, in foals and dogs. Among the clinical signs are watery diarrhea, dehydration, **acidosis**, and frequently, death.

Enterotoxins and pilus antigens are the two most prominent virulence factors thus far identified for ETEC. Two enterotoxins, one heat-stable (ST) and one heat-labile (LT), are produced by enterotoxigenic strains of *E. coli;* not all cultures produce both of these plasmid-based enterotoxins. The majority of strains produce ST, followed by those producing both ST and LT, and last, those exclusively producing LT. The ST is further divided into STa and STb, and the LT is subdivided into LT-I and LT-II. The action of ST or LT toxin can be demonstrated in ligated intestinal segments, certain cell cultures, and suckling mice. The enterotoxin producers do not ordinarily invade, but their enterotoxin is adsorbed to epithelial cells in the jejunum and ileum. The LT stimulates adenyl cyclase, resulting in conversion of adenosine triphophate to cyclic AMP. Cyclic AMP induces the excretion of Cl^- and inhibits the adsorption of Na^+, causing great fluid losses. Likewise, STa affects a guanylate cyclase, resulting in ion

Table 16.1　Some Properties of Two Enterotoxins of *Escherichia coli*

	Heat-Stable	Heat-Labile
Calves	Most cases	Few cases
Pigs	Most cases	Most cases
Molecule	Very small peptide	Large protein
Heat stability	Resists 121°C/15 minutes	Destroyed by 60°C/30 minutes
Antigenicity	Negative	Positive
Antibody neutralization	Generally negative	Positive
Onset time and duration (ligated rabbit ileal loop)	Rapid and short	Slow and long
Adenyl cyclase activation	No	Yes
Guanylate cyclase activation	Yes	No
Tissue culture assay	Negative	Positive
Suckling mouse assay	Positive	Negative

and fluid losses to the lumen of the intestine. The two enterotoxins can be differentiated on the basis of their toxic, immunologic, physical, and chemical characteristics. Some of the properties of the two different enterotoxins are given in Table 16.1.

The letter K ordinarily stands for the surface or envelope antigen of enterobacteria (referred to further on). K88, K99, and other designations currently stand for different pilus antigens. Colonization of the small intestine by enterotoxigenic strains of *E. coli* depends on these pili. K88, K99, 987P, and F41 cultures of ETEC are associated with enterotoxigenic diarrhea in swine; K99 and F41 cultures with diarrhea in calves; and K99 with diarrhea in lambs. Other pilus types may also be involved with the aforementioned animals.

On occassion, some strains of ETEC produce an adhesion known as "curli" that binds extracellular matrix proteins. The production of curli is thought to increase the range of the age of susceptibility in animals concurrently infected with ETEC and rotavirus or cryptosporidia.

The pilus antigens of ETEC that cause diarrhea in humans are referred to as colonization factor antigens (CFAs). At present, the three antigenically distinct CFAs in ETEC are CFA/I, CFA/II, and CFA/IV. These pilus antigens are antigenically distinct from those that are found on ETECs of animals. Finally, the ETEC produce a variety of **mannose-resistant adhesins**.

Invasive Disease

As a general rule, the acute infections of neonatal animals characterized by bacteremia or septicemia are mainly caused by invasive strains of *E. coli*. The mode of infection is primarily by ingestion or via an *E. coli*–contaminated umbilicus. An inadequate intake of colostrum is particularly predisposing. Invasive strains cause colisepticemia or septicemic colibacillosis, a frequent disease of calves (first week of life) and a less frequent infection of lambs, piglets, and puppies.

Death usually ensues in the absence of treatment. Invasive strains attach to mucosal cells of the small intestine, penetrate the intestinal wall, and enter the lymphatics.

There may follow bacteremia or septicemia and endotoxemia. The strains involved belong to a few serotypes.

EIEC commonly possess the C531A adhesin and fimbrial antigen F17. EIEC strains have both chromosomal and plasmid (on the invasiveness plasmid) genes that are essential for disease production. Virulence properties include production of capsules, outer membrane proteins, siderophores, and repeats in structural toxin family of hemolysins (except strains isolated from foals). The presence of capsules aids in serum resistance and escape from phagocytosis. Outer membrane proteins of special importance are those associated with the uptake and transport of iron into the bacterial cell. These include the ferrichrome receptor (78 kDa) and the aerobactin receptor (74 kDa), both of which act as "**gated porins.**" Protection can be provided to animals with antibody against these receptors. However, *E. coli* will preferentially take up iron from hemoglobin.

There are a variety of siderophores (iron-obtaining proteins) associated with *E. coli*. There are essentially three types of siderophores associated with iron uptake in *E. coli*:

- First is enterobactin (enterochelin), which is capable of removing iron from iron-binding proteins and transporting it inside the bacterial cell. It takes the product of seven genes to make this siderophore. However, this siderophore can only be used once, as it is cleaved in the process of removing the iron.
- Second is the siderophore aerobactin, which can be differentiated from enterobactin by its inability to be bound by serum albumin and because it can be reused by the cell.
- Last, *E. coli* is capable of using non-native siderophores such as those of fungi, siderophores ferrichrome, and coprogen rhodororulic acid. In addition, *E. coli* can use citrate to obtain iron.

There are two basic types of hemolysins associated with EIEC: the alpha- and beta-hemolysins. The alpha-hemolysin is heat-labile, and the gene for the hemolysin can be of either chromosomal or plasmid origin. The hemolysin lyses red blood cells, as well as phagocytic cells, early in the growth phase of the bacteria and requires calcium ions. It functions as a pore-forming cytolysin, compromising the integrity of the red blood cell plasma membrane. Furthermore, the alpha-hemolysin is the most potent leucocidin known, and in sublytic concentrations, it has been observed to inhibit antigen processing and presentation by macrophages. The other hemolysin, beta-hemolysin, has not been well-characterized, but it has a range of activities similar to that of alpha-hemolysin.

EIEC is not common in farm animals. Invasiveness of *E. coli* strains can be detected by the capacity of a strain to cause keratoconjunctivitis in the eye of a guinea pig (Sereny test) or by its capacity to penetrate cells in tissue culture. In colisepticemia, enteroinvasive strains can be cultured from fresh blood and vital organs.

Nonenterotoxigenic Diarrheas

The term EPEC is used rather loosely in veterinary medicine to refer to *E. coli* strains that cause intestinal infection in all domestic animals. By definition, EPEC refers to specific serogroups recognized as causing diarrheal syndromes of humans, including serogroups O26, O111, and O128. In animals, these strains, called attaching and effacing strains, attach to small intestinal epithelial cells and cause effacement of the microvilli.

Mechanisms by which these strains produce lesions are not fully understood. However, certain plasmid-coded virulence factors are known to be involved. One of the features associated with the EPEC stains is a unique pilus that aggregates into bundles to bind to intestinal epithelial cells. Once bound to the intestinal cell, the EPEC strains secrete signaling proteins that activate a **tyrosine kinase**, resulting in the rearrangement of cytoskeletal proteins and causing the effacement of the microvilli. Diarrhea is the result of increased intracellular calcium levels and the production of protein kinase C, which results in the loss of Cl^- and water from the intestinal epithelial cells. EPEC strains lack the invasiveness of EIEC strains.

Certain strains of *E. coli* (EHEC) produce shiga-like toxins (verotoxins) that are active in Vero (monkey kidney cells) and HeLa cells. The type 2 variant of verotoxin is suspected to play a role in the pathogenesis of edema disease in pigs and diarrhea in calves and rabbits. These *E. coli* strains attach to and efface the microvilli of the gut epithelium. They are also referred to as verotoxigenic *E. coli* (VTEC) or attaching and effacing *E. coli* (AEEC).

More than 57 serotypes of EHEC have been recognized in humans and animals. EHEC strains do not synthesize LTs or STs, and they are not enteroinvasive. They colonize the intestinal mucosa by intimate attachment to and effacement of microvilli. Plasmid coded pili and verotoxins are the two most important virulence factors of these strains. Verotoxin types 1 and 2 are synonymous with shiga-like toxins I and II.

Some strains of EHEC produce enterohemolysin (60 kDa), which is distinctly different than the alpha- and beta-hemolysins described earlier. Its production has been correlated with the production of vero- and shiga-like toxins. Enterohemolysin is cell associated and is produced in later phases of growth. Similar to alpha-hemolysin, it is a pore-forming cytolysin; however, its production is phage mediated.

Both the EPEC and EHEC strains produce an adhesin known as intimin, which plays a major role in the adherence of these strains. Intimin is an outer membrane protein that causes the "intimate" attachment of the *E. coli* with the intestinal epithelial cells, whereas that mediated by fimbriae is a loose attachment. Intimin mediates the phosphorylation of tryosine residues of host cell proteins and reorganizes **cytoskeletal elements**.

Evidence for the presence of enteroaggregative *E. coli* as pathogens in domestic animals is currently lacking. Cytotoxin necrotizing factor–producing *E. coli* are infrequently associated with diarrhea in calves, pigs, and humans. Toxin and pili are thought to be the most important virulence factors of these strains.

It is of interest that most of the attaching and effacing strains produce urease. Production of the shiga-like toxin can be tested for in Vero cell cultures. DNA probes for the genes encoding toxins 1 and 2 are used in public health laboratories and are available commercially. The characteristic changes involving the mucosal epithelium are seen in histological sections.

Edema Disease

Edema disease is an acute, frequently fatal enterotoxemia of weaned pigs. A number of theories have been put forward to account for the occurrence of the disease in a particular herd, but none has been confirmed. The disease is characterized by edema, both subcutaneous and subserosal, caused by particular hemolytic serotypes (O antigens 139 and 141) of *E. coli* capable of producing shiga toxin (vero cytotoxin) II e. This toxin is similar to shiga toxin II; however, it binds to cells possessing a **Gb4** (globotetraosyl ceramide) **receptor**. As a result, shiga toxin II e binds to different groups of cells than shiga toxin II does. The genes associated with shiga toxin II e are located on the chromosome of at least four serotypes of *E. coli*. The disease is peracute, affecting particularly healthy piglets. The mortality rate ranges from 30% to 90%.

Diagnosis is usually based on history, clinical signs, and necropsy findings. Although testing is not carried out routinely, the shiga-like toxin can be detected in Vero cells and in an assay in mice.

Antimicrobial treatment is of value if administered in time. Drugs are selected based on susceptibility tests. Monitoring of feed intake after weaning is thought to be helpful.

Colibacillosis in Chickens and Turkeys

Escherichia coli infections are important in turkeys and chickens. The organism enters the bloodstream via the respiratory tract and causes an acute septicemia. Other conditions associated with colibacillosis in chickens and turkeys include air-sacculitis, fibrinopurulent serositis, synovitis, cellulitis, panophthalmitis, and salpingitis.

Other Infections

Escherichia coli is a frequent opportunist causing a wide variety of infections in domestic animals, including mastitis, particularly in cattle; urinary tract infections (bacteriuria, cystitis, and pyelonephritis) in all animals; abortion; wound infections; arthritis; metritis; meningitis; canine otitis externa; septicemia; pneumonia; and other infections.

It is of interest that virulent *E. coli* causing urinary tract infections in humans are restricted to a small number of O serogroups. These isolates have large blocks of genes, called pathogenicity-associated islands. Among their virulence factors are specific adhesions including **p-pili**, pore-forming hemolysin, cytotoxic necrotizing factor, a siderophore aerobactin, and an autotransported protease.

Antigenic Nature and Serology

Identification of the serotypes and pilus (fimbrial) antigens of this species is carried out routinely in most veterinary diagnostic laboratories. Serotyping could be of value in identifying serotypes that are frequently enterotoxin producers.

The antigens used to designate serotypes are as follows:

- **Somatic or O antigens.** Designated by Arabic numerals; for example, O133.
- **K (surface or envelope) antigens.** There are more than 80 different K antigens. They are designated by a letter and an Arabic number; for example, K4.
- **H or flagellar antigens.** Designated by H followed by an Arabic number; for example, H2. If there are no flagella, it is designated NM (nonmotile).

An example of a complete designation is O111:K4:H2.

SOME ENTEROBACTERIA OF LESSER SIGNIFICANCE

Klebsiella

Strains have been recovered from various animal infections, including pneumonia and suppurative infections in foals; cervicitis and metritis in mares; mastitis in cows; wound infections; urinary infections, particularly in dogs; and septicemia and pneumonia in dogs. Most of the strains recovered from clinical specimens are *K. pneumoniae*. *Klebsiella* organisms are associated with wood products used as bedding for cattle and have been implicated as the cause of a frequent, severe mastitis in cows.

Many capsule types of *Klebsiella* have been identified and many have been causally associated with metritis in mares. *Klebsiella* capsular typing is not carried out routinely in veterinary diagnostic laboratories.

Shigella

Members of this group are not important as causes of disease in domestic animals. All species cause dysentery in humans and other primates. Unlike the salmonellae, they do not cause systemic disease. *Shigella* species are closely related to *E. coli*.

Edwardsiella

Edwardsiella tarda is recovered occasionally from the intestinal tract of animals and humans. A few opportunistic infections have been reported in humans and animals. *Edwardsiella tarda* has been implicated as the cause of diarrhea, wound infections, and sepsis in animals and humans. *Edwardsiella tarda* and *E. ictaluri* are common pathogens of catfish.

Enterobacter

Strains of this group, *Klebsiella*, and *E. coli* are referred to as coliforms. Strains of *Enterobacter* are only occasionally incriminated in animal disease. *Enterobacter cloacae* and *E. aerogenes* are opportunistic pathogens. The most common infection they produce is bovine mastitis. *Enterobacter sakazaki* is known occasionally to cause meningitis and sepsis in human neonates.

Proteus

Proteus mirabilis has been implicated in a variety of sporadic infections of dogs, cats, cattle, fowl and other animals. Urinary tract infections caused by *P. mirabilis* are frequent in dogs and cats. In these species and in humans, *P. mirabilis* infection can lead to the formation of struvite or apatite stones in the kidney. Urease produced by the bacteria catalyzes the production of such stones. *Proteus* species are occasionally involved in ear infections in dogs and cats, and it is thought they may be involved in diarrhea in young mink, lambs, calves, goats, and puppies.

Plesiomonas

Plesiomonas shigelloides (formerly *Aeromonas shigelloides*) is the only species in the genus. It is a facultatively anaerobic, gram-negative rod with polar flagella. Nonmotile strains have been recognized occasionally from clinical specimens. This species occurs widely in water, fish, and other aquatic animals. *Plesiomonas shigelloides* produces oxidase and catalase and ferments glucose. The organism grows well on the common laboratory media at 37°C and is nonhemolytic on blood agar. The minimum and maximum growth temperatures are 8° and 42°C, respectively. The organism has been recovered from the gut of fish and from a variety of animals, including cattle, goats, dogs, cats, monkeys, swine, snakes, and toads. It has been implicated only rarely in infection of domestic animals.

Plesiomonas shigelloides causes diarrhea in humans associated with travel. Most infections are thought to result from drinking contaminated water or eating raw seafood. Cellulitis, septicemia, and meningitis also have been reported in humans. *Plesiomonas shigelloides* produces heat-labile and heat-stable enterotoxins. Their exact role in pathogenesis is not known.

Serratia

The one species of significance in infections is *Serratia marcescens*, which may produce a red pigment. It is responsible for infrequent cases of bovine mastitis and other uncommon sporadic infections in domestic animals. It also causes septicemia in chickens and is thought to cause infections in geckos and tortoises.

Morganella

Morganella morganii (formerly *Proteus morganii*) is a well-recognized human pathogen. It has been associated with ear and urinary tract infection in dogs and cats.

Providencia

Species of this genus rarely cause animal infections. *Providencia heimbachae* has been isolated from penguin feces and from an aborted bovine fetus; its significance is not known.

GENERAL

Resistance

Like most vegetative forms of bacteria, enterobacteria are not especially resistant to physical and chemical influences (disinfectants). Sunlight and desiccation kill them readily; freezing does not.

Laboratory Diagnosis

Tissues, feces, portion of intestine, urine, milk, blood, and other clinical materials are submitted for culture. The organisms grow well on ordinary unenriched culture media. Selective media are available that favor the growth of some genera; for example, Brilliant Green Agar and Mac-Conkey Agar (see Table 16.2).

The colonies of the various enterobacteria usually look much the same on blood agar; however, occasional strains are mucoid and some are hemolytic. Colonies on selective media show considerable differences among genera; these are helpful in presumptive identification.

After observing the kinds and numbers of colonies, several are inoculated in triple sugar iron (TSI) agar. This medium is used to detect fermentation of lactose, sucrose, and glucose and production of H_2S and gas. Among the tests used for identification are the IMViC reactions (indole, methyl red, Voges-Proskauer [acetyl-methyl carbinol], citrate [utilization]) and the other reactions listed in Table 16.3. The definitive identification of many species of the enterobacteria require many biochemical tests. However, cultures of *E. coli* and *Salmonella* can be presumptively identified on the basis of their TSI reactions and their appearance on selective media.

Some *Proteus* species may spread or swarm over the agar plate; swarming is inhibited if the agar is increased to 4%.

The following laboratory procedures are employed for the detection of fimbrial antigens and enterotoxins:

- Demonstration of fimbrial antigens using a latex agglutination test and specific antisera in a slide agglutination test.
- An ELISA for the detection of fimbrial antigen in fecal extract.
- A fluorescent antibody test for the detection of fimbriae in smears from the ileal mucosa.
- An ELISA using monoclonal antibodies for detection of ST and LT toxins.
- DNA probes for the genes encoding the ST and LT toxins.

Immune Response

The predominant immune response in *E. coli* infections is humoral and occurs at the site of attachment. This humoral response occurs against the bacteria directly or to the products such as colonization factors and toxins. In neonates, some of this immunity can be obtained through the transfer of antibodies via colostrum and milk.

T a b l e   1 6 . 2   Appearance of Important Enterobacteria on Selective Media

Enterobacteria	Brilliant Green Agar	MacConkey Agar	Heckton Enteric Agar

Coliforms:
  Escherichia coli
  Enterobacter
  Klebsiella
	Growth inhibited generally. If present, are yellowish-green.	Grow and are red. *Enterobacter* and *Klebsiella* may be larger and mucoid.	Grow and are yellow-orange or yellow-green. *Enterobacter* and *Klebsiella* may be larger and mucoid.

Proteus	Grow, do not spread; yellowish-green. Sucrose-negative; strains are colorless.	Grow and may spread. Colorless.	Grow; may spread, colorless; H_2S-positive strains are black.
Salmonella	Grow. Red because of peptone hydrolysis.	Grow; colorless.	Grow; H_2S-positive strains are black; H_2S-negative strains are colorless.

Table 16.3   Differentiation of Some Important Genra of Enterobacteriaceae*

	Escherichia	Salmonella	Klebsiella	Proteus	Enterobacter	Citrobacter	Yersinia
Motility	+	+	−	+	+	+	−
TSI† slant	A	Alk	A	Alk	A	Alk (A)	Alk
TSI† butt	AG	A; GV	AG	AG	AG	AG	A
Glucose	+	+	+	+	+	+	+
Sucrose	V	−	+	V	+	V	−
Lactose	+	−	+	−	+	+	−
H₂S	−	V	−	+	−	−	−
Urease	−	−	V	+	−	−	−
VP‡	−	−	+	−	+	−	+V
Arginine	−	V	−	−	V	V	−
Lysine	+	+	+	−	V	−	−
Ornithine	V	+	−	V	+	V	−V
Phenylalanine	−	−	−	+	−	−	−

*Results: +, positive; V, variable; −, most strains negative; A, acid (yellow); G = gas; Alk, alkaline.
†Triple sugar iron agar.
‡Voges–Proskaur reaction.

Treatment and Prevention

Treatment will depend on the nature of the *E. coli* infection. In general, treatment involves restoration of loss of fluid and electrolytes and administration of antimicrobial drugs. Susceptibility tests are indicated, as *E. coli* strains are frequently resistant to a number of drugs. Gentamycin, trimethoprim-sulfas, enrofloxacin, apramycin, ceftiofur, tetracyclines, chloramphenicol, ampicillin, neomycin, and amoxicillin have been effective. Resistance is usually plasmid-based, and the plasmids involved are transported among enteric organisms primarily by conjugation. Included in the plasmid (R factor) is the resistance transfer factor and genes for resistance to several drugs. The three main mechanisms whereby *E. coli* can develop or acquire resistance to antibiotics are discussed in Chapter 8.

Dehydration requires the administration of electrolytic fluids, and hypogammaglobulinemia indicates the need for supplemental colostrum or bovine gammaglobulin.

Escherichia coli bacterins are used to immunize cows and sows to prevent disease in their young. Because of antigenic heterogeneity, however, they are considered to be of limited value. Pilus vaccines have been developed and appear to be of value. Sows have been given field cultures of "pathogenic" *E. coli* orally. *Escherichia coli* antigens are combined with rotavirus antigens in some products. Cows and sows exposed to pathogenic *E. coli* may provide protective antibodies to their neonates.

Sound management practices including provision of ample colostrum and warm, clean quarters for the newborns are important.

Public Health Significance

Several toxin-producing strains of *E. coli* are recognized as important food-borne pathogens. Not all of these strains have an animal origin.

The EHEC serotype O157:H7 is associated with hemorrhagic colitis and hemolytic uremic syndrome in humans, of which there have been more than 20,000 cases and about 250 deaths annually in the United States. The principal source of this serotype is contaminated, insufficiently cooked meat, particularly ground beef. It is estimated that serotype O157:H7 is carried in the intestine of up to 40% of cattle. This serotype does not produce disease in cattle. Meat is mainly contaminated by contact with feces during slaughter. *Escherichia coli* O157:H7 can grow in the human intestine and thus can contaminate swimming pools, resulting in multiple water-borne infections.

The potent toxins produced by this EHEC serotype are responsible for the hemorrhagic diarrhea and renal failure.

It is of interest that O157:H7 has retained the genetic backbone of *E. coli* but has added an additional 1387 genes, including 200 "islands" of potentially pathogenic genes. Many virulence factors are similar to those found in other pathogens, and it is thought that they were acquired by **horizontal gene transfer**. It has been suggested that the recent appearance of these pathogenic strains may have been the result of modern farming methods and food handling practices.

GLOSSARY

acidosis Refers to a condition of decreased alkalinity of tissue and blood, accompanied by various signs including vomiting and general malaise.

cytoskeletal elements Refers to the cytoskeleton or scaffold of eukaryotic cells; for example, microtubules, microfilaments, and intermediate filaments.

"gated porins" Specific proteins that can act as gates (channels or pores) into the cell for specific substances.

Gb4 receptor Refers to the globotetraosyl ceramide receptor located on the surface of some eukaryotic cells. The gene encoding this receptor in humans is located on chromosome 4.

horizontal gene transfer Movement of genetic information from one cell to another (not an offspring).

mannose-resistant adhesins Adhesins that are capable of binding in the presence of large quantities of mannose, in contrast to those that are unable to bind, as mannose will block their ability to do so.

p-pili Refers to periplasmic pili.

tyrosine kinase One of a group of enzymes that preferentially phosphorylates the tyrosine residues of particular proteins. Typically observed in cell signaling mechanisms.

17 Enterobacteriaceae II: *Salmonella* and *Yersinia*

The basic characteristics of members of the family Enterobacteriaciae were given in the previous chapter. The important genera *Salmonella* and *Yersinia*, which also belong in this family, are discussed in this chapter.

SALMONELLA

Salmonellae occur frequently and worldwide as intestinal pathogens of animals and humans. The forms of salmonellosis seen in animals are principally septicemia and acute, subacute, and chronic enteritis. An asymptomatic carrier state is common. The forms seen in humans are principally gastroenteritis (food poisoning), enteric fever (typhoid fever), and septicemia or bacteremia. Unlike the other enteric bacteria, except for *Yersinia*, the salmonellae are facultative intracellular parasites.

More than 2400 different serotypes or serovars have been identified, all of which are potentially pathogenic, causing sporadic infections as well as outbreaks with fatalities.

Classification

Several proposals have been put forward to reclassify the *Salmonella–Arizona* group. The proposal that is widely used recognizes the following three species:

- **Salmonella choleraesuis.** One serotype or serovar; host preference, swine.
- **Salmonella typhi.** One serotype; host, humans.
- **Salmonella enteritidis.** About 2000 serotypes, each of which is given a species name; infects animals and humans.

The practice generally followed is to refer to each serotype as a species. Some serotypes are given species names based on their geographic origin; for example, *Salmonella dublin*. The *Salmonella* serotypes or serovars can be subdivided into biovars based on differences in biochemical patterns within a serovar; for example, *S. choleraesuis* biovar *kunzendorf*. Biovars are usually identified in reference laboratories.

The following antigens are employed in the identification of serotypes:

- **Somatic or O antigens.** Designated by Arabic numerals; group classification is based on several of these antigens.

- **Flagellar antigens.** Phase 1: designated by small letters of the alphabet, more or less specific for the salmonella. Isolates must be in this phase before they can be typed. Phase 2: designated by Arabic numerals; less specific and duplicated in other bacterial species.
- **K antigens (capsular or envelope).** "Vi" antigen, "M" antigen, and so forth. These antigens may interfere with agglutinability of O antisera.

An example of a complete designation is *Salmonella typhimurium*, 1,4,5,12:i:1,2. Major antigens are separated by colons, and the components of an antigen are separated by commas. The system used for the identification of serotypes is the Kauffmann–White scheme.

In most veterinary diagnostic laboratories, the salmonella isolates are examined serologically to determine their group. Group identification is based on the possession of certain somatic or O antigens. *Salmonella* O antisera are available commercially for each group. The procedure is a simple slide agglutination test. It is usual to test an isolate first against a polyvalent O serum covering important groups. If this is positive, then tests are conducted with the individual group sera. Serotypes within a group have a common antigenic determinant. There are additional groups, but most clinical isolates from humans and animals are found in groups B through E.

Important species within each serogroup are shown in Table 17.1.

Determination of the serotype may be carried out in reference laboratories. In certain situations, for example, significant outbreaks, determination of the serotype is important.

Host Predilection

Although many *Salmonella* species are capable of causing disease in domestic animals, a relatively small number are responsible for most infections. They are as follows:

- **Cattle.** *S. typhimurium, Salmonella newport, S. dublin.*
- **Sheep and goats.** *S. typhimurium, S. dublin, Salmonella montivideo, Salmonella anatum.*
- **Swine.** *S. choleraesuis, S. typhimurium.*
- **Horses.** *S. typhimurium, S. enteritidis, S. newport, S. anatum, Salmonella arizonae, Salmonella angona.*
- **Dogs and cats.** *S. typhimurium.*

Table 17.1 Important Diseases Caused by *Salmonella*

Serogroup	Species or Serovars	Disease
A	*S. paratyphi* A	Paratyphoid fever in humans.
B	*S. schottmuelleri*	Paratyphoid fever in humans.
	S. typhimurium	Gastroenteritis in humans; most prevalent species causing infection in various animal species.
	S. agona	Various infections in horses and other animals.
	S. abortus—equi	Abortion in mares and jennets.
	S. abortus—bovis	Abortion in cattle.
	S. abortus—ovis	Abortion in sheep.
C_1	*S. choleresuis*	Enteritis in pigs; frequent secondary invader in hog cholera; infections in humans.
	S. typhisuis	Infections in young pigs.
	S. montevideo	Infections in cattle and pigs primarily.
C_2	*S. newport*	Infections in humans, various animals, and especially cattle.
D_1	*S. enteritidis*	Infections in various animals; gastroenteritis in humans.
	S. gallinarum	Fowl typhoid, an acute intestinal disease of young chickens and turkeys.
	S. pullorum	Severe intestinal infections of chicks and poults (pullorum); chronic infections in older fowl.
	S. typhi	Typhoid fever in humans.
	S. dublin	Severe infections in cattle
E_1	*S. anatum*	Keel disease in ducklings.
	S. muenster	Infections in cattle primarily.

Salmonellosis in poultry is discussed separately below.

Pathogenesis

Infection is almost always by ingestion of contaminated food and water. The origin of contamination is frequently other shedding animals, including rodents and birds. The disease is sometimes endemic on farms and in stables and clinics. Young and debilitated animals are particularly susceptible. The incidence of infection is often high, but the occurrence of clinical disease is low. Stresses resulting from transport, crowding, parturition, and surgery may precipitate clinical disease.

The salmonellae infect epithelial cells lining the ileum and colon and are taken up by macrophages in which many are able to survive. The virulence factors involved in *Salmonella* infections are numerous and complex. Among them are the following:

- At least three toxins are elaborated: endotoxin, enterotoxin, and cytotoxin. The latter acts by inhibiting host cell protein synthesis and permitting Ca^{2+} to escape from host cells.
- Contributing to adherence are surface polysaccharide O antigen, flagellar H antigen, and fimbriae.
- The capsular Vi polysaccharide of *S. typhi* inhibits complement binding and, thus, antibody-mediated killing.
- At least 10 proteins encoded by *Salmonella* genes are involved in invasion. These genes encode a surface adhesin and proteins responsible for assembly of surface appendages used for host-cell binding.
- Proteins encoded by other *Salmonella* genes neutralize toxic oxygen products of macrophages.

Antibacterial **defensins** produced by macrophages are neutralized by other *Salmonella* proteins. These proteins make possible the intracellular growth and survival of salmonellae.
- Virulence factors involved in persistence and spread of some *Salmonella* species have been associated with plasmids.
- In addition, salmonellae produce iron-chelating proteins, siderophores, that sequester iron and thus contribute to bacterial growth.

The following are important features in the pathogenesis of strains causing enterocolitis and diarrhea:

- Ingestion of salmonellae.
- Colonization of the lower intestine with mucosal invasion. Cytotoxin produced.
- Acute inflammation with or without ulceration. Prostaglandin synthesis, enterotoxin production, and proinflammatory cytokines synthesized by epithelial cell are responsible for acute inflammation and possible damage to the mucosa. Feces may contain blood, mucus, and neutrophils.
- With invasion of the mucosa, adenylate cyclase is activated, and the resulting increase in cyclic AMP induces secretion that may result in marked fluid increase in the bowel and diarrhea.
- Intestinal infections may lead to bacteremia or septicemia, with death or localization in internal organs.

Pathogenicity

- **Cattle.** Endemic on farms with sporadic cases; outbreaks related to various stresses; septicemia in neonates and acute enteritis in older calves.

- **Sheep and goats.** In the former, acute enteritis with occasional septicemia; abortions; acute enteritis in adult goats and septicemia in neonates.
- **Swine.** Septicemia, chronic enteritis, and acute enteritis with pneumonia; important secondary pathogen in hog cholera.
- **Horses.** Sporadic cases after stresses, for example, surgery and transport; outbreaks in stables and clinics with variable syndromes and many carriers; septicemia in neonatal foals.
- **Dogs and cats.** Up to 5% of dogs and cats carry *Salmonella*; however, clinical disease is infrequent. Cats are generally resistant to infection, but outbreaks occur in kittens. When disease occurs in dogs and cats, it is usually related to various stresses or immunosuppression. All clinical syndromes of salmonellosis are seen with sometimes localization and abscessation in internal organs.

Treatment and Control

There is the view that antimicrobial treatment should only be administered to animals with acute salmonellosis, in that treatment may prolong the carrier state and lead to the emergence of resistant strains. All isolates should be subjected to antimicrobial susceptibility tests, as many strains are multiply resistant. The kind and method of treatment (oral or parenteral) will depend on such considerations as the animal species, the severity of the disease, and the number of animals involved. Some drugs that have been effective are tetracyclines, chloramphenicol, trimethoprim-sulfonamides, ampicillin, amoxicillin, floroquinolones, and third-generation cephalosporins.

Control measures involve preventing the exposure of the presumably uninfected animals from sources of the infection; that is, fomites, contaminated food and water, and shedding individuals. This is difficult and involves segregation of the affected animals and the introduction of only uninfected animals. When possible, avoid stresses.

Immunity to salmonellosis is probably predominantly cell-mediated, and thus, the value of bacterins is questionable. Attenuated live *S. typhimurium* and *S. dublin* vaccines are used in cattle. Various salmonellae, such as *S. choleraesuis* and *S. typhimurium*, are incorporated in bacterins, alone or with other bacteria. A vaccine containing live attenuated *S. choleraesuis* is being used currently. A *S. dublin* bacterin is used to prevent salmonellosis in calves.

Public Health Significance

The carrier state may be considerable in domestic (including poultry) and wild animals; turtles and other pets may also shed salmonellae. Human patients, both sick and convalescent, and subclinical carriers may shed organisms. Other sources are feces of humans and animals; whole eggs, especially duck eggs; egg products; meat and meat products; poultry; and fertilizers and animal feeds prepared from bones, fishmeal, and meat.

Infections and epidemics are usually traceable to various food products derived from meat, eggs, milk, and poultry. Other means of infection derive from food and water contaminated with rodent feces, from infected food handlers, and from contaminated equipment and utensils. Sporadic cases occur from direct contact with an infected animal or person.

Salmonelloses of Poultry

The salmonelloses of poultry are of great economic importance. They are discussed briefly here.

PULLORUM DISEASE. This is an acute, usually fatal disease of chicks (under 3 weeks of age) and young turkeys. It is caused by *Salmonella pullorum* and characterized by either a whitish or yellowish diarrhea or, in the peracute form, no apparent clinical signs. Adult chickens and other avian species are occasionally infected. Survivors may become carriers with infected ovaries. Transmission is mainly via the egg.

The disease has been eradicated from most commercial flocks. This has been accomplished by testing breeding stock with agglutination procedures and removing reactors. Antimicrobial drugs are not employed for treatment or control.

FOWL TYPHOID. This is an acute disease of chickens, turkeys, ducks, geese, and wild birds caused by *Salmonella gallinarum*, which is closely related to *S. pullorum*. *Salmonella gallinarum* is egg-transmitted and, although it can infect chicks and poults, producing an infection resembling pullorum, it is most important as a cause of severe salmonellosis in mature flocks.

The disease is controlled like pullorum disease by the testing of breeding stock. Live avirulent and killed vaccines are used for prevention.

ARIZONA INFECTION. This is an acute or chronic egg-transmitted disease mainly of turkeys caused by serotypes of *S. arizonae*. The disease tends to persist in flocks, affecting mainly poults 3–4 weeks of age. Various drugs have been used to treat infected poults. *Salmonella arizonae* has been kept to low levels in breeding flocks by treating eggs at hatcheries with antibiotics. Strict sanitation in hatcheries is important in control.

PARATYPHOID INFECTIONS. These are infections caused by various salmonellae; for example, *S. typhimurium* (most common), *S. enteritidis*, *Salmonella heidelberg*, and more than a dozen others. The prevalence of species varies geographically and with the avian species. Both domestic and wild species are affected, and the severity of infections varies from subclinical to acute. Mortality is highest amongst young birds.

Antimicrobial drugs are used to reduce losses, but they are unable to eliminate the disease. Turkeys are injected with antibiotics after hatching to prevent the disease. With strict sanitary measures and the use of antimicrobials, losses can be controlled, but infections persist in flocks.

YERSINIA

This genus of enterobacteria includes 10 species, of which *Yersinia pestis*, *Yersinia pseudotuberculosis*, and *Yersinia enterocolitica* are pathogenic for animals and humans. The organism *Yersinia ruckeri*, whose taxonomic position is unclear, is a pathogen of fish. Yersiniae are gram-negative or gram variable, non-spore-forming, facultatively anaerobic rods or coccobacilli. All species except *Y. pestis* are motile at 22°–30°C, and their optimum temperature for growth is 25°–28°C.

The nonpathogenic *Yersinia* are important because they occur in clinical materials and could be mistaken for the pathogenic species. They are *Yersinia frederiksenii*, *Yersinia intermedia*, *Yersinia kristenii*, *Yersinia bercovieri*, *Yersinia mollaretii*, *Yersinia rodhei*, *Yersinia aldovae*, and *Yersinia ruckeri*.

The reservoir of *Y. pestis*, the cause of human plague, is wild rodents. The habitat of *Y. pseudotuberculosis* and *Y. enterocolitica* is the intestine of domestic and wild animals and birds. All three species cause disease in humans and animals, although domestic animal infections by *Y. pestis* are rare.

YERSINIA PESTIS

Although plague is an important human disease, it is of minor significance in domestic animals, and thus, only its main features are provided here.

General Features of Plague

Plague is fundamentally a disease of rats and other wild rodents. Humans and domestic and wild animals are considered accidental hosts.

The disease is transmitted by fleas, which become infected from rats or other rodents in which the disease is bubonic and similar to that seen in humans. The organisms ingested by the flea multiply in the gut. When the flea bites, the aspirated blood containing *Y. pestis* from the flea is regurgitated into the bite wound. The term used for infected lymph nodes is buboes. The bubonic form can give rise to the pneumonic form, which is highly contagious and usually fatal if not treated sufficiently early. Both the bubonic and pneumonic forms of plague in humans can be epidemic.

Sylvatic plague occurs in wild rodents other than rats. At least 38 species of wild rodents, including marmots and squirrels, have been found to be susceptible. Fleas, very infrequently, transmit plague from rodents to humans. Sylvatic plague has given rise to outbreaks of the bubonic disease and, rarely, pneumonic plague.

Between 1910 and 1951, 523 cases of bubonic plague in humans were reported in the United States, and the fatality rate was 65%. Outbreaks have occurred in California, Louisiana, Florida, Texas, and Washington. In addition, sporadic cases have been reported from Arizona, Idaho, New Mexico, Nevada, Oregon, and Utah. Fortunately, many of the foci of sylvatic plague are situated in sparsely populated and isolated rural districts where the fleas of wild rodents do not have the opportunity to bite humans.

Pathogenesis

All three important *Yersinia* species are facultative intracellular parasites. Within a few hours of the fleabite, *Y. pestis* organisms are carried to regional lymph nodes, where they multiply rapidly. Many are destroyed by neutrophils, but many of those phagocytized by macrophages survive and multiply. Some protection against phagocytosis is provided by the protein-complex capsule. All virulent strains have a 72-kb plasmid with genes that encode V-W antigens and outer membrane proteins (Yops), which contribute to extracellular (antiphagocytic) and intracellular survival. The lipopolysaccharide (LPS) of *Y. pestis* is thought to be responsible for hemorrhage, vascular collapse, and focal necrosis. The role of the highly mouse-toxic murine toxin in plague is not clear.

Pathogenicity (Animals)

Plague has been reported rarely in dogs, cats, camels, elephants, buffaloes, deer, and some other animals.

The disease is seen occasionally in cats in regions of sylvatic plague. Cats usually acquire the disease from eating dead rodents. The disease is rare in dogs. Characteristics of the disease are high fever; lethargy; swelling and abscessation of lymph nodes, particularly around the head and neck; and a mortality of about 50% in the absence of treatment.

Diagnosis

Although veterinarians can encounter plague in various animal species, they are most likely to see it in cats. Although plague in cats is dealt with in the text that follows, the general principles also apply to other animals. The possibility of feline plague should be kept in mind in areas of the sylvatic disease. Cats showing lymphadenopathy with abscesses should be particularly suspect.

Special precautions, including flea treatment and the use of gloves and masks, should be taken if plague is suspected. Exudate from abscesses should be sent to a special laboratory equipped to deal with the diagnosis of this dangerous pathogen. The location of such laboratories can be obtained in the United States through the Public Health Service.

The animal should be treated for fleas and kept under strict isolation pending the results of the laboratory examination. A mask and gloves should be used when handling the animal. Laboratory procedures and animal inoculations should be carried out in special facilities of the U.S. Public Health Service.

The organism can be identified by specific fluorescent antibody staining of lymph node aspirates. It can also be isolated from blood and tissues without difficulty. Unlike the other yersiniae, it is nonmotile.

Treatment

Animals suspected of plague infection, if not killed, must be kept under strict isolation with great care exercised to prevent infection.

Abscesses (buboes) should be lanced and drained. Streptomycin, doxycycline, gentamycin, or chloramphenicol are effective if administered early.

Public Health Significance

The plague agent is highly infectious for humans, and great care must be taken to avoid exposure to potentially infected animals (clinical materials) and fleas. In several feline cases, there has been transmission to humans; one veterinarian is reported to have died. Some of the ways by which humans can be infected are

- Exposure to infected fleas on rodents brought home by cats.
- Exposure to infected fleas carried by dogs and cats.
- Direct contact with infected dogs, cats, and possibly other animals.
- Fleas from infected rats and other rodents.

Vaccination and chemoprophylaxis are useful for preventing plague in humans who have been exposed.

Control

Control of disease transmission largely depends on control of sylvatic reservoirs. The use of insecticides should precede the elimination of rodents, for otherwise, the dislodged fleas seek human hosts.

Control fleas and prevent cats from hunting in endemic areas.

YERSINIA PSEUDOTUBERCULOSIS AND YERSINIA ENTEROCOLITICA

Yersinia pseudotuberculosis is very closely related to *Y. pestis*. It is mainly an animal pathogen; human infections are rare. *Yersinia enterocolitica* is a pathogen of both animals and humans. The habitat of both is the intestinal tract of domestic and wild animals and birds. Important sources are food and water contaminated by animal and bird feces. Transmission is mainly by ingestion of contaminated food and water.

Pathogenesis

Following ingestion, both species adhere to mainly the ileal mucosa, where they multiply and invade epithelial lining cells, **M cells**, and macrophages with concentration in mesenteric nodes and Peyer's patches. By rather complex processes, infected epithelia may become phagocytic. There is an intense inflammatory reaction, and in some instances, organisms spread to other sites.

The three pathogenic species share a number of the same virulence factors, including expression of V-W (so-

matic antigens) and Yops antigens referred to under *Y. pestis* above. The genes for these antigens are expressed at 37°C in the presence of low Ca^{2+} concentration. In addition to these plasmid genes, there are chromosomal genes; for example, *inv* (invasin), which encodes an outer membrane protein that mediates adherence and cell invasion, and the *ail* (adherence invasion locus) gene, which encodes another outer membrane protein with a similar function. Additional virulence factors that enable organisms to survive in macrophages have been described. LPS is thought to have a role in the production of some of the lesions of yersiniosis.

Pathogenicity

Yersinia pseudotuberculosis produces pseudotuberculosis (caseous abscesses) in various rodents, guinea pigs, cats, chinchilla, and turkeys; epididymo-orchitis of rams; abortion in goats; and occasional infections in swine, cattle, sheep, deer, buffaloes, and other wild animals and birds. The infection in animals initially involves the mesenteric nodes and Peyer's patches, with occasional spread from the caseous abscesses in the mesenteric nodes to the liver and spleen particularly.

Infrequent infections simulating typhoid and appendicitis (mesenteric adenitis) occur in humans.

The reservoir of *Y. enterocolitica* is domestic and wild animals. It has been isolated from chinchilla, hares, deer, rabbits, dogs, pigs, horses, mink, various avian species, goats, cattle, sheep, water, and milk. The organism has been recovered from a considerable percentage (25%) of mesenteric nodes of swine and also from tongues (35%).

The infections in animals resemble those caused by *Y. pseudotuberculosis* but are less frequent. Ileitis, gastroenteritis, and mesenteric adenitis are the most common disease processes.

This organism, an important human pathogen, causes gastroenteritis, bloody diarrhea, mesenteric adenitis, and other infections in humans.

Most strains produce a heat-stable enterotoxin.

Isolation and Identification

It should be kept in mind that animals may shed yersiniae in their feces; thus, isolation alone may not warrant a diagnosis. The organisms grow well on blood agar and MacConkey agar at room temperature. If the number of organisms is small, it is advisable to use a "cold enrichment" procedure like that used for *Listeria monocytogenes*.

Yersinia enterocolitica and *Y. pseudotuberculosis* are motile at 22°–25°C; *Y. pestis* is not. The nonpathogenic yersiniae must be considered in identification as they occur in feces. Final species identification is based upon biochemical tests; a commercial test strip is available.

There are six serotypes of *Y. pseudotuberculosis*. More than 90% of infections in humans and animals are caused by O-group 1 strains. There are six biotypes of *Y. enterocolitica* and more than 50 serotypes. Their identification is important in that only some serotypes are considered pathogenic. It is of interest that serogroup O:9 cross-reacts with *Brucella* species to yield identical titers and thus may give rise to false *Brucella* agglutination reactions.

Treatment and Control

Long-acting tetracyclines, trimethoprim-sulfonamides, aminoglycosides, and chloramphenicol have been effective.

Because of the ubiquity of these yersiniae, control in animals is usually not feasible. Stresses should be avoided and sources of infection isolated or eliminated.

GLOSSARY

defensins Small, cationic, bactericidal peptides generated by phagocytes, such as neutrophils and macrophages.

M cells Also known as microfold cells. M cells are specific cells of the intestinal epithelium near lymphoid follicles that endocytose a variety of protein and peptide antigens. The endocytosed antigens are then directly transported into the underlying tissue, where they are taken up by macrophages. Note that the antigens are not degraded by the M cells, but merely transported to the regional macrophages.

18 *Actinobacillus* and *Haemophilus*

These genera share the family Pasteurellaceae with *Pasteurella* and *Mannheimia*. Species of the genus *Actinobacillus* are gram-negative, nonmotile, small rods and coccobacilli. They are non-spore-forming, facultatively anaerobic, and fermentative and require complex nutrients for growth. Some of them are commensals on the mucous membranes of the respiratory and genitourinary tracts. Infections may be endogenous or exogenous.

More than a dozen species have been designated. The following cause significant disease in animals:

- ***Actinobacillus lignieresii.*** Causes actinobacillosis in cattle and sheep.
- ***Actinobacillus equuli.*** Causes foal septicemia.
- ***Actinobacillus pleuropnemoniae.*** Causes contagious pleuropneumonia of pigs.
- ***Actinobacillus seminis.*** Causes epididymitis in young rams (a disease resembling that caused by *Brucella ovis*) and purulent polyarthritis and gangrenous mastitis in sheep.
- ***Actinobacillus actinoides.*** Causes pneumonia in calves and seminal vesiculitis in bulls. It is probably identical to *Haemophilus somnus*.
- ***Actinobacillus salpingitidis.*** Found in the oviduct and respiratory tract of chickens, *A. salpingitidis* occasionally causes **salpingitis** and peritonitis.
- ***Actinobacillus suis.*** Causes septicemia and other infectious processes in pigs.
- ***Actinobacillus capsulatus.*** Causes arthritis in rabbits.

The following species are of minor significance: *Actinobacillus ureae* (formerly *Pasteurella ureae*) is recovered from humans and its occurrence in animals is questionable; *Actinobacillus minor*, *Actinobacillus indolicus*, and *Actinobacillus porcinus* are commensals of the upper respiratory tract of pigs; *Actinobacillus muris* has been recovered from mice, *Actinobacillus scotiae* from porpoises, *Actinobacillus delphinicola* from sea mammals, *Actinobacillus succinogenes* from the bovine rumen, and *A. rosii* from the vagina of postparturient sows.

Actinobacillus actinomycetemcomitans has been renamed *Haemophilus actinomycetemcomitans* (see below).

All of these organisms probably occur as commensals, giving rise on occasion to exogenous and endogenous infections.

ACTINOBACILLUS LIGNIERESII

Actinobacillus lignieresii is worldwide in distribution and occurs as a commensal in the alimentary tract of cattle. Six serotypes (somatic antigens) have been identified. Their occurrence correlates with geographic and host species origin.

The organism usually produces a sporadic, endogenous disease, but on occasion, several animals in a herd may be infected. It gains entrance to the oral mucosa through injuries.

Pathogenicity

Actinobacillosis is seen most commonly in cattle, less commonly in sheep, and rarely in pigs, dogs, and humans. Lesions usually consist of multiple, granulomatous abscesses. In cattle and sheep, these occur most frequently around the head and neck region. The lesion commences as a firm nodule that eventually ulcerates and discharges a viscous, white-to-faintly-green pus that contains small granules. The granules are greyish-white and usually less than 1 mm in diameter. By comparison, the sulfur granules of bovine actinomycosis are several millimeters in diameter.

Unlike bovine actinomycosis, the infection is spread via the lymphatics. Lesions may involve the tongue (wooden tongue), lungs, and less frequently, other internal organs. Rarely, granulomatous abscesses occur in the udder of the sow.

Little is known about the immune response in this disease. The granulomatous nature of the lesions suggests a strong component of cellular immunity.

Direct Examination

Small, gram-negative rods are demonstrable within granules. The granules are examined in the same manner as those from actinomycosis: wash, examine granule under a coverslip in 10% NaOH, prepare smear and stain. The granules in actinobacillosis are small (~1 mm) and grey or white.

Laboratory Diagnosis

Pus and necrotic material from early, nondischarging lesions are submitted.

Actinobacillus lignieresii can be recovered consistently if clinical material is seeded onto serum or blood agar and incubated at 37°C; 10% CO_2 stimulates growth.

Small, translucent, smooth, and glistening colonies resembling those of nonmucoid *Pasteurella multocida* are evident in 24–48 hours. Stained smears disclose small gram-negative rods or coccobacilli.

The organism grows on MacConkey agar and is usually nonhemolytic and catalase- and urease-positive. It is identified definitively by biochemical criteria.

Treatment

Advanced cases are not usually treated. In early cases, surgical drainage along with a broad-spectrum antibiotic or a sulfonamide is employed. Potassium iodide given orally is useful in reducing inflammation. Treatment must be prolonged.

Public Health Significance

Several cases of an acute, suppurative bronchopneumonia and infected horse- and sheep-bite wounds have been reported in humans.

ACTINOBACILLUS EQUULI

This organism is commonly found in the intestinal tract of horses.

The mode of infection is by ingestion or inhalation. It may also be via the umbilicus or across the placenta. *Strongylus* larvae may carry the organism into arteries.

Pathogenicity

Many foals develop *A. equuli* infection disease within a few hours or days of birth. Those dying within 24 hours of life have a severe enteritis. Those living for several days may develop a purulent nephritis, meningitis, pneumonia, or septic arthritis (called joint-ill or sleepy foal disease).

The following manifestations may be seen in older horses: lameness caused by purulent arthritis, infected aneurysms leading in some instances to systemic involvement, infrequent abortion, nephritis, peritonitis (colic), and endocarditis.

Septic arthritis, endocarditis, suppurative nephritis, septicemia, and mastitis are occasionally seen in swine.

To date, very little is known about the virulence factors of *A. equuli*. Recent data indicate that *A. equuli* may possess toxins similar to the Apx toxin family of *A. pleuropneumoniae*, which may play a role in pathogenesis.

Laboratory Diagnosis

Affected tissues, purulent material, feces, and blood are submitted.

The organism grows well on blood and MacConkey agar. The colonies of fresh isolates are rough in appearance but mucoid in character, probably because of a mucinous capsule. They may lose their mucoid character on transfer. The organism is usually catalase-negative and urease-positive; some strains are beta-hemolytic. Final identification is based on several biochemical characteristics including fermentation of carbohydrates.

Treatment and Control

Good sanitation at parturition, with disinfection of the umbilicus, is important. Prophylactic treatment of all foals shortly after birth with penicillin and streptomycin or tetracyclines has been effective. The nature and location of the infection must be considered in treatment of adult horses. Drugs that have been effective are chloramphenicol, tetracyclines, ampicillin, third-generation cephalosporins, and trimethoprim-sulfonamide.

Immunization is not practiced, and little is known about the immunology of the infection. Maternal antibodies in the colostrum are important in protecting foals. Strains are antigenically heterogeneous.

ACTINOBACILLUS PLEUROPNEUMONIAE

Formerly *Haemophilus pleuropneumoniae*.

The disease *A. pleuropneumoniae* causes, swine pleuropneumonia, is of great economic importance.

It is a commensal of the upper respiratory tract of some pigs. The organism is transmitted by direct and indirect contact, and infection is via the respiratory tract and most commonly by inhalation.

Pathogenicity and Pathogenesis

The morbidity and mortality of swine pleuropneumonia is usually very high in newly infected pigs of all age groups; however, the disease is seen most frequently in pigs 2–6 months of age. Acute, subacute, and chronic respiratory infections are seen. The acute form is characterized by a severe fibrinous pleuropneumonia. The chronic form, which often occurs in feeders, is characterized by pleurisy, pleural adhesions, and **pulmonary sequestration** and abscessation.

It has been hypothesized that antigen (endotoxin)-antibody complexes damage blood vessel endothelium and result in vasculitis, thrombosis with consequent edema, necrosis, infarction, and hemorrhage.

The capsular polysaccharides divide *A. pleuropneumoniae* into a number of serotypes. The capsule has antiphagocytic properties, allowing the organism to evade some of the host immune responses. The lipopolysaccharide is associated with adherence of the organism to the cells of the porcine respiratory tract.

In addition to lipopolysaccharide and the capsule, cytotoxins and other outer membrane proteins have a role in virulence and pathogenesis. The cytotoxins belong to RTX (repeats in structural toxin) cytolysin family. These pore-forming toxins are hemolytic (resemble the alpha hemolysin of *Escherichia coli*). They are heat-labile, immunogenic, and thought to be responsible for the severe lesions. They are also considered to be major virulence factors that form pores in the membranes of phagocytes, such as macrophages. Furthermore, they can stimulate the lethal oxidative burst of phagocytes, resulting in damage to host cells from the extracellular release of oxygen radicals. With regard to iron acquisition, *A. pleuropneumoniae* will bind only porcine **transferrin**, and it is unable to use other transferrins. This trait is associated with the host-species specificity of the organism. In addition, *A. pleuropneumoniae* expresses receptors for porcine hemoglobin and ferrichrome.

Antigenic Nature

There are two biotypes, one of which requires nicotinamide adenine dinucleotide (NAD) for growth. This biotype consists of 12 major serotypes and two subtypes. The biotype not requiring NAD consists of two or three serotypes. Serotypes are based on differences in capsular polysaccharide antigens. Serotypes 1, 5, and 7 are most common in North America. Serologic tests, for example, enzyme-linked immunosorbent assay (ELISA) and complement fixation, are used in surveys, epidemiological studies, and efforts at elimination of the disease from herds.

Laboratory Diagnosis

Actinobacillus pleuropneumoniae grows well on blood or serum-enriched agar. Most strains require the V factor (NAD), which can be supplied by yeast extract or a staphylococcus streak. When the V factor is required, the organism grows only alongside the staphylococcus. Two colony types may be seen, a round, "waxy" type and a flat, soft, glistening variety; both types are hemolytic. A positive CAMP reaction is seen with a β-toxin-producing staphylococcus (see Chapter 24).

The characteristic cellular and colonial morphology, along with the V factor requirement and a positive CAMP reaction, strongly indicates *A. pleuropneumoniae*, biotype 1. Definitive identification is generally based on various biochemical characteristics. A rapid latex agglutination procedure has been developed for identification of capsular antigens.

Immunity

Immunity in swine pleuropneumonia is predominantly humoral. Maternal immunity protects neonates for 5–9 weeks. Capsular antigens elicit protective antibodies. Bacterins confer homologous protection and reduce mortality, but they do not completely prevent chronic pulmonary lesions. Polyvalent bacterins only elicit antibodies against the particular serotypes contained in the bacterin. In contrast, natural infection and aerosol exposure provide cross-serotype protection. A live attenuated vaccine and a recombinant vaccine are of value; both are noncapsulated.

Treatment and Control

The treatment of chronic cases is ineffective. *Actinobacillus pleuropneumoniae* is susceptible to many antimicrobial drugs including tetracyclines, chloramphenicol, spectinomycin, erythromycin, nitrofurazone, ampicillin, trimethoprim-sulfonamides, gentamycin, and penicillin G. Medicated feed or water is used in treatment of in-contact pigs. Antimicrobial susceptibility tests should be carried out because drug-resistant strains are encountered.

When feasible, affected animals should be separated from the nonaffected animals. Isolation and preventive treatment of newly introduced animals is recommended. Shade and measures to reduce face flies and other insects, for example, the use of insecticide tags, are helpful.

ACTINOBACILLUS SUIS

Actinobacillus suis is worldwide in distribution and occurs as a commensal in the tonsils and on mucous membranes of the respiratory and genital tracts of pigs. Route of infection is probably via the upper digestive or respiratory tracts and the umbilicus. Bacteremia or septicemia may occur from the initial infection.

Actinobacillus suis is most frequently associated with acute septicemia in young pigs (less than 6 months of age.) The organism has also been implicated in arthritis, pneumonia, pericarditis, nephritis, meningitis, and metritis in older pigs.

A cytotoxin in the RTX family, similar to the cytotoxin or hemolysin of *A. pleuropneumoniae*, has been described. Its role in pathogenesis is not clear.

The laboratory diagnosis and treatment of *A. suis* infections is essentially similar to that of *A. pleuropneumoniae*.

HAEMOPHILUS

Species of the genus *Haemophilus* are small, pleomorphic, gram-negative rods. They are oxidase-positive, nonmotile, facultatively anaerobic, and with one exception (*Haemophilus somnus*), require the X or V factor or both. Many of the haemophili produce capsules, although noncapsulated strains exist.

More than a dozen species of animal and human origin are recognized. They occur as commensals on mucous membranes of the genital, upper digestive, and respiratory tracts. Some are potential pathogens. Except for *H. somnus*, they require one or both of the following factors for growth:

- **X factor.** A requirement for the iron porphyrin, hemin; supplied by blood agar or chocolate agar.
- **V factor.** NAD or one of its riboside precursors; supplied by fresh yeast extract, staphylococcal growth, or chocolate agar.

The hosts and X and V factor requirements of some important species are given in Table 18.1.

The mode of infection is most frequently by inhalation. Fomites may be involved. Infections may be endogenous or exogenous.

Haemophilus spp. are fragile and sensitive to sunlight and drying and are readily killed by common disinfectants. Specimens should, preferably, be submitted on dry ice as soon as possible after collection.

Generally speaking, the virulence of *Haemophilus* spp. is related to the presence of the polysaccharide capsule. *Haemophilus influenzae* possess a polysaccharide capsule of which there are six serotypes: A, B, C, D, E, and F. Of these, capsular serotype B is the most virulent strain because of the presence of the capsular polysaccharide PRP (polyribose ribitol phosphate).

HAEMOPHILUS SOMNUS

The disease syndromes caused by *H. somnus* are given the name *H. somnus* disease complex.

Pathogenesis and Pathogenicity

Virulence is associated with capsule (polysaccharide) formation, and it is likely that endotoxin has an important role. Young or previously unexposed animals are most susceptible. Various stresses such as crowding, extremes of temperature, and transport may be contributory to disease.

The four principal syndromes that characterize the *H. somnus* disease complex are

- Respiratory involvement, with fibrinopurulent bronchopneumonia and bacteremia or septicemia. The following syndromes derive from the initial respiratory infection and bacteremia.
- Localization in the central nervous system, with **thromboembolic** meningoencephalitis (TEM) resulting from vasculitis of meningeal vessels.
- Fibrinous pleuritis and arthritis.
- Genital infection with vaginitis, endometritis, and cervicitis.

More than one syndrome may be seen in the same animal. Other infections caused by *H. somnus* are tracheitis, laryngitis, mastitis, conjunctivitis, otitis, sporadic abortion, and myocardial and muscular necrosis.

The neural manifestation of the disease and the acute septicemic form are usually fatal. Not all animals in the herd are affected. Outbreaks are often associated with stress and are frequently seen in feedlot cattle. Asymptomatic carriers are common. It is not clear whether the absence of clinical signs in carriers is the result of a difference in the host response or of a difference in the virulence of isolates. In some instances, the carrier isolates appear to be less virulent than those from diseased animals.

In addition to the antiphagocytic activity of capsules, virulence factors include *H. somnus* lipooligosaccharide (LOS), released in membrane fibrils and blebs, which has been observed to stimulate apoptosis in bovine endothelial cells. The LOS of *H. somnus* undergoes a phenomenon known as antigenic phase variation, which is thought to aid in the ability of the bacterium to evade the host immune response. In addition, *H. somnus* produces an immunoglobulin-binding protein that has been observed to preferentially bind immunoglobulins of the IgG2b isotype in cattle.

Histophilus ovis and *Haemophilus agni* are now considered identical to *H. somnus*. They are commensals of the genital tract of sheep and have been reported as causes of epididymitis and orchitis in rams and pneumonia, mastitis, myositis, polyarthritis, meningitis, and septicemia in sheep.

HAEMOPHILUS PARASUIS

Haemophilus parasuis is a secondary invader in swine influenza, enzootic pneumonia, and other pneumonias.

It is the primary agent of Glasser's disease, a worldwide disease of young pigs, characterized by a **polyserositis** and, occasionally, by meningitis. The signs and lesions resemble those of polyserositis caused by *Mycoplasma hyorhinis*. Stresses such as transport, cold, and weaning predispose to the disease. The disease may be mild with low morbidity or severe with considerable mortality in particularly susceptible pigs.

Haemophilus parasuis is one cause of infectious arthritis and pneumonia in older pigs.

HAEMOPHILUS PARAGALLINARUM

Haemophilus paragallinarum is the cause of infectious coryza of chickens. This disease has both acute and chronic forms and is characterized by nasal discharge, sneezing, and swelling of the face. The morbidity rate is high and the mortality rate is low. It is mainly a disease of pullets and layers; broilers are occasionally affected. There is often significant economic loss because of the reduction in growth and egg production. Recovered chickens may carry and shed the organism for long periods.

Three serovars, A, B, and C, occur, and bacterins must contain the serovar(s) likely to be encountered.

OTHER *HAEMOPHILUS* SPECIES

Haemophilus haemoglobinophilus

Haemophilus haemoglobinophilus is a commensal of the lower genital tract of dogs. It has been implicated in cystitis in dogs and may have a role in canine neonatal and genital infections. It requires the X factor.

Haemophilus felis

Haemophilus felis is a commensal of the nasopharynx of apparently normal cats. It requires CO_2 and V factor for growth.

Haemophilus influenzaemurium

Haemophilus influenzaemurium is a commensal of mice; it has been implicated as a cause of cystitis and respiratory infections in mice. It requires the X factor.

Haemophilus paracuniculus

Haemophilus paracuniculus, which requires the V factor, has been isolated from the intestine of rabbits. Its significance is not known.

Haemophilus piscium

Haemophilus piscium is the cause of ulcer disease in trout, an infection characterized by ulcers of the gills and mouth. Its identity as an *Haemophilus* species is uncertain.

A number of *Haemophilus* species cause infections in humans. *Haemophilus influenzae*, the most studied species, causes meningitis, otitis, bronchopneumia, pericarditis, and other infections, particularly in the young. *Haemophilus ducreyi* is the cause of chancroid (genital ulceration), which occurs most commonly in tropical regions but also occasionally in North America.

GENERAL

Specimens

Haemophilus spp. are fragile and do not survive long when removed from the host. Clinical material is best frozen (dry ice preferred) and delivered to the laboratory within 24 hours. Refrigeration and transport media may not be sufficient to assure viability.

Laboratory Diagnosis

Specimens for isolation of *H. somnus* are collected from lesions, including those in the brain. Organisms can be recovered from semen samples and preputial washings of healthy bulls. Isolation can be made on media supplemented with blood and yeast in an atmosphere of 10% CO_2. *Haemophilus somnus* does not grow initially without CO_2. It does not require either the X or V factor. Definitive identification requires a number of biochemical tests.

The other species of *Haemophilus* of animal origin will grow on blood agar, with a *Staphylococcus* streak (growth) providing the V factor. Blood agar supplies sufficient hemin; chocolate agar supplies both X and V factors. If *Haemophilus* is suspected, blood plates with a *Staphylococcus* streak should be incubated in an atmosphere containing 10% CO_2. Plates are incubated for 24–48 hours. Small dewdrop colonies appear after 24 hours of incubation. If the V factor is required, the small colonies will appear near the *Staphylococcus* streak (satellite growth).

For practical purposes, identification is based on morphologic and colonial characteristics, X or V factor requirements and host, lesions, and clinical signs (see Table 18.1). Species can be identified definitively, using a number of biochemical tests; however, because of the fastidious growth requirements of these organisms, such tests are not carried out routinely in the diagnostic laboratory.

Immunity

Specific capsular antibodies are considered important in virulence and in elicitation of protection. Immunity to *Haemophilus* spp., is thought to be predominantly humoral. Most species are antigenically heterogeneous. A number of serotypes of *H. somnus*, *H. parasuis*, and *H. paragallinarum* have been identified.

HAEMOPHILUS SOMNUS. Agglutination, ELISA, and complement-fixation tests are used in serological surveys for *H. somnus* exposure and infection. Bacterins, which must contain the pertinent serotypes, reduce the severity of infections.

HAEMOPHILUS PARAGALLINARUM. Serological tests, including agglutination, ELISA, and agar gel precipitation tests, are used to detect birds carrying this organism. Bacterins are used to prevent infectious coryza. Three serovars, A, B, and C, occur, and bacterins must contain the serovar(s) likely to be encountered.

Treatment

Haemophilus spp. are susceptible to a wide spectrum of antimicrobial drugs. If feasible, susceptibility tests should be carried out as resistant strains may be encountered.

Table 18.1   X and V Factor Requirements of Significant *Haemophilus* species and Their Principal Diseases

Species	Requirement for		Principal Hosts and Diseases
	X	**V**	
Haemophilus parasuis	−	+	Swine: Glasser's disease (polyserositis), respiratory second invader, arthritis
Haemophilus haemoglobinophilis	+	−	Dogs: Cystitis, genital and neonatal infections
Haemophilus paragallinarum	−	+	Chickens: Infectious coryza
Haemophilus somnus	−	−	Cattle: Respiratory infection, septicemia, neurologic and genital infections
			Sheep: Septicemia, genital infections, epididymitis, mastitis, arthritis, and other infections

HAEMOPHILUS SOMNUS.   Animals with clinical signs are separated and treated with penicillin and streptomycin or oxytetracycline. Treatment is usually effective if begun early. Cattle with TEM that are not recumbent are treated with oxytetracycline, florfenicol, or trimethoprim-sulfadoxine.

HAEMOPHILUS PARASUIS.   Avoidance of stresses is important. The following drugs have been effective: ampicillin, penicillin, ceftiofur, florfenicol, enrofloxacin, and trimethoprim-sulfonamide.

HAEMOPHILUS PARAGALLINARUM.   Infectious coryza is controlled in large flocks by elimination of the affected chickens with thorough disinfection. Among the drugs used are erythromycin, sulfonamides, oxytetracycline, other tetracyclines, and fluoroquinolones. Drugs are usually administered in water or feed.

GLOSSARY

polyserositis Inflammation of the serous membranes; namely, the pleura, peritoneum, and pericardium.

pulmonary sequestration Loss of connection of lung tissue with the pulmonary veins and the bronchial tree.

salpingitis Inflammation of a fallopian or eustachian tube.

thromboembolic Associated with thromboembolism, which is the blocking of a blood vessel by a fragment or particle that has broken away from a blood clot at a particular location.

transferrin A beta globulin in blood plasma, which can combine with ferric ions and thus transport iron throughout the body.

19 *Pasteurella* and *Mannheimia*

Species of the genera *Pasteurella* and *Mannheimia* of the family Pasteurellaceae are small gram-negative rods or coccobacilli. They are nonmotile, non-spore-forming, facultatively anaerobic, oxidase positive, and fermentative. Most are commensals on the mucous membranes of the upper respiratory and digestive tracts of domestic and wild animals.

The species included in the genera *Pasteurella* and *Mannheimia* are listed below.

MOST IMPORTANT SPECIES FROM A DISEASE STANDPOINT

Pasteurella multocida

Three subspecies have been proposed, namely,

- ***P. multocida* subsp. *multocida*.** Contains most of the strains that cause significant disease in domestic animals.
- ***P. multocida* subsp. *septica*.** Recovered from various sources, including dogs, cats, birds, and human beings. Important in wound infections that result when people are bitten by dogs and cats.
- ***P. multocida* subsp. *gallicida*.** Recovered from avian species and may occasionally cause fowl cholera.

These three subspecies are differentiated in the laboratory by minor differences in biochemical tests. The iden-

tification of these subspecies may be useful in epidemiologic and research studies, but their recognition is of little significance for practitioners. Most diagnostic laboratories will probably continue to use the name *P. multocida* without naming the subspecies.

Pasteurella haemolytica

- ***P. haemolytica*, biotype A.** This important species has been moved to the genus *Mannheimia* and is now named *Mannheimia haemolytica*. Information on its occurrence and disease significance is given in Table 19.1.
- ***P. haemolytica*, biotype T.** Renamed *Pasteurella trehalosi*. Information on its occurrence and disease significance is given in Table 19.1.

More detail is provided for the above species further in the chapter.

SPECIES OF LESSER IMPORTANCE

- ***Pasteurella granulomatis*.** This species has been renamed *Mannheimia granulomatis*. It is associated with a severe, progressive, fibrogranulomatous disease of cattle in southern Brazil. Lesions caused by ***Dermatobia hominis*** may initiate the disease process.

Table 19.1 Differential features of *Mannheimia haemolytica* and *Pasteurella trehalosi*

	M. haemolytica	*P. trehalosi*
Fermentation		
arabinose	+	−
trehalose	−	+
salacin	−	+
xylose	+	−
lactose	+	−
Susceptibility to penicillin	High (except serotype 2)	Low
Serotypes	1,2,5,6,7,8,9,11,12,13,14,16	3,4,10,15
Principal location in normal host	Nasopharynx	Tonsils
Principal disease association	Pneumonia in cattle and sheep; septicemia in nursing lambs	Septicemia in feeder lambs

- *Pasteurella pneumotropica.* This organism can be recovered from the nasopharynx of some guinea pigs, rats, hamsters, mice, dogs, and cats. It is usually a secondary invader in pneumonic disease in mice and rats and has been implicated in enteritis of hamsters. It is not a significant pathogen in dogs and cats. It resembles *P. multocida* culturally, but it can be distinguished biochemically.
- *Pasteurella dagmatis.* This is a commensal organism of the oro- and nasopharynx of dogs and cats. In human beings, it causes local and systemic infections resulting from animal bites. These strains had been previously designated a variety of *P. pneumotropica.*
- *Pasteurella gallinarum.* Commensal in upper respiratory tract of chickens; occasionally causes low-grade respiratory infections in chickens.
- *Pasteurella canis.* This species includes many of the formerly *P. multocida*–like strains from canine mouths and dog-bite infections.
- *Pasteurella stomatis.* This species has been recovered from the respiratory tracts of dogs and cats. Many of the *Pasteurella* strains recovered from cats, and some recovered from dogs, are *P. multocida* (subsp. *multocida* or subsp. *septica*). *Pasteurella* species have a low capacity for causing disease in dogs and cats. They are usually secondary invaders and involved in mixed infections.
- *Pasteurella anatis.* This species has been recovered from the intestinal tracts of ducks.
- *Pasteurella langaaensis.* It has been isolated from the respiratory tracts of normal chickens.
- *Pasteurella avium* and *Pasteurella volantium.* These have been recovered from the respiratory tracts of normal chickens.
- *Pasteurella caballi.* This aerogenic species has been isolated from equine clinical specimens. It is a commensal of the upper respiratory tract of horses and was considered to have a causal role in some upper respiratory infections, pneumonia, peritonitis, and a mesenteric abscess.
- *Pasteurella lymphangitis.* Causes an uncommon lymphangitis in cattle.
- *Pasteurella mairi.* Recovered from porcine aborted fetuses.
- *Pasteurella testudinis.* A commensal in the respiratory tract of turtles.
- *Pasteurella aerogenes.* A commensal in the intestine of swine; rarely pathogenic.
- *Pasteurella bettyae* (**CDC group HB-5**). The reservoir of this species is not known. It has been associated with a variety of human infections.
- *Pasteurella anatipestifer.* This organism has been renamed *Riemerella anatipestifer* (see Chapter 34).

Three additional species of *Mannheimia* have been designated, but there significance in animal disease appears to be minor.

DISTRIBUTION AND HABITAT

Pasteurella and *Mannheimia* organisms are distributed worldwide. Most occur as commensals on the mucous membrane of the upper respiratory and digestive passages of animals. The carrier rate of the more pathogenic species is usually lower than that of the less pathogenic species.

LABORATORY DIAGNOSIS

This is essentially the same for all species and is outlined below in detail for *P. multocida.* The various species are identified on the basis of differences in biochemical reactions.

TREATMENT

Antimicrobial susceptibility tests should be carried out if isolates are deemed significant. The treatment relating to the important species of *Pasteurella* and *Mannheimia* is discussed below.

PASTEURELLA MULTOCIDA

Infection may be acquired by direct or indirect contact, inhalation, ingestion, and via fomites and wounds.

Pathogenesis

As in other gram-negative infections, endotoxins no doubt play a role in pathogenesis. Various environmental stresses are important in predisposition to infection. Passage of the infecting agent from animal to animal results in enhancement of virulence. *Pasteurella multocida* is a frequent secondary invader in pneumonic disease; however, it may also be a primary cause of disease, as in fowl cholera and epizootic hemorrhagic septicemia. When it is primary, septicemia frequently occurs.

A thermolabile toxin is produced mainly by capsular D strains recovered from swine and other animals. Some investigators think that the toxigenic cultures alone, or together with *Bordetella bronchiseptica,* cause atrophic rhinitis of swine. It is thought that *B. bronchiseptica* infection of the turbinate mucosa facilitates colonization by toxigenic strains of *P. multocida.* Toxigenic strains of *P. multocida* have been isolated from disease in humans.

Among the properties of the *P. multocida* toxin are the following:

- It is mainly cell-associated and appears to be released when bacteria die.
- It is a heat-labile polypeptide with molecular weight 125,000–160,000.
- It produces necrosis (dermonecrotic) when inoculated into the skin of the guinea pig.
- It is immunogenic and lethal for mice.

The gene encoding for the toxin has been cloned and expressed in *Escherichia coli*. The recombinant toxin had properties comparable to those of the original purified toxin.

Also important in pathogenesis is the polysaccharide capsule, which with some serotypes, consists of hyaluronic acid. The serotype B:2 produces hyaluronidase, and some strains produce neurominidase. The outer membranes of virulent strains are toxic for phagocytes.

Pathogenicity

The diseases associated with *P. multocida* are too numerous to review fully. It may be a primary agent, but more frequently, it is a secondary invader when resistance of the animal is reduced by various stresses. It may be secondary to a primary virus, mycoplasma, or other bacterium.

Pasteurella multocida is a primary or, more frequently, a secondary invader in pneumonia of cattle, swine, sheep, goats, and other species. As a secondary invader, it is frequently involved in bovine pneumonic pasteurellosis and in enzootic pneumonia of pigs. As mentioned earlier, toxin-producing strains, alone or with *Bordetella bronchiseptica*, cause the important economic disease of swine, atrophic rhinitis. This is a widespread, economically important disease characterized by an inflammation of the nasal mucosa, leading often to atrophy of the turbinate bones and distortion of the nasal septum that sometimes results in shortening or twisting of the upper jaw. Prognathism (jutting of the lower jaw) is a common sign. Other signs of this chronic infection are coughing, sneezing, and weight loss.

It causes fowl cholera, a widespread, contagious disease of domestic and wild birds. It begins as a septicemia or bacteremia with a high mortality. Many surviving birds have localized infections (chronic fowl cholera) and serve as sources of infection for other birds. Turkeys are more susceptible than chickens, and losses in commercial flocks can be large.

Two serotypes of *P. multocida* cause hemorrhagic septicemia, an acute disease principally of cattle and water buffalo in tropical and subtropical regions excluding Australia, North and South America (except for bison in the United States), and most countries of Europe. The disease is an acute septicemia characterized by a rapid course, swollen and hemorrhagic lymph nodes, and numerous subserous petechial hemorrhages. The morbidity rate varies considerably, but the mortality is high. Hemorrhagic septicemia caused by other serotypes occurs infrequently in wild ruminants, such as deer and elk.

Pasteurella multocida is one of the causes of the pleuropneumonia form of "snuffles" in rabbits; it is a cause of severe mastitis of cattle and sheep, and it is responsible for a variety of sporadic infections in animals, including encephalitis, meningitis, and abortion.

Direct Examination

Bipolar organisms can be demonstrated in blood smears in septicemias. This is of minor significance except as an aid in the diagnosis of hemorrhagic septicemia.

Laboratory Diagnosis

Specimens are selected according to the location of the infectious process. The organisms survive well in transport media and in refrigerated and frozen tissues.

Definitive diagnosis is based on isolation and identification of *P. multocida*. Good primary growth requires media enriched with serum or blood. Colonies appear after incubation for 24 hours at 37°C in air or in an atmosphere of 6%–8% CO_2. They are usually of moderate size, round, and grayish. Some strains produce large mucoid colonies. Fresh cultures have a characteristic odor.

Smears reveal small, gram-negative rods and coccobacilli. Marked pleomorphism is not uncommon.

Of special significance are nonmotility, indole production, lack of hemolysis, and production of oxidase. In contrast, *M. haemolytica* is beta-hemolytic and indole-negative and grows on MacConkey agar. Definitive identification is based on biochemical tests (Table 19.2).

Mice and rabbits are susceptible to most strains. Lethal infections develop within one or several days. Mouse inoculation is occasionally used to recover *P. multocida* from heavily contaminated specimens, including nasal swabs from pigs.

The laboratory diagnosis of other *Pasteurella* spp. is essentially similar to that just described for *P. multocida*.

Antigenic Nature

Types A, B, D, E, and F have been identified on the basis of differences in capsular substances (polysaccharides).

- **Type A.** Causes fowl cholera, pneumonia, and many other infections of various animals.
- **Type B.** Causes epizootic hemorrhagic septicemia in Asia, the Middle East, and southern Europe.
- **Type D.** Recovered relatively infrequently from various infections in many animals, but frequently from pneumonia and atrophic rhinitis in swine.
- **Type E.** Causes hemorrhagic septicemia in Africa.
- **Type F.** Recovered from turkeys; its role in disease is not yet clear.

Capsular types may be subdivided further into somatic types (at least 16) on the basis of serologic differences in lipopolysaccharides (somatic or O antigens). A serotype is designated by the capsular type, followed by the number representing the somatic type; for example, serotype B:2 is the cause of hemorrhagic septicemia in many regions, and E:2 causes the same disease in Africa. Different varieties within a serotype can be identified by deoxyribonucleic acid (DNA) fingerprinting, and thus, this procedure can be useful in epidemiological studies.

Treatment

Susceptibility tests are important, as antimicrobial resistance is frequent in *P. multocida* and *M. haemolytica*; it is less common in other pasteurellae. The resistance-encoding genes occur on plasmids. The following antibacterial drugs are used: penicillin G, tetracyclines, sulfonamides,

Table 19.2   Differentiation of Important *Pasteurella* and *Mannheimia* Species

Species	Beta-hemolysis	Ornithine	Indole	Urease	Trehalose	Maltose	D-Xylose	L-Arabinose	Mannitol	Sorbitol	Dulcitol
Pasteurella multocida	–	–	+	–	V*	–	+	–	+	+	–
Pasteurella dagmatis	–	–	+	+	+	+	–	–	–	–	–
Pasteurella gallinarum	–	–	–	–	+	+	–	–	–	–	–
Pasteurella canis	–	+	V	–	V	–	V	–	–	–	–
Pasteurella langaaensis	–	–	–	–	+	–	–	–	+	–	–
Pasteurella stomatis	–	–	+	–	–	–	–	–	–	–	–
Pasteurella trehalosi	+	–	–	–	+	+	–	–	+	+	–
Mannheimia haemolytica	+	–	–	–	–	+	+	+	+	+	–

*–, negative; +, positive, V, variable.

chloramphenicol, florfenicol (related to chloramphenicol but safer), ceftiofur (naxel), spectinomycin, and tilmicosin. Sulfaquinoxaline and other sulfonamides, quinolones, tetracyclines, and penicillin are used for fowl cholera. Antimicrobial drugs are administered in feed and water to poultry and swine.

Various treatment strategies are used for atrophic rhinitis; for example, antimicrobial drugs are given to sows prior to farrowing, to newborn pigs, and to newly weaned pigs, as well as to growing pigs. Administration is usually by feed or water. The drugs most commonly used are sulfonamides, ceftiofur, tylosin, and tetracyclines.

It does not seem possible to keep herds entirely free of infectious atrophic rhinitis. When the clinical disease is prevalent and severe, vaccination, antimicrobial treatment, and separation of new stock are applied in the interest of control.

Immunity

Immunity is predominantly humoral. Pasteur's first vaccine was developed to prevent fowl cholera. It was an attenuated strain that was not altogether satisfactory. In recent years, vaccines consisting of live attenuated strains, administered in drinking water, have been employed to prevent fowl cholera. Several live attenuated vaccines are being employed to prevent pneumonic pasteurellosis in cattle with varying degrees of success.

Whole-broth killed cultures (bacterins) with a high concentration of organisms, some containing adjuvants, have been used widely to prevent the following *P. multocida* infections:

- **Fowl cholera.** The causal serotypes must be present in the bacterin.
- **Bovine pneumonic pasteurellosis.** Caused mainly by *M. haemolytica*, and sometimes the viruses para-influenza-3 and infectious bovine rhinotracheitis virus are involved.

- **Pneumonia in sheep.** Caused by *M. haemolytica*.
- **Hemorrhagic septicemia.** Caused by serotype B:2 or serotype E:2 strains.

A live, intranasal, heterotypical (serotype B:3,4) vaccine is being used experimentally to prevent hemorrhagic septicemia.

Public Health Significance

Because dogs and cats harbor these organisms in their mouths as commensals, humans and various animals are infected by bites. A wide variety of infections, directly or indirectly derived from animals, have been reported in humans, including sinusitis, pneumonia, peritonitis, urinary tract infection, endocarditis, otitis, meningitis, abscesses, cellulitis, tonsillitis, appendicitis, bacteremia, and septicemia. Human infections, rarely fatal, are most often secondary to some primary disease process.

PASTEURELLA TREHALOSI

Formerly *P. haemolytica*, biotype T. Two different biotypes of *P. haemolytica* had been identified, biotype A and biotype T. They differed in several characteristics, including pathogenicity, antigenic nature, and biochemical activity (Table 19.1). The name *P. trehalosi* has been proposed for *P. haemolytica*, biotype T.

MANNHEIMIA HAEMOLYTICA

Formerly *Pasteurella haemolytica*, biotype A (Table 19.1).

Pathogenesis and Pathogenicity

Pasteurella trehalosi and *M. haemolytica* elaborate a soluble cytotoxin (leukotoxin) that kills alveolar macrophages and other leukocytes of ruminants, thus breaching the lung's primary defense mechanism. Some properties of the cytotoxin are the following: It is produced by all strains of *M. haemolytica* and *P. trehalosi*; it is a thermolabile protein of relatively large molecular weight; it resembles the alpha-hemolysin of *E. coli*; and it is immunogenic. The DNA fragment responsible for leukotoxin has been successfully cloned in *E. coli*. There is considerable evidence that the cytotoxin plays an important role in the pathogenesis of pneumonia in ruminants.

Mannheimia haemolytica has a primary or secondary role in pneumonia of cattle, goats, and sheep and is frequently recovered from the bronchopneumonic lungs of cattle with pneumonic pasteurellosis (shipping fever). Other important diseases in which this organism is involved are mastitis of ewes and septicemia of nursing lambs. *Pasteurella trehalosi* causes septicemia in feeder lambs.

Laboratory animals are refractory to experimental infection.

Laboratory Diagnosis

Direct examination is of limited value.

Media containing serum or blood are required for good growth of both species. Colonies are round, grayish, and usually somewhat smaller than those of *P. multocida*. They are usually surrounded by a zone of beta-hemolysis. This zone varies considerably and may be no larger than the colony, and thus, it is not apparent unless the colony is removed. Bovine blood is more suitable than that of sheep or horses for the demonstration of hemolysis.

Smears from colonies disclose small gram-negative rods or coccobacilli. They are beta-hemolytic, indole-negative, nonmotile, and grow on MacConkey agar. Additional biochemical test are required for definitive identification (Table 19.2).

Treatment

Treatment is essentially the same as that for *P. multocida*. Susceptibility testing is important in that multiple drug resistance is encountered.

Antigenic Nature and Immunity

Mannheimia haemolytica and *P. trehalosi* are antigenically heterogeneous and somewhat resemble *P. multocida* in that they have capsular and somatic varieties. The somatic antigens are so complex that serotypes are designated according to differences in capsular substances. Type 1 is the most common type encountered in bovine pneumonia. There are 16 serotypes of *M. haemolytica* based on capsular antigens. These antigens are recognized by an indirect hemagglutination procedure (Table 19.1).

Immunity is thought to be predominantly humoral.

Bacterins containing both *M. haemolytica* and *P. multocida* are widely used in cattle and sheep, although their value is questionable. Claims of efficacy in the prevention of bovine pneumonic pasteurellosis have been made for several live and subunit vaccines.

PASTEURELLA HAEMOLYTICA–LIKE ORGANISMS FROM POULTRY AND SWINE

Distinct varieties of "*P. haemolytica*" can cause infrequent low-grade infections in poultry and swine. They frequently can be recovered from the upper respiratory tract of chickens and turkeys. "*P. haemolytica*" of chicken, turkey, and swine origin differ in certain biochemical characteristics from the conventional ruminant strains, and in addition, the former strains have not yet been serotyped. The taxonomic position of these "atypical" strains is not yet clear. They are referred to as *P. haemolytica*–like. Some produce leukotoxin.

GLOSSARY

Dermatobia hominis This tropical warble fly is an important parasite of cattle in South America. Its larval stages are found in many animals including cattle, sheep, goats, swine, rabbits, dogs, cats, and humans.

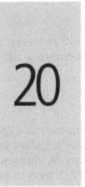

20 | Lawsonia, Campylobacter, Arcobacter, and Helicobacter

It is of interest that *Lawsonia intracellularis* is the only species of the genus that belongs in the Family Desulfovibrionaceae of sulfate- and sulfur-reducing bacteria. These organisms are found in aquatic habitats and waterlogged soil. *Arcobacter* and *Campylobacter* are similar in morphology but belong in a different section of δ-Proteobacteria.

Lawsonia intracellularis is a slender, curved, microaerophilic, obligate intracellular, gram-negative rod. Before being adequately characterized, it was referred to as *ileal symbiont intracellularis*. It can be grown in cultures of intestinal epithelial cells (enterocytes) and other cell lines, but not in cell-free media. It is now considered the primary cause of the common swine disease proliferative enteropathy or proliferative enteritis; however, other bacteria, for example, clostridia, *Escherichia coli* and *Bacteroides*, are considered to have a necessary ancillary role.

Lawsonia intracellularis has been confirmed as the cause of intestinal disease in a wide range of animal and avian species. Whether or not there are differences in the strains from different animal species is not yet known. Proliferative intestinal lesions can be readily produced experimentally in pigs, hamsters and mice.

LAWSONIA INTRACELLULARIS

There is an absence of knowledge relating to adhesins, receptors, and attachment, and the mechanisms of entry of *L. intracellularis* to enterocytes. The organisms can multiply rapidly in the cytoplasm of enterocytes and avoid the harmful effects of phagosomal fusion. Little is know of the immune response to this organism.

The organism is passed in the feces in small numbers, and the mode of infection is ingestion.

Pathogenicity

Proliferative enteropathy is most often seen in weaned pigs up to 12 weeks of age. Invasion of enterocytes results in their proliferation with loss of normal villus structure and replacement with glandular epithelium. There is little inflamation, and lesions are mainly confined to the terminal ileum; they may be focal or diffuse. The cardinal sign is diarrhea with a reduction in weight gain. The disease may be mild, with pigs recovering without treatment. Some pigs may develop necrotic enteritis, followed by emaciation. With acute hemorrhagic enteropathy and necrotic enteritis, the disease is frequently fatal.

The gross lesions, which mainly involve the terminal ileum, are thickening of the wall, areas of hemorrhagic or necrotic enteritis with tarry feces, and clotted blood in the lumen.

There have been increasing reports of proliferative enteropathy in horses, although its extent and significance is not yet clear.

Laboratory Diagnosis

Ordinarily, the diagnosis is based on the gross lesions.

The small rods of *L. intracellularis* can be demonstrated in impression smears from biopsies or smears from scrapings of lesions stained by the modified acid-fast stain and by silver stains such as the Warthin–Starry.

The organisms and characteristic tissue changes can be seen in histopathologic sections of lesions and biopsies.

Culture of the organism in enterocytes is generally impracticable.

Treatment

The antimicrobial agents, tylosin, tiamulin, lincomycin, tetracyclines, and carbadox, administered in the feed, have been effective.

Efforts should be directed toward preventing exposure to infectious feces, fomites, and contaminated quarters.

CAMPYLOBACTER

Campylobacter organisms are S-shaped, spirally curved (one or more spirals), gram-negative, pleomorphic rods. They are motile by a single polar flagellum at one or both ends, microaerophilic (3%–5% CO_2), aerobic or anaerobic, and oxidase-positive. They do not use carbohydrates.

Eighteen species are recognized, but only two species, *Campylobacter fetus* (with two subspecies) and *Campylobacter jejuni* are frankly pathogenic for animals. The generally nonpathogenic *Campylobacter* spp. are found on the mucous membrane of the genital and intestinal tracts. These will be discussed later with *C. jejuni*.

CAMPYLOBACTER FETUS

Strains of *C. fetus* comprise two subspecies, *C. fetus* subsp. *fetus* and *C. fetus* subsp. *venerealis*, both of which occur widely.

Both subspecies possess a surface protein capsule. This high–molecular weight surface array protein is essential for virulence. It mediates resistance to serum killing and to phagocytosis by preventing the binding of serum C3b. Additional virulence factors have yet to be identified.

Subspecies *venerealis*

This subspecies is the cause of bovine genital campylobacteriosis. In this disease, the organism can be found in the preputial cavity of the asymptomatic bull and the genital tract of the cow and heifer. The mode of infection is venereal; organisms are present in the semen of infected bulls. The placenta and fetus may be invaded with occasional abortion at 5–8 months. If birth occurs, the newborn may only live for a few hours. In some individuals, the embryo may die and be resorbed. The infected placenta is usually hemorrhagic and edematous. The uterine infection causes a metritis that results in infertility, and the organism may be shed from the uterus for varying periods. The result is usually an appreciably delayed calving season.

Subspecies *fetus*

This organism occurs in the intestine of cattle and sheep and in the genital tract of infected sheep and cattle. The mode of infection is ingestion, directly or via fomites, but not venereally from the ram. After ingestion, there is hematogenous spread with infection of the uterine mucosa. It may cause abortion in cattle (sporadic) and in sheep (multiple). The placenta and fetus may be infected, with abortions occurring late in pregnancy; fetuses may undergo autolysis, and there may be stillbirths. After expelling the fetus, ewes may develop metritis.

The placenta may be hemorrhagic and edematous. Necrotic foci in the fetal liver are characteristic.

Specimens

Special methods are employed for the collection of cervical mucus and preputial secretions for culture. Fetal stomach contents, fetal tissues, and placenta may also be cultured. It is important that clinical materials be fresh. *Campylobacter* spp., do not survive outside the host for more than several hours unless protected from drying and sunshine.

Filtration may be used to aid recovery; *Campylobacter* can pass through a 0.65-μm membrane filter.

Direct Examination

Campylobacter fetus can be demonstrated (presumptively) in the fetal stomach contents by negative staining and by phase or dark-field microscopy. A fluorescent antibody reagent can be used to identify *C. fetus* in preputial washings, cervical mucus, and fetal stomach contents. A polymerase chain reaction (PCR) procedure has been used to detect subsp. *venerealis* in semen.

Immune Response

Nonspecific defenses, such as gastric acidity and intestinal transit time, are thought to be important, as *C. jejuni* can be killed by hydrochloric acid. Neutrophils and macrophages are often observed in the feces of infected individuals, suggesting they too may play a role in the elimination of the organism from the host. Specific immunity, involving intestinal IgA and systemic antibodies (IgM and IgG), develops. Whether this antibody response eliminates the infection or protects against reinfection is not known. However, it has been noted that immunocompromised individuals and hypogammaglobulinemic individuals have a higher risk of severe, recurrent, or bacteremic infections.

In the case of *C. fetus*, the 99-kDa protein of the S-layer protein is the immunodominant antigen. Although their role is not known, development of humoral immunity is similar to that described for *C. jejuni*.

Laboratory Diagnosis

Blood agar (*Brucella* agar base) containing antibiotics to reduce growth of contaminants is satisfactory. For optimal recovery, plates are incubated at 37°C in an atmosphere of 10% CO_2, 5% O_2, and 85% N_2. Gas-generation packs are available to provide the desired atmosphere.

Fine pinpoint colonies are seen after 3–6 days of incubation. Smears reveal small, gram-negative rods that assume various forms, short and long, both curved and S-shaped. Long, wavy filaments may be seen in some cultures.

A fluorescent antibody procedure will identify *C. fetus*. A presumptive identification of subspecies is often made based on history and source of isolates. Definitive identification is based on a number of phenotypic tests.

Isolates of *Campylobacter* spp. have been identified based on 16S ribosomal RNA gene sequences. More recently, fluorescent amplified fragment length polymorphism (AFLP) fingerprinting, using the 16S rRNA sequences, has been found to be very specific in identifying various *Campylobacter* spp.

Cervical and vaginal mucus agglutination tests are used but are only moderately reliable. Other serologic procedures, including an enzyme-linked immunosorbent assay

(ELISA) for antibodies in vaginal secretion, have been developed but are not routinely used.

Treatment and Prevention

The *C. fetus* subspecies are susceptible to a number of antibiotics, but treatment is not usually feasible. Losses caused by the bovine disease may be reduced with penicillin and streptomycin. Irrigation of the uterus and prepuce with streptomycin is sometimes carried out. Tetracycline administered in feed or by injection may be of prophylactic value and may reduce the number of ovine abortion.

Bacterins composed of killed *C. fetus* subsp. *venerealis* combined with adjuvants such as oil, alum, or related compounds are of some value in cattle, but immunity is of short duration. Vaccination has been used in an effort to eliminate the carrier state in bulls. Bacterins are also used to prevent the ovine disease.

To prevent *C. fetus* subsp. *venerealis* infection, semen for artificial insemination is routinely treated with streptomycin and penicillin. Using only artificial insemination will result in eventual elimination of *C. fetus* subsp. *venerealis*. Infected bulls should not be used to provide semen. *Campylobacter fetus* subsp. *venerealis* can be eliminated from a herd, but subsp. *fetus* cannot.

Public Health Significance

Campylobacter fetus subsp. *fetus* causes infrequent human infections, but not *C. fetus* subsp. *venerealis*. Those exposed to cattle and sheep are most likely to be infected; for example, veterinarians, farmers, packing house workers, and others associated with cattle and sheep. Among the infections seen are bacteremia, septic arthritis, endocarditis, septic abortions, peritonitis, salpingitis, meningitis, and thrombophlebitis. Patients with underlying disease, such as HIV infection, are particularly susceptible, and the prognosis may not be favorable.

INFREQUENTLY PATHOGENIC SPECIES

These include the following species with their sources (usually fecal):

- *Campylobacter coli:* Pigs and poultry; human infections.
- *Campylobacter concisus:* Human infections.
- *Campylobacter helveticus:* Dogs and cats.
- *Campylobacter hyoileri:* Pigs.
- *Campylobacter hyointestinalis:* Pigs; human infections
- *Campylobacter jejuni* subsp. *doylei:* Human infections; has only been recovered from humans.
- *Campylobacter mucosalis:* Pigs; human infections.
- *Campylobacter lari:* Gulls and other avian species, dogs, and cats; human infections.
- *Campylobacter upsaliensis:* Dogs; human infections.

- *Campylobacter sputorum* bivar *bubulus:* Cattle and sheep; human infections.
- *Campylobacter sputorum* bivar *fecalis:* Cattle and sheep: intestinal and genital tracts.
- *Campylobacter sputorum* bivar *sputorum:* Cattle and sheep: genital tract; human infections.

The human infections referred to above are opportunistic. They include, but are not limited to, wound infections, diarrhea, proctitis, endocarditis, gastroenteritis, meningitis, sepsis, abscesses, and periodontal disease. Several additional species of nonpathogenic *Campylobacter* spp., whose names have not been given, are recovered from the feces of domestic animals and birds. They also are infrequent causes of human infections.

CAMPYLOBACTER JEJUNI

Campylobacter jejuni occurs frequently as a commensal in the intestinal tract of many species of domestic and wild animals, including birds, poultry, dogs, and cats.

Pathogenesis and Pathogenicity

Virulence factors associated with *C. jejuni* include adhesin, endotoxin, cytotoxin, and enterotoxin. Invasiveness has been associated with flagella and adhesin, which allow bacterial colonization. Furthermore, *C. jejuni* is capable of survival in the phagosomes. The lipopolysaccharide is a potent endotoxin. Enterotoxin is similar to cholera toxin in that it activates adenylate cyclase, thus increasing intracellular levels of cyclic AMP. This results in large fluid loss into the lumen of the intestine, resulting in diarrhea. The production of cytotoxin results in local tissue destruction and abscess formation.

Because many animals are carriers of *C. jejuni*, it is often difficult to determine the significance of the organism in individuals with diarrhea. Observing large numbers of morphologically characteristic organisms in stained smears from rectal scrapings indicates pathogenic significance.

Campylobacter jejuni causes infections characterized by diarrhea and enterocolitis in dogs, cats, sheep, goats, calves, laboratory animals, mink, ferrets, and other animals. Infections are more severe in younger animals.

The organism also causes, infrequently, abortion in bitches, ewes, and cows and mastitis in cows.

Campylobacter jejuni is the cause of avian infectious hepatitis of chickens and turkeys. This is a widespread infection, which is usually benign. However, on occasion it affects flocks with a low mortality, high morbidity, and chronic course with loss of condition; hemorrhagic and necrotic changes are seen in the liver. Treatment is not usually feasible.

Campylobacter jejuni occasionally infects companion and exotic birds. Erythromycin in the drinking water is an effective treatment.

CAMPYLOBACTER COLI

Campylobacter coli occurs as a commensal in the intestinal tract of poultry and swine. Although it produces a heat-labile enterotoxin, it is rarely pathogenic. It is easily confused with *C. jejuni.*

CAMPYLOBACTER UPSALIENSIS

This species has been recovered from feces of both healthy and diarrheic dogs and cats and from feces of healthy children.

Laboratory Diagnosis

Isolation and cultivation of the species just discussed is essentially the same as described above for the subspecies of *C. fetus,* except that the incubation temperature is 42°C.

Special measures such as filtration, the use of antibiotics in primary media, and below-surface sampling are used to reduce contaminants.

Growth is slow, and colonies of the various species resemble (in size and morphology) those of *C. fetus.* They are slightly mucoid in appearance and are grey to pink or yellowish grey in color.

In avian hepatitis, the characteristic morphology and motility of *C. jejuni* can be demonstrated in bile by phase microscopy. This organism grows readily in a candle jar.

Campylobacters recovered from feces are not usually speciated. They are presumptively identified on the basis of colonial growth, characteristic morphology, and motility. Definitive identification of the various species is based on growth characteristics, biochemical tests, and 16S rRNA gene sequences.

Species-specific deoxyribonucleic acid (DNA) probes are being used in some diagnostic laboratories for the identification of campylobacters recovered from feces. The fluorescent AFLP fingerprinting, using the 16S rRNA sequences, has been found to be very specific in identifying various *Campylobacter* spp.

A commercial latex agglutination test is available for the identification of *C. jejuni, C. coli,* and other *Campylobacter* spp. An ELISA is available for the serodiagnosis of *C. jejuni* infection.

Treatment

Given the self-limiting character of many of the infections, treatment may not be necessary. Because of the prevalence of resistance, susceptibility tests are recommended. Erythromycin and tylosin have been effective. Resistance has been encountered to tetracylines and quinolones.

Public Health Significance

Campylobacter jejuni is the most frequent pathogen recovered from diarrheic stools associated with gastroenteritis in humans. The sources of the organism are many, including milk, poultry carcasses, feces of animal and human carriers, food and water contaminated by feces, and dog and cat feces with or without diarrhea. The course is usually 1–7 days with fever, abdominal pain, nausea, vomiting, and watery diarrhea with or without blood in the stool. Most infections are asymptomatic. Disseminated infections may occur in immunosuppressed individuals.

Campylobacter coli, C. hyointestinalis, and *C. upsaliensis* cause infrequent foodborne diarrheic infections. Human infections caused by other infrequently pathogenic *Campylobacter* spp. are referred to above.

ARCOBACTER

Arcobacters are *Campylobacter*-like, and the genus is in the family Campylobacteriaceae. They are gram-negative, curved, S-shaped or helical, aerotolerant, motile rods.

Their habitat, except for one species, is the intestinal tract of some animals, including poultry, where they are present usually as harmless commensals. Four species are recognized. *Arcobacter butzleri, Arcobacter cryaerophilis,* and *Arcobacter skirrowii* are associated with diarrhetic illness and reproductive disease in livestock. *Arcobacter cryaerophilis* has been implicated as an important cause of infertility and late-term abortions in swine.

The fourth species, *Arcobacter nitrofigilis,* occurs in roots of a plant and is not pathogenic for animals.

Arcobacter butzleri has been recovered from human patients with bacteremia, peritonitis, endocarditis, and diarrhea. *Arcobacter cryaerophilis* has been isolated from human patients with diarrhea and bacteremia.

Arcobacters grow on the same media that support the growth of campylobacters. Media are incubated in a microaerobic atmosphere at 37°C. Filtration is used to remove contaminating bacteria when feces are being examined. Definitive identification requires phenotypic tests. DNA-based identification, such as PCR, may facilitate identification.

As yet, there is little information available on treatment. Selection of drugs should be based on the results of susceptibility tests.

HELICOBACTER

Organisms of the genus *Helicobacter* resemble campylobacters and were previously classified in the genus *Campylobacter.* They are gram-negative, spiral and curved, motile (several sheathed flagella) and microaerophilic. At least 19 species of *Helicobacter* have been named, and all occur in the stomach or intestine of animals and humans worldwide.

Helicobacter spp. are carried in the stomach or intestine of many animals without causing apparent disease. They live beneath the mucous coating, where the pH may reach 7.4. It is estimated that the carrier rate of *Helicobacter pylori* for humans is ~50%. It is thought that the inflammatory response, the accumulation of T cells, and the growth of *Helicobacter* lead to gastritis and sometimes gastric ulcers.

Increasing age is considered a factor in infection; however, there is little information on susceptibility and resistance. There appears to be no protective immunity after infection.

Transmission is considered to be mainly fecal/oral and oral/oral.

They occur in the gastric mucus layer, and their capacity to break down urea with the production of ammonia and carbon dioxide with the consequent raising of the pH contributes to their survival.

The virulence factors of *Helicobacter* include adhesin, flagella, cytotoxin, urease, acid-inhibitory protein, mucinase, catalase, superoxide dismutase, vacuolating cytotoxin (Vac A), and cytotoxin-associated gene (*Cag A*).

Pathogenicity

Helicobacter pylori is capable of causing chronic gastritis, mainly in the antrum of the stomach, and duodenitis and duodenal ulcer disease in humans. Gastric ulcer disease and gastric adenocarcinoma have been epidemiologically associated with this organism. This species has the potential to cause similar disease in cats. Other species implicated in gastric disease in humans are *Helicobacter canis, Helicobacter felis, Helicobacter rappini, Helicobacter bilis,* and *Helicobacter heilmannii (Helicobacter bizzozeronii).*

There has been much debate about the pathogenic significance of these organisms in dogs and cats. Evidence suggests that they can cause gastritis and more serious disease in both species.

Species implicated in gastric disease in cats are *H. felis, H. pylori, H. canis,* and *H. heilmannii.*

Species with the potential to cause gastric disease in dogs are *H. felis, H. canis, H. bilis, Helicobacter salomonis,* and *H. rappini.*

The following clinical signs have been attributed to *Helicobacter* infections in dogs and cats: vomiting, regurgitation, abdominal pain, fever, diarrhea, anorexia, weight loss, and poor condition.

Laboratory Diagnosis

Isolation and identification or demonstration of characteristic helical organisms, along with evidence of gastritis, warrants a diagnosis. Evidence of urease is supportive.

Scrapings of the gastric mucosa are examined under phase microscopy for motile, helical-shaped organisms. These organisms can also be seen in smears and stained sections of gastric biopsies taken from areas of gastritis. Preparations may also be examined by electron microscopy.

The isolation and identification of species of helicobacters are complex and are not attempted in most veterinary diagnostic laboratories. They are microaerophilic, oxidase positive, do not use carbohydrates, and with the exception of *H. canis,* are catalase positive. Skirrow's medium and chocolate agar with the addition of antibiotics are used for isolation. Incubation for up to a week may be required for appreciable growth.

Helicobacter heilmannii, the most common species in dogs and cats, has not been cultured on artificial media; *H. felis* is difficult to isolate and identify.

Most of the species considered to be pathogenic elaborate urease, and a urease test can be performed on biopsy material. A kit is available commercially. A breath test (for urease) similar to that used for human infections has been described for dogs.

An ELISA is used to determine the antibody response, and enzyme immune assays are used to detect antigen in feces.

PCR is not practical for the routine diagnosis of *H. pylori*. It may be useful in detection of the organism when testing stool or drinking water.

Treatment

For dogs and cats, metronidazole with amoxicillin or metronidazole with tetracycline, and both combinations with bismuth sub salicylate (Pepto-Bismol) per os, in divided doses for 2–3 weeks have been effective. Amoxicillin with omeprazole (inhibits gastric acid secretion) is used; cimetidine is also used to reduce gastric acid. The drugs mentioned above will greatly reduce the number of gastric bacteria in dogs and cats, but recurrence of infection appears to be common.

Public Health Significance

It is assumed that some species occurring in dogs and cats and other animals may be transmissible to humans.

21 *Clostridium*

The clostridia and relatives are the first bacteria listed in Volume 3 of *Bergey's Manual* (2nd edition). They are described as "The Low G+C Gram Positives." They are large, usually gram-positive (young cultures particularly), spore-forming rods. Included in the genus are obligate anaerobes as well as aerotolerant species. Spores are not formed in the presence of air. The genus, which contains more than 100 species, is heterogeneous and will probably be divided into several phylogenetic clusters.

GENERAL

Only a few species cause diseases in man and animals. They can be divided into four major groups according to the kind of disease they produce:

- The histotoxic clostridia cause a variety of tissue (often muscle) infections, frequently following wounds or other trauma. Examples are blackleg and malignant edema.
- The hepatotoxic clostridia produce their toxins in the liver and cause the diseases bacillary hemoglobinuria and black disease.
- The enterotoxigenic clostridia produce mainly enterotoxemia and food poisoning, although they are occasionally histotoxic.
- The neurotoxic clostridia cause disease by the production of the potent exotoxins (neurotoxins) of tetanus and botulism.

Habitat

Clostridia are free-living saprophytes, distributed widely in the soil. They persist in ecologic niches with a suitably low oxidation-reduction potential. Some species are more prevalent in some geographic areas. Several species commonly occur in the intestinal tract.

Mode of Infection

Although most important clostridial infections are acquired by ingestion or via wounds, some arise endogenously.

INGESTION. Blackleg (cattle), botulism (food), enterotoxemia, bacillary hemoglobinuria, and black disease are acquired by ingestion.

WOUNDS. *Clostridium tetani, Clostridium chauvoei* (sheep), *Clostridium septicum,* and other gas gangrene (myonecrosis) organisms infect wounds.

Morphology

The disease-producing clostridia (Fig. 21.1) are motile (except for *C. perfringens*) and nonencapsulated. They are relatively large rods with rounded ends, occurring singly in short chains or as long filaments.

Endospores may be located centrally, subterminally, or terminally.

Cultivation

Most grow well on blood agar in an atmosphere devoid of oxygen, in cooked meat medium, and in thioglycolate broth. Oxygen is toxic in varying degrees to the clostridia. Some species are aerotolerant, whereas others, such as *Clostridium novyi*, are particularly sensitive to oxygen. Most laboratories incubate plate media in anaerobic jars. Some larger laboratories have anaerobic glove boxes for work with anaerobes in general. Colonies are 1–3 mm in diameter, round or slightly irregular, slightly raised, granular, and transparent or translucent, with fine filamentous margins. The growth of some species swarms on moist agar media. The colonies of *Clostridium perfringens* are round with a characteristic double zone of hemolysis on blood agar. Special media are employed for toxin production.

Isolation and Identification: General

The isolation and identification of clostridial species is laborious and time-consuming. After obtaining pure cultures, a battery of biochemical tests is required for identification. Special anaerobic media systems are available commercially for the identification of clostridial species. The availability of fluorescent antibody (FA) reagents for the identification of several species from

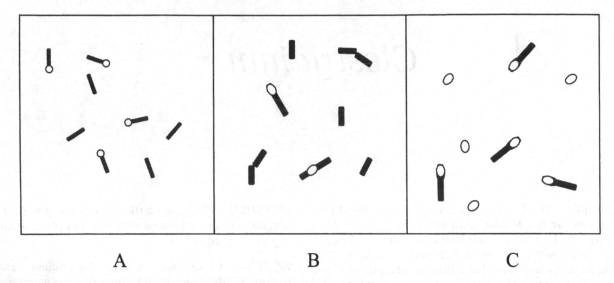

FIGURE 21.1   Morphology of *Clostridium* spp. **(A)** *Clostridium tetani*, both sporing ("drumstick") and nonsporing bacilli. **(B)** *Clostridium perfringens*; note that sporing bacilli are rarely seen except when grown on special media. **(C)** *Clostridium sporogenes*, with both endospores and spores lacking a vegetative cell.

smears has obviated the need for conventional laboratory procedures.

Precise identification can be made by gas–liquid chromatographic analysis of metabolic products, but this is beyond the scope of most diagnostic laboratories.

Resistance

The endospores of clostridia are highly resistant to various physical and chemical agents, including disinfectants. In this respect, they are similar to the spores produced by *Bacillus anthracis*, in that 30 minutes of boiling may be required to kill the spores of *Clostridium botulinum*; autoclaving at 121°C for 20 minutes is lethal. The vegetative forms of the clostridia are susceptible to common disinfectants.

CLOSTRIDIUM CHAUVOEI

Clostridium chauvoei is the cause of blackleg.

Occurrence

Clostridium chauvoei is widespread in soils, but it is more prevalent in certain geographic areas. It is found in the intestine and in normal tissues of some animals, including the livers of some apparently normal dogs and cattle. It is not as common in the soil as are some other clostridia.

Toxins

The following toxins have been identified:

- Alpha toxin: Hemolysin, necrotoxin.
- Beta toxin: Deoxyribonuclease.
- Gamma toxin: Hyaluronidase.
- Delta toxin: Hemolysin.

Pathogenesis

In blackleg, *C. chauvoei* is thought to enter the animal by ingestion or to be endogenous. The pathogen is carried by the blood to damaged muscle tissue, where it multiplies if conditions are anaerobic. *Clostridium chauvoei* may enter wounds along with other organisms. The mixed infection and necrotic tissue provide an anaerobic milieu for *C. chauvoei*, which multiplies and produces its exotoxins and other metabolites. Bacteremia usually occurs late in the disease.

Pathogenicity

Blackleg in ruminants affects cattle (usually 4 months to 3 years of age) via ingestion; it may be endogenous. It affects sheep and goats via wounds. The lesion is not always easy to find: It is dry and dark and has gas bubbles and a rancid odor. There may be a bacteremia. The onset is sudden—animals may be found dead without premonitory signs; there is initial fever, depression, acute lameness, and death.

Specimens

The specimens should be fresh and from affected muscles. Because clostridia of the types that cause gas gangrene invade tissues from the intestine shortly after death, isolation or demonstration of these organisms is not always significant. This is especially so with *C. septicum* and *C. perfringens*.

Laboratory Diagnosis

Isolation and identification is laborious and not usually carried out. A reliable direct FA procedure is available for identification of organisms in tissues or cultures. Animal inoculation: guinea pigs die within 48 hours; however, rabbits are resistant.

Treatment and Control

When an outbreak occurs, all cattle in the susceptible age range should be vaccinated and treated prophylactically with penicillin. Treatment of clinical cases is usually unsuccessful.

Formalinized whole-broth cultures, usually alum precipitated, are used to produce lifelong immunity in cattle and sheep. Protection is both antibacterial and antitoxic. A soluble heat-labile protective antigen is associated with the alpha toxin. Recovery from disease renders animals immune for life. A commonly used double bacterin contains *C. chauvoei* and *C. septicum*. Some products also contain *C. novyi* type A, *Clostridium sordellii*, or both and *C. perfringens*.

CLOSTRIDIUM SEPTICUM

Clostridium septicum causes malignant edema and braxy.

Occurrence

The organism occurs worldwide and is found in the intestine and soil.

Toxins

The following toxins have been identified:

- Alpha toxin: Lethal, lecithinase, necrotizing and hemolytic.
- Beta toxin: A deoxyribonuclease and leukocidal.
- Gamma toxin: Hyaluronidase.
- Delta toxin: Hemolyzing and necrotizing factor.

Pathogenicity

The pathogenesis of *C. septicum* infection is similar to that of gangrene caused by *C. chauvoei*. It affects, sporadically, horses, cattle, sheep, pigs, and occasionally other animals with an emphysematous, necrotic myositis or gas gangrene. The common portals of entry are wounds and compound fractures. A large, expanding swelling involves skeletal muscles pits on pressure, is gelatinous and red, and has little gas. Malignant edema may result from injuries to the vulva during parturition. Clinical signs include high fever, anorexia, depression, and lameness depending on the location of the lesions.

In sheep, the highly fatal disease braxy is associated with eating frozen succulent feed. It produces necrotic lesions and hemorrhagic edema of the abomasal and duodenal walls. It is mainly a European disease, although cases have been reported in the United States.

Clostridium septicum causes an infrequent gangrenous dermatitis in chickens.

Specimens

Specimens should be fresh and from affected muscles.

Laboratory Diagnosis

Isolation and identification is not usually carried out. An FA procedure similar to that used for *C. chauvoei* is available. Animal inoculation is lethal for guinea pigs and rabbits. Long chains of filaments are seen in impression smears from the tissues of guinea pigs and rabbits. Other clostridia that occasionally cause gas gangrene, such as *C. novyi*, type A (FA available), *C. sordellii*, and *C. perfringens*, type A, are isolated and identified by conventional procedures.

Treatment and Control

To be successful, treatment with penicillin or broad-spectrum antibiotics must be early in the disease. Local administration of penicillin into affected muscle may limit spread of the lesion.

Clostridium septicum is included in some multiple-component bacterins. A *C. chauvoei/C. septicum* bacterin, referred to above, to prevent blackleg is widely used in cattle and sheep to prevent both diseases.

CLOSTRIDIUM HAEMOLYTICUM

Also known as *Clostridium novyi*, type D. *Clostridium haemolyticum* causes bacillary hemoglobinuria.

Occurrence

Clostridium haemolyticum is probably present worldwide, wherever liver flukes occur. In the United States, it is found predominantly in the mountain valleys of Nevada, Montana, and several other western states, as well as along the Gulf of Mexico. Apparently it is not abundant in either the intestine or soil. Subclinical infections may occur in some animals, which may serve as carriers that shed organisms via the intestinal tract.

Toxins

Lecithinase C is produced that is lethal, necrotizing, and hemolytic. It resembles the beta toxin of *C. novyi* type B (black disease). Other minor toxins are produced.

Pathogenicity and Pathogenesis

Infection with *C. haemolyticum* is limited to cattle and sheep, in which it causes bacillary hemoglobinuria or red water. The mode of infection is by ingestion, with the organism probably reaching the liver hematogenously. Liver flukes result in infarction of branches of the portal vein. The spores can germinate and grow in the damaged anaerobic tissue, where they produce their toxin. The infarct is usually 5–20 cm in diameter. The disease does not appear in areas where conditions are not favorable for the flukes or the snails.

Death is apparently brought about by lysis of erythrocytes by the toxin, and the animal perishes of anoxia. The disease appears to be produced by a single enzyme, lecithinase C, acting on a single substrate, the lecithoprotein complex of the surface of the erythrocyte.

Specimens

Specimens should be taken from affected liver tissue.

Laboratory Diagnosis

Isolation and identification is laborious. An FA procedure is available.

Treatment and Control

Penicillin and broad-spectrum antibiotics are effective if given early in bacillary hemoglobinuria.

The disease may be controlled by elimination of liver flukes through destruction of snails. Formalized alum-precipitated whole-broth cultures are used to produce an active immunity. Immunity is of relatively short duration, and animals at risk should be vaccinated every 6 months.

CLOSTRIDIUM NOVYI

Synonym

Also known as *Clostridium oedematiens*. There are three types other than *C. novyi* type D or the *C. haemolyticum* just discussed. They are

- Type A: Causes gas gangrene and is found worldwide in humans, cattle, and sheep; causes big head in rams.
- Type B: Causes black disease and has been reported in sheep in Oregon, Colorado, Montana, and worldwide; potentially found wherever liver flukes occur.
- Type C: Causes osteomyelitis and has been reported in water buffaloes in Indonesia.

Occurrence

Types A and B are found in the intestine and livers of animals, and type A occurs commonly in soil.

Toxins

Several exotoxins are produced, including some with lethal and necrotizing properties. Type B, *C. novyi* produces alpha and beta toxins. The beta toxin, like the beta toxin of *C. haemolyticum*, is lecithicinase C. The alpha toxin is phage mediated. Types A and B differ antigenically; serum protection tests in animals distinguish them.

Pathogenicity

Type A, which causes gas gangrene initiated in wounds, is found alone or in mixed infections with *C. chauvoei*, *C. septicum*, or *C. sordellii*. It is also seen in "big head," a disease of rams characterized by significant edematous swelling of the head and neck. Damage caused by butting allows entrance of the organism to the subcutis of the head. Big head may be caused by other clostridia.

Type B causes black disease or infectious necrotic hepatitis in sheep and, occasionally, cattle. The mode of infection is oral, with the organism (spores) being carried to the liver via the blood. This is a localized infection of the liver, initiated in local tissue destruction resulting from the migration of young liver flukes.

Toxin is produced in the local lesion and absorbed into the circulating blood, eventually producing death in a course as short as 2–3 days. Signs include anorexia and profound depression. Recovery is rare. Intense congestion of the blood vessels of the skin may result in the skin's blackening. Cutaneous edema resulting from impairment of the heart may be present; it is usually sterile.

Specimens

Specimens should be taken from affected liver tissue.

Laboratory Diagnosis

Clostridium novyi type B is fastidious, and isolation and identification is difficult. The FA procedure does not distinguish between types.

Types A and C are isolated and identified by conventional procedures.

Treatment and Control

Treatment is of little value in black disease.

The disease is controlled by elimination of liver flukes by destruction of snails.

Formalinized bacterin and toxoid are of value. Type A is included in some bacterins for the prevention of gas gangrene infections.

CLOSTRIDIUM PERFRINGENS

Clostridium perfringens causes enterotoxemia.

Occurrence

Clostridium perfringens, type A, is probably more widespread than any other potentially pathogenic bacterium. It is present in air, soil, dust, and manure and in the water of lakes, streams, and rivers. It has been isolated from vegetables, milk, cheese, canned food, fresh meat, shellfish, and mollusks. It is constantly present in the intestinal contents of humans and animals and in their environment.

Types B, C, D, and E strains are found less commonly in the intestinal tracts of animals.

Toxins

The major toxins of *C. perfringens* and their characteristics are

- Alpha: Lethal, lecithinase, hemolytic, necrotizing; principal lethal toxin.
- Beta: Lethal, necrotizing; responsible for partial loss of the mucosa.
- Epsilon: Lethal, **permease**; a protoxin converted to toxin by proteolytic enzymes.
- Iota: Lethal, dermonecrotoxic, **adenosine diphophate (ADP)-ribosylating**, formed as a protoxin and subsequently activated by proteolytic digestion.

The species is divided into types A, B, C, D, and E on the basis of immunologic differences in the four major lethal necrotic toxins, alpha, beta, epsilon, and iota, as determined by protection tests in animals. The distribution of these major toxins relative to the type of *C. perfringens* is shown in Table 21.1.

Collaginase, a proteolytic enzyme, is produced by all types and is responsible for the digestion and liquefaction of collagen in connective tissue. Hyaluronidase, which hydrolyzes hyaluronic acid, the ground substance of tissues, is produced by many strains.

A deoxyribonuclease is produced by all types except type B, but it is not considered important in pathogenesis.

Enterotoxin (molecular weight [MW] ~34,000) is produced primarily by type A strains; other types may or may not produce it. Enterotoxigenic type A strains rank second to *Salmonella* as the cause of food poisoning in humans in the United States.

Pathogenicity

TYPE A. This is most widespread type. It has been implicated as the cause of necrotic enteritis in poultry and dogs and also an infrequent hemorrhagic enteritis in dogs; the cause of enterotoxemia and colitis in horses, diarrhea in pigs, wound infection leading to gas gangrene in animals and humans, and food poisoning in humans (diarrhea 6–24 hours after eating meat; not serious).

TYPE B. This type causes dysentery in lambs up to 3 weeks of age (lamb dysentery), which is primarily an enterotoxemia with significant enteritis and extensive ulceration. It does not occur in the United States or Australia.

This type also causes enterotoxemia in calves, sheep, goats, and foals.

TYPE C. It produces struck, an acute intoxication in adult sheep in England and Wales, and hemorrhagic enteritis in neonatal calves, foals, lambs, piglets, and chickens. Enterotoxemia has been reported in adult goats. It is also responsible for enteritis necroticans, a serious disease of humans.

TYPE D. This type causes enterotoxemia, "overeating disease," or "pulpy kidney" disease in sheep and goats of all ages, but particularly in feedlot sheep. It is a true toxemia with little evidence of enteritis. Epsilon toxin is apparently produced in the upper intestine, and the protoxin is activated by tryptic enzymes.

TYPE E. This type has been reported to cause hemorrhagic enteritis in calves in the United Kingdom. The iota toxin has been reported to cause enteritis in rabbits.

Specimens

Specimens should be fresh, small intestinal content. Refrigerate.

Laboratory Diagnosis

In cases of enterotoxemia, many large, gram-positive organisms usually are seen in smears from the small intestine.

First, determine whether the intestinal content is toxic for mice intravenously. If it is, mice are injected with mixtures of sterile (filtered) or antibiotic-treated intestinal contents and *C. perfringens*–type antitoxins. The tests also may be carried out in the skin of guinea pigs. The type of *C. perfringens* involved is determined by the protection or neutralization pattern observed (see Table 21.2).

These neutralization tests are cumbersome and expensive to perform and are not carried out routinely in diagnostic laboratories. There is evidence that an enzyme-linked immunosorbent assay (ELISA) can be used in lieu of the neutralization procedures.

Table 21.1 Occurrence of Major Toxins among Types of *Clostridium perfringens*

C. perfringens type	Toxin			
	Alpha	Beta	Epsilon	Iota
A*	+	−	−	−
B	+	+	+	−
C*	+	+	−	−
D	+	−	+	−
E	+	−	−	+

*Also produces enterotoxin.

Table 21.2 Pattern of Neutralization Reactions in Mice or Guinea Pigs between *Clostridium perfringens* Toxins (Intestinal Content) and Antitoxins

Intestinal Content Type	Major Lethal Toxins	Antitoxins				
		A	B	C	D	E
A	Alpha	+	+	+	+	+
B	Alpha, beta, epsilon	−	+	−	−	−
C	Alpha, beta	−	+	+	−	−
D	Alpha, epsilon	−	+	−	+	−
E	Alpha, iota	−	−	−	−	+

Note: +, toxin neutralized, mice protected; −, no neutralization, mice die.

Isolation and identification can also be carried out. All toxigenic strains of *C. perfringens* produce the lethal alpha toxin (lecithinase), which can be identified by the Nagler reaction or procedure. In this test, *C. perfringens*, elaborating the alpha toxin (lecithinase), produces an opalescence around the organism's growth in an egg-yolk agar. This opalescence is prevented by the presence of an anti–alpha toxin serum. The type is determined by animal protection or neutralization tests using toxin produced (if toxic) in a broth culture. Not all strains are toxigenic.

Clostridium perfringens produces few spores, unless grown on special media, and is nonmotile. It produces a characteristic double zone of hemolysis on blood agar, caused by two toxins. The narrow, clear zone next to the colony is produced by theta toxin, and the alpha toxin causes the partial, larger, outer zone. Although characteristic, stormy fermentation in milk is not specific for *C. perfringens*. Definitive identification can be carried out by the conventional means referred to earlier.

Deoxyribonucleic acid probes specific for genes that are responsible for toxins are currently being evaluated. A latex test for detecting type A enterotoxin is available commercially.

Treatment and Control

Given the severity of the disease, antimicrobial treatment is not usually effective.

Good management and feeding practices are important in prevention.

Antitoxins prepared in horses hyperimmunized against toxins produced by *C. perfringens* types B, C, and D are available. Passive immunization is protective for no longer than 2–3 weeks.

Active immunization is practiced principally in sheep. Formalinized whole-broth cultures prepared from strains of types C and D are used to produce an active immunity. Immunity may not last for more than 6–12 months.

Toxoids and bacterins are used to protect against types B, C, and D enterotoxemia of lambs. Ewes are given two doses of toxoid 6 weeks before lambing. Lambs may be immunized with bacterin or toxoid during the first week of life, if ewes were not immunized, and before entering feedlots.

Clostridium perfringens antigens are sometimes included in multivalent clostridial bacterins.

CLOSTRIDIUM TETANI

Occurrence

Spores of *C. tetani* are found throughout the world. The organism may be part of the normal flora of the soil, especially in the eastern part of the United States. It is less common west of the Mississippi River. It frequently has been isolated from the intestinal tract of animals. It is probably not more common in horse manure. The horse, however, is more subject to hoof injuries and is quite susceptible to tetanus. Humans and horses are most suscepti-

ble, followed by pigs. Cattle and sheep are next; it is rare in dogs, and cats and poultry are resistant.

Toxin

Tetanospasmin or neurotoxin is one of the most powerful exotoxins known. This heat-labile protein (MW 150,000) is produced by growing cells and released during autolysis. The neurotoxin is responsible for the characteristic spastic paralysis of tetanus.

The neurotoxin (tetanospasmin) is highly toxic when injected parenterally; however, it is harmless when administered by mouth. Animal species vary in their susceptibility to the toxin. Horses and humans are the most susceptible. One milligram of pure toxin contains about 100 million mouse-lethal doses.

Toxin is elaborated at the site of infection and passes along the axis cylinders of the motor neurons of the spinal cord and medulla. The toxin binds almost irreversibly to the gangliosides of nerve cells, and for this reason, antitoxin may not be effective. All strains produce only one antigenic type of neurotoxin. The toxin acts at the inhibitory synapse, where it blocks the normal function of the inhibitory transmitter. This results in excitation of the central nervous system.

Pathogenicity

Spores usually germinate in dirty and neglected wounds with some necrosis (lowered oxidation reduction potential); infection is usually mixed. Toxin is elaborated at the wound site after spores germinate, grow, and autolyse. Docking and castration wounds, umbilical infections (tetanus neonatorum), parturition (puerperal tetanus), dehorning, and ringing are among the circumstances that can contribute to tetanus in animals.

Tetanus is sometimes described as ascending or descending based on the movement and distribution of the toxin. Descending tetanus is the most common form seen in horses and humans. The first sign to appear in horses involves the nictitating membrane, followed by involvement of the muscles of the fore and hind limbs.

Tetanus is characterized clinically by convulsive contractions of voluntary muscles. In fatal cases, muscles throughout the body become involved. When death occurs, it results from spastic paralysis of muscles involved in respiration. In nonfatal tetanus, the spasms involve fewer muscles and gradually regress.

Specimens

Specimens should be material from the wound site.

Laboratory Diagnosis

This is almost always based on clinical signs. Isolation of the organism is not usually attempted. Organisms cannot always be demonstrated. Not all cultures of *C. tetani* are toxin producers. Characteristic "drumstick" spores (terminal) are produced. Swarming is seen in agar cultures.

Treatment and Prophylaxis

If indicated, surgical debridement of the wound or probable site of infection should be carried out. Antitoxin and penicillin are administered for prophylaxis. Toxoid may be administered at another site.

There is no effective and specific treatment for tetanus. Administration of antimicrobial drugs and antitoxin is of limited or no value. Active immunization with toxoid should be carried out. Nursing care with appropriate tranquilizers and sedation to prevent tetanic seizures is important. Mortality may be as high as 50% in generalized tetanus in horses and humans.

Recovery from tetanus does not usually confer permanent immunity because so little toxin is produced.

CLOSTRIDIUM BOTULINUM

Occurrence

Spores of *C. botulinum* are frequently encountered in the soil. Ordinarily it does not take up residence in the intestine. However, some cases of infant botulism have occurred in which the toxin has been produced in the stomach or intestine. The type of *C. botulinum* may vary from one geographic area to another.

Toxins

Like other clostridial toxins, the exotoxins of *C. botulinum* are heat-labile proteins (100°C for 10 minutes).

Seven types of neurotoxin (A, B, C, D, E, F, G) have been identified on the basis of antigenic differences. The toxins have been purified and are the most potent toxic substances known. One milligram of neurotoxin contains more than 120 million mouse-lethal doses. Less than 1 μg of toxic polypeptide preparation is lethal for man. The toxins, usually produced in foods, are absorbed from the intestinal tract. The toxin is released when the organisms die and undergo autolysis. Unlike most other toxins, they are resistant to peptic and tryptic digestion.

After absorption, the toxin is transported to susceptible neurons via the bloodstream. It appears to be specifically directed to the peripheral nerves and does not affect other body cells. It does not abolish conduction in the motor nerves but, rather, prevents the passage of impulses from the nerve to the muscle. The toxin acts by blocking the release of acetylcholine at synapses and neuromuscular junctions. There is no evidence that the toxin affects the nerve cells of the brain. The paralysis is flaccid in contrast to the spastic paralysis of tetanus. Paralysis is ascending, and death is caused by circulatory failure and respiratory paralysis, as a result of the action of the toxin on motor nerves.

Pathogenicity

The principal media for the production of botulinum toxins are various spoiled foods, such as canned vegetables, forage, meat, and fish. The toxin also may be produced in animal carcasses that dogs, chickens, and other animals may eat. There are considerable differences in the potency of the various types of toxin.

Botulism in mink (types A, B, and C) has been traced to spoiled meat, including whale meat. Types A, B, E and F are the principal causes of human botulism. Type A strains are implicated in botulism in mink and chickens. Type B botulism occurs in cattle and horses.

The name toxicoinfectious botulism has been given to the form of botulism in which the organism grows in tissues or organs and produces its toxin. Included in this category are infant botulism and wound botulism. It has been suggested that shaker foal syndrome is a manifestation of toxicoinfectious botulism, with type A or B growing in such foci as gastric ulcers, abscesses, liver necrosis, or various necrotic lesions.

Type C botulism occurs in cattle, sheep, turtles, chickens ("limberneck"), and wild fowl, particularly water fowl that have eaten rotting vegetation. Forage (spoiled oat, hay, silage) poisoning of horses has been attributed to type C botulism.

Type C (alpha) primarily affects birds and turtles. Type C (beta) toxicosis is seen mainly in cattle, sheep, and horses. This variety of C is not neurotoxic but affects vascular permeability and has enterotoxic activity.

Type D botulism causes "lamziekte" or "loin disease" in cattle with pica (phosphorus deficiency) in South Africa, Texas, South America, and probably other regions. The toxin is produced in bones and tissues of dead animals as a result of the growth of *C. botulinum* in carcasses. Hungry animals eat toxin-containing bones and tissue. The disease is seen most frequently during droughts, when the pasture is poor. Sheep are also susceptible to this toxin type.

Type G, which has been given the name *C. argentinense*, is not yet considered to cause botulism.

Many clinical diagnoses of botulism are not confirmed in the laboratory.

Specimens

Specimens that should be suspected are food, meat, forage, urine, and serum.

Laboratory Diagnosis

Extracts of food or forage are inoculated into guinea pigs or mice to determine whether or not toxin is present. If this material is toxic, protection tests are carried out using the extract and type antitoxins in guinea pigs or mice to determine the type involved. Food is fed to the test species. The organism often can be recovered from food and typed. If the level of toxin is high in an animal, it sometimes can be demonstrated in urine and serum by mouse inoculation.

Treatment and Control

Treatment of botulism requires early tracheotomy and intravenous administration of antitoxin. Animals that have consumed toxin and have not developed clinical signs should, if feasible, be given the appropriate antitoxin.

Immunization is not widely practiced in the United States. Toxoids have been used principally in cattle and mink, with success in some parts of the world. Bivalent or trivalent antitoxins are available for prophylactic use. They are of questionable value after clinical signs have appeared.

Control involves avoiding spoiled or otherwise suspicious food. Cooking at 100°C for 10 minutes destroys the toxin.

CLOSTRIDIUM PILIFORME

Formerly *Bacillus piliformis*, this interesting gram-negative, intracellular organism, the cause of Tyzzer's disease, is now included in the genus *Clostridium* based on 16S rRNA sequence analysis.

Pathogenicity

The organism probably occurs frequently in the intestine of rodents. Under circumstances of stress such as experimentation, cortisone treatment, or thymectomy, it causes enteritis, colitis, and hepatitis. The latter is evidenced by livers with diffusely distributed pale grey necrotic foci. Organisms are probably carried to the liver from intestinal infection. The disease may occur sporadically or as a serious epizootic in mice, rats, gerbils, hamsters, rabbits, and monkeys. Sporadic infections have been reported in the cat, dog, foal, fox, coyote, and calf.

Laboratory Diagnosis

Smears are made from the necrotic foci in the liver and stained with Giemsa. Long, slender organisms are seen in the cytoplasm of hepatic cells. Very long, thin, tortuous filaments are sometimes seen as well as short bacillary forms and occasionally filaments with moniliform swellings. Tapering and beading of the filaments are characteristic features. The organisms are motile by peritrichous flagella and have subterminal spores that are difficult to see in tissue sections. A diagnosis is usually made on the basis of smears and characteristic lesions in the liver.

What presumably are subclinical infections can be detected with a complement-fixation test. A fluorescent antibody has been used to identify organisms in smears.

The organism has not been cultivated on artificial media but it can be cultivated in the yolk sac of embryonated chicken eggs and in cell cultures.

Treatment and Control

Broad-spectrum antibiotics in the drinking water reduce losses in outbreaks in laboratory animals. The organism is also susceptible to penicillin, ampicillin, and erythromycin. The course of the disease is so short (~3 days) that treatment of clinical cases is rarely successful.

While cleaning and disinfecting, it should be kept in mind that the spores of *C. piliformes* are somewhat resistant. A temperature of 80°C will kill them in 30 minutes.

CLOSTRIDIUM DIFFICILE

This organism is responsible for pseudomembranous colitis in humans and enterocolitis in laboratory animals on prolonged antibiotic regimens. It is considered to be one probable cause of frequently fatal clostridia-associated enterocolitis of horses and hemorrhagic necrotizing enterocolitis in swine and foals. It has also been considered a possible cause of chronic diarrhea in dogs.

It is probably worldwide in occurrence. The organism is present in the intestine of some humans and animals.

Toxins

Two antigenically different toxins, A (enterotoxin) and B (cytotoxin), have been identified. Toxin B is more potent than A; both are cytotoxic and found in fecal specimens.

Laboratory Diagnosis

An ELISA is used to detect toxin in the human disease. Vast numbers of large gram-positive rods are seen in smears from intestinal content or feces. The organism is isolated on a special selective agar and identified. With pure cultures, it can be determined whether or not an isolate is a toxin producer. However, it should be kept in mind that individuals without clinical signs may be carriers of toxigenic strains. A diagnosis is based on both microbiological and pathologic findings.

Treatment and Control

Vancomycin is the preferred treatment; an alternative but less effective drug is metronamidazole. Vaccines or bacterins are not available.

OTHER CLOSTRIDIA

Clostridium spiroforme

This organism is considered to be the cause of spontaneous and antibiotic-associated diarrhea and colitis in rabbits and guinea pigs.

Clostridium sordellii

This organism has been reported to cause gas gangrene in cattle, enterotoxemia in cattle and foals, and big head (discussed earlier) in young rams.

Clostridium colinum

This species is the cause of an acute or chronic ulcerative enteritis of quail, young turkeys, grouse, partridge, and other game birds.

Clostridium sporogenes

Although ordinarily a nonpathogen, *C. sporogenes* occurs occasionally along with other bacteria in clostridial gas gangrene, causes enterotoxemia in rabbits, and is possibly involved in the causation of cerebrocortical necrosis (polioencephalomalacia) of ruminants by virtue of its production of thiaminase in the intestine and rumen.

Clostridium villosum

This organism has been isolated from fight wounds and pyothorax in cats. It is probably part of the normal oral flora of the cat.

GLOSSARY

ADP ribosylation Addition of ribose to the ADP molecule.
permease An enzyme that allows the movement of a substance into cells.

22   Mycoplasmas

Mycoplasmas are the smallest and simplest free-living organisms known. They are considered to have evolved (degenerative gene deletion) from gram-positive bacteria and are phylogenetically most closely related to clostridia. Their genomes are small, 500 to 1000 genes, and consist of a circular double-stranded deoxyribonucleic acid (DNA) molecule. They are in the class Mollicutes and include the genera listed in Table 22.1. Only species of the genera *Mycoplasma* and *Ureaplasma* are significant animal pathogens. Species of both genera require cholesterol for growth, a unique characteristic for prokaryotes, and ureaplasmas are distinctive in that they hydrolyze urea.

These organisms have no rigid cell wall and consequently are plastic and highly pleomorphic. They are bound by a limiting trilayered membrane consisting of membrane proteins, lipoproteins, and glycolipids and occur in a variety of forms including pear-shaped cells and filamentous structures. Some divide by binary fission, whereas others have a reproductive cycle, unlike conventional bacteria. In the latter case, elongated forms break up into round forms that are able to pass through a 0.15-μm filter. Most species use either glucose or arginine as their major source of energy and are nutritionally fastidious.

Some occur as commensals on mucous membranes of the upper respiratory tract and digestive tract, the genital tract, and in the bovine udder and are nonpathogenic. Some species are frankly pathogenic, and others are opportunists.

GENERAL

Structure

Mycoplasmas in Giemsa-stained smears are seen as coccobacilli, coccal forms, ring forms, and spirals. They are difficult to demonstrate in and from tissues. Coccoid forms range in size from 0.2 to 0.3 μm in diameter, and there is considerable variation in size of other forms. They can readily pass a 0.45-μm membrane filter. Dark-field and phase contrast microscopy are recommended for studying the morphology of mycoplasmas in liquid media. Shapes of cells are distorted when examinations involve smears and conventional staining.

The genome of mycoplasmas and ureaplasmas is a circular, double-stranded DNA molecule. That it has less genetic information than the genome of bacteria is indicated by its low guanine-plus-cytosine content. DNA analysis does not support the theory that the L forms of bacteria (referred to below) are related to mycoplasmas.

Some mycoplasmas, such as *Mycoplasma pneumoniae* and *Mycoplasma genitalium*, possess unique attachment organelles, shaped as a tapered tip. *Mycoplasma pneumoniae*, a human respiratory tract pathogen, adheres to the respiratory epithelium primarily through this attachment organelle.

Cultivation

Disease-producing mycoplasmas require cholesterol or related sterols for growth, and they are unable to synthesize

Table 22.1   Some Important Features of Mycoplasmas

Genus	Number of species	Require sterols	Presence of lipoglycans	Characteristics
Mycoplasma	110	+	+	Many pathogenic species; facultative anaerobes
Anaeroplasma	4	+/−	+	Found in bovine and ovine rumen; obligate anaerobes
Spiroplasma	33	+	−	Spiral-to-corkscrew-shaped cells; pathogenic for plants
Ureaplasma	6	+	−	Coccoid cells; strong urease reaction; animal and plant pathogens
Acholeplasma	16	−	+	Mainly nonpathogenic; facultative anaerobes
Asteroleptoplasma	1	−	+	Obligate anaerobe; found in bovine and ovine rumen
Entomoplasma	5	−	?	Facultative anaerobe; insect and plant pathogen
Mesoplasma	13	−	?	Ecologically and phylogenetically related to *Entomoplasma*

Note: +, positive or needed; −, negative or not required; +/−, variable; ?, not known.

purines and pyrimidines—thus the requirement for complex media. They are usually grown on media consisting of beef infusion, peptone, 20% horse serum, and yeast extract; agar is added to make a solid medium. Inhibitors of bacterial growth, which may be included, are penicillin and thallium acetate. Additives, such as mucin, may be required for the growth of some species.

Parasitic mycoplasmas contain 10%–20% lipid and possess a relatively low content of nucleic acids as compared with bacteria. Most grow aerobically, but some require nitrogen with 5%–10% CO_2. They can be grown in chicken embryos and cell cultures. In fact, they are frequent contaminants in cell cultures and may be difficult to eliminate.

Colony Morphology

After 2–6 days of aerobic incubation at 37°C, colonies on solid media are 10–600 μm in diameter. Under low-power magnification, colonies appear transparent and flat and often resemble a fried egg. The latter appearance is caused by the central growth into the agar. The growth into the agar makes it difficult to remove colonies from the agar surface.

Cell wall–defective bacterial forms produce colonies on agar that resemble those of mycoplasmas. They are referred to as L forms, or L-phase variants. They often revert to typical bacteria and are not genetically related to mycoplasmas. L forms do not require sterols for growth, and the morphologic elements in colonies are larger than those of mycoplasmas. Although their disease significance is uncertain, they may account for persistence of bacteria in tissues.

Agar cultures are transferred by pushing a block of agar, colony side down, over another plate with a glass rod. Blocks with colonies are dropped into broth. Care must be taken to obtain pure cultures.

Ureaplasmas produce smaller colonies than other mycoplasmas and, unlike the latter, they can hydrolyze urea. Interestingly, adenosine triphophate is generated through an electrochemical gradient generated by the ammonia produced during the intracellular hydrolysis of urea. Special procedures are required for the cultivation and maintenance of ureaplasmas.

Pathogenesis

The mode of infection is most frequently by inhalation. Infection may be endogenous or exogenous.

It is known that some species attach to cells by specific receptors; for a number of species, the host cell attachment is mediated by sialic acid moieties. Intimate contact with host cells is necessary for assimilation of vital nutrients, including growth factors, and nucleic acid precursors that mycoplasmas cannot synthesize. The small size and plastic nature of these organisms enable them to adapt to the shape and contours of host cell surfaces.

A high–molecular weight protein has been identified as an important adhesin. Some mycoplasmas have a predilection for infecting mesenchymal cells lining serous cavities and joints; others parasitize tissues of the respiratory tract, including the lungs. Their attachment to cells

of the respiratory tract may result in destruction of cilia predisposing to secondary bacterial infection.

Species show considerable host specificity. They are generally considered to be extracellular parasites, although there is evidence that some may also be intracellular. *Mycoplasma neurolyticum* produces a membrane-associated toxin. The fibrinous exudate frequently present in infections protects them from antibody and antimicrobial drugs and contributes to chronicity. Bacterial secondary invaders are not uncommon.

Aside from the neurotoxin of *M. neurolyticum*, the mechanisms by which mycoplasmas cause disease are poorly understood. It is thought that a galactan capsule produced by *Mycoplasma mycoides* has a pathogenic role. Cytotoxic glycoproteins and proteins have been isolated from the membranes of several species. Among the products produced during growth by some species are capsular carbohydrate, hemolysins, proteolytic enzymes, ammonia, and endonucleases. It is suggested that accumulation of mycoplasmal metabolites may contribute to cytopathic effects and tissue damage.

Infections are frequently chronic and low grade. Various stresses predispose to these infections. Experimental disease is often difficult to produce.

Pathogenicity

There are a large number of mycoplasmas (species) associated with animals. They are listed along with host and disease status in Table 22.2. The most important species causing disease in domestic animals are discussed below.

Immune Response

The immune response is predominantly humoral. As in bacterial infections, IgM and IgA are present initially, followed by IgG. IgM and IgG antibodies are mycoplasmacidal and may persist for many months. IgA antibodies are temporary; they block the adherence of mycoplasmas to host cells. Some mycoplasmas have been reported to exhibit antigenic variation of major surface protein antigens, allowing the pathogen to evade the host immune system.

Various procedures are used to detect and measure antibodies, including agglutination, agar gel precipitation, complement fixation, enzyme-linked immunosorbent assay (ELISA), and counterimmunoelectrophoresis.

AVIAN MYCOPLASMAS

The significant avian species and other species are listed below.

Mycoplasma gallisepticum (MG)

This is the primary cause of chronic respiratory disease and air sac disease of chickens, turkeys, and other fowl; infectious sinusitis of turkeys; and synovitis. MG is of major eco-

Table 22.2 Mycoplasmas and Associated Animal Diseases (Excluding Poultry)

Animal	*Mycoplasma/Ureaplasma*	Disease
Cattle	M. alkalescens	Mastitis, arthritis
	M. bovigenitalium	Mastitis, arthritis
	M. bovirhinis	Mastitis
	M. bovis	Pneumonia, various infections
	M. bovoculi	Keratoconjunctivitis
	M. californicum	Mastitis, arthritis
	M. canadense	Mastitis
	M. dispar	Mastitis, arthritis
	M. mycoides subsp. mycoides (sc)*	Contagious pleuropneumonia
	U. diversum	Vulvovaginitis, infertility, abortion
Swine	M. hyopneumoniae	Enzootic pneumonia
	M. hyorhinis	Polyserositis, arthritis
	M. hyosynoviae	Polyarthritis
Sheep	M. agalactiae	Contagious agalactia
	M. capricolum subsp. capricolum	Septicemia, pneumonia, mastitis, arthritis
	M. conjunctivae	Keratoconjunctivitis
	M. mycoides subsp. mycoides (lc)*	Pleuropneumonia, septicemia, arthritis
	M. ovipneumoniae	Pneumonia
Goats	M. agalactiae	Contagious agalactia
	M. capricolum subsp. capricolum	Septicemia, pneumonia, mastitis, arthritis
	M. capricolum subsp. carpripneumoniae	Contagious pleuropneumonia
	M. conjunctivae	Keratoconjunctivitis
	M. mycoides subsp. capri	Pleuropneumonia, septicemia, arthritis
	M. mycoides subsp. mycoides (lc)	Pleuropneumonia, septicemia, arthritis
	M. putrefaciens	Mastitis, arthritis
Horses	M. equigenitalium	Abortion
	M. felis	Pleuritis
Dogs	M. canis	Urogenital tract infections
	M. cynos	Pneumonia
	M. spumans	Arthritis
Cats	M. felis	Conjunctivitis
	M. gateae	Arthritis
Mice	M. neurolyticum	Conjunctivitis, neurological infections
	M. pulmonis	Respiratory infections
Rats	M. arthritidis	Arthritis
	M. pulmonis	Respiratory and genital tract infections

*sc = small colony; lc = large colony.

nomic importance, resulting in reduced egg production, poor growth, and death. Egg transmission is of major importance. Spread is also by direct and indirect contact.

It is beta-hemolytic, ferments a number of carbohydrates, and agglutinates chicken red cells.

Mycoplasma synoviae

This species is considered the cause of infectious synovitis of chickens and turkeys. Although all synovial membranes may be affected, the lesions involving the hock and wing joints are most apparent. *Mycoplasma synoviae* has been isolated from the respiratory tracts of normal chickens and turkeys. Transmission is by eggs, aerosol, and direct contact.

It is pathogenic for chicken embryos and ferments glucose and maltose, but not lactose, sucrose, or mannitol.

Mycoplasma meleagridis

Mycoplasma meleagridis causes airsacculitis of turkeys. Transmission is by eggs and then laterally to poults. Fomites may also contribute to spread. It is isolated from semen, vagina, bursa of Fabricius, air sacs, lungs, trachea, and sinuses. Egg hatchability may be reduced.

It is nonhemolytic and does not ferment glucose.

Mycoplasma iowae

This species is recovered from turkeys and chickens, in which it is considered a potential pathogen. It can cause exudative airsacculitis, toe and leg deformities in young poults, and decreased egg hatchability.

The following avian species are not considered pathogenic: *Mycoplasma gallinarum*, *Mycoplasma pullorum*, *Mycoplasma gallinaceum*, *Mycoplasma columbinasale*, *Mycoplasma iners*, and *Acholeplasma laidlawii*. *Mycoplasma anatis* has been associated with sinusitis in ducks.

MYCOPLASMAS OF SWINE

Mycoplasma hyorhinis

This mycoplasma causes polyserositis and arthritis in young pigs and is a secondary invader in rhinitis and pneumonia. It is frequently found in the upper respiratory tract.

Mycoplasma hyosynoviae

This mycoplasma causes arthritis in young and feeder pigs; it is frequently found in the upper respiratory tract.

Mycoplasma hyopneumoniae

Mycoplasma hyopneumoniae is the primary cause of enzootic pneumonia of swine, the most widespread pneumonic disease of swine. Ordinarily, it is a mild, chronic disease with effects mainly reflected in delayed weight gains. As a result of various stresses the pneumonia, usually complicated by *Pasteurella multocida*, can become severe.

Mycoplasma floculare

A commensal of the upper respiratory tract, which is sometimes isolated with *M. hyopneumoniae*, *M. floculare* is of low or questionable pathogenicity.

Several additional species of questionable disease significance are listed in Table 22.2.

MYCOPLASMAS OF CATTLE

Mycoplasma mycoides subsp. *mycoides* (small colony type) causes contagious bovine pleuropneumonia (CBPP), a major plague of cattle that is enzootic in parts of Africa and Asia. CBPP is a highly contagious disease characterized by septicemia, frequently followed by localization in the thorax with extensive suppurative lesions involving the lungs, pleura, and pericardium.

Like many other mycoplasmas, *M. bovis* can be found as a commensal in the respiratory and genitral tracts. It is a frequent cause of a severe mastitis, arthritis, and less frequently, genital infections. *Mycoplasma califoricum*, *Mycoplasma canadense*, and occasionally *Mycoplasma bovigenitalum* and *Mycoplasma alkalescens* have also been implicated as causes of a severe, often destructive mastitis that is difficult to treat. It occurs most frequently when management and sanitation has been lax.

Mycoplasma bovigenitalum and *Ureaplasma diversum* are commensals of the genital tract that are considered the cause of granular vulvitis and vaginitis, endometritis with reduced fertility, and on occasion, abortion; in the male, they are the cause of seminal vesiculitis.

Mycoplasma bovis is frequently isolated along with other pathogens in bovine respiratory disease. Its significance is not clear. Another respiratory commensal, *Mycoplasma dispar*, causes a mild respiratory infection in calves.

The other mycoplasmas recovered from cattle are listed in Table 22.2.

MYCOPLASMAS OF SHEEP AND GOATS

Several species of *Mycoplasma* cause important diseases of sheep and goats.

Contagious caprine pleuropneumonia (CCP) is an acute serofibrinous pleurisy and pneumonia that may involve an entire lobe. It is characterized by red and grey hepatization with characteristic hemorrhagic infarction. A severe arthritis may be a sequela of a bacteremia. CCP has been attributed to *M. mycoides* subsp. *capripneumoniae*, and *M. mycoides* subsp. *mycoides* (large colony). It occurs in Europe, Asia, and Africa, and there is evidence that it exists in the United States.

The "small colony" form of *M. mycoides* subsp. *mycoides* is the causative agent of contagious bovine pleuropneumonia, referred to earlier.

Contagious agalactia is an acute, subacute, or chronic disease of sheep and goats caused by *Mycoplasma agalactiae* (other mycoplasmas, namely, *M. mycoides* subsp. *mycoides*—large colony—and *Mycoplasma capricolum*, are claimed to cause similar syndromes). It is characterized by bacteremia (after ingestion), with localization and inflammatory activity in the udder, uterus, joints (arthritis), and eyes (conjunctivitis). There is interstitial mastitis that without treatment may lead to extensive fibrosis. Contagious agalactia occurs in Mediterranean countries and some regions of Europe, Africa, and Asia.

Polyarthritis in sheep and goats is probably the most common and geographically widespread mycoplasmosis in these species. It is most often caused by *M. capricolum*.

Mycoplasma ovipneumoniae is found as a commensal of the respiratory and genital tracts of sheep and goats. It is considered to produce primary infection in the lung that may become complicated by secondary invaders such as *Mannheimia haemolytica*.

Keratoconjunctivitis in sheep and goats is a worldwide disease caused by *Mycoplasma conjunctivae*.

M. mycoides subsp. *mycoides* (large colony) has been reported to cause epizootics in kids characterized by septicemia, polyarthritis, and pneumonia, with high morbidity and mortality rates. The organism is usually acquired from the milk of shedding females.

Other disease manifestations that have been mycoplasma-associated are enzootic pneumonia, arthritis, conjunctivitis, vulvovaginitis, infertility, and central nervous system disorders (See Table 22.2).

MYCOPLASMAS OF HORSES

A number of species have been isolated from various specimens from horses; except for *Mycoplasma felis*, they have not yet been considered pathogenic. There is convincing evidence that *M. felis*, a commensal in the equine upper respiratory tract, causes a pleuritis, which ordinarily resolves spontaneously.

MYCOPLASMAS OF DOGS

Mycoplasma cynos is considered a cause of a rapidly spreading respiratory infection involving the lungs. By itself it may have little significance, but in combination with other bacteria and viruses, it may cause a severe pneumonia. Several other species have also been associated with respiratory infections. *Mycoplasma canis* and *Mycoplasma spumans* are reported to cause canine urinary tract infections including urethritis, balanoposthitis, cystitis, vaginitis, nephritis, and endometritis.

Other species whose significance is uncertain that are recovered from the dog are *Mycoplasma maculosum*, *Mycoplasma edwardii*, *Mycoplasma molare*, and *Mycoplasma opalescens*.

MYCOPLASMAS OF CATS

Mycoplasmas occur commonly as commensals in cats. They have been recovered from a wide variety of infections but their pathogenic significance is still largely speculative. *Mycoplasma felis* is considered the cause of a mucoid conjunctivitis. *Mycoplasma gateae*, *Mycoplasma feliminutum*, and *M. felis* have been implicated in feline pneumonia. *Mycoplasma gatae* is considered a cause of polyathritis.

MYCOPLASMAS OF OTHER SPECIES

Most of the mycoplasmas that have been recovered from domestic animals, rats, mice, and guinea pigs are listed in Table 22.2.

GENERAL

Specimens

Mycoplasma are more fragile than bacteria because of the absence of a cell wall. They are readily killed by drying, sunshine, and chemical disinfection.

Their particular fragility must be considered in the submission of specimens. They should be refrigerated and delivered to the laboratory within 48 hours. Mycoplasmas in tissues can be preserved for longer periods by freezing, preferably on dry ice.

Laboratory Diagnosis

The association of a culture with a lesion is suggestive of a particular organism; for example, a mycoplasma recovered from polyserositis in a young pig would probably be *M. hyorhinis*.

The cultivation of mycoplasmas is discussed above. Definitive diagnosis is usually based on isolation and identification or detection of the mycoplasmas in tissues by a fluorescent antibody procedure. Diagnostic DNA probes and amplification of specific genomic mycoplasmal sequences by polymerase chain reaction (PCR) are currently being developed. Precise identification is sometimes difficult and may require the help of a reference laboratory. The following approaches have been used for identification

- An agglutination procedure is used to identify avian mycoplasmas and sometimes other species. Other serological procedures such as complement-fixation and ELISA have been used for antigen recognition.
- Direct and indirect fluorescent antibody staining is used to identify organisms in smears and colonies on plates.
- Growth inhibition tests: specific antisera inhibit growth of homologous immunotypes (species). Small discs containing serum are placed on inoculated agar plates. A positive test is indicated by an absence of growth around the disc. This is a particularly useful procedure, but antisera are not always available. Monoclonal antibodies are available for some species.
- Other criteria: fermentation of sugars, colony characteristics, pathogenicity, hemagglutination,

tetrazolium reduction, hemolysis; species-specific DNA probes have been developed for identification of some mycoplasmas; species-specific PCR procedures have and are being developed for identification. The growth of *Ureaplasma* is inhibited by thallium acetate.

A number of serologic procedures including complement-fixation, agar gel immunodiffusion, and ELISA are used to detect antibodies to mycoplasmas.

Treatment

Antimicrobials that are active against the cell wall are ineffective against mycoplasmas. Because in vitro susceptibility tests are difficult to perform, evidence for efficacy of drugs is based mainly on experience. Drugs that have been most effective are erythromycin, tylosin, tiamulin, azithromycin, clarithromycin, and fluorquinolones. Tetracyclines, kanamycin, gentamycin and chloramphenicol, and lincosamide are also employed. Treatment should be administered for up to 3 weeks, as response is slow. Resistance to tylosin and tetracyclines has been reported.

Control

Flocks have been established that are free of avian mycoplasmas. Chickens providing eggs must be negative to cultural and serologic procedures. Chicks and eggs are screened so that the flocks are maintained free of mycoplasmas. Dipping hatching eggs in an antibiotic solution has been effective in producing chicks free of *M. gallisepticum*.

Herds of pigs free of swine mycoplasmas and other important viral and bacterial pathogens (specific pathogen–free pigs) have been established from caesarian-delivered pigs raised in isolation.

Immunization

Cattle are vaccinated with a live attenuated *M. mycoides* subsp. *mycoides* strain to prevent contagious bovine pleuropneumonia.

Live, attenuated, and inactivated vaccines give partial protection against losses in egg production and infections caused by *M. gallisepticum*. Vaccines against enzootic pneumonia of pigs are now available commercially.

23   *Erysipelothrix* and *Bacillus*

The genus *Erysipelothrix* is included in the section "Mollicutes of The Low G + C Gram Positives." The Bacilli and Lactobacilli are in a different section of this large group of gram-positive non-spore-forming rods.

ERYSIPELOTHRIX

Erysipelothrix organisms are small, nonmotile, catalase-negative, fermentative, facultatively anaerobic rods that grow in the range of 15°–45°C.

Erysipelothrix has two species, *Erysipelothrix rhusiopathiaae* and *Erysipelothrix tonsillarum*. *Erysipelothrix rhusiopathiae* is found widely in nature, is carried by a number of animals, and is an important pathogen of mainly swine and poultry. It causes an occasional and not usually serious infection in humans called erysipeloid. *Erysipelothrix tonsillarum* closely resembles *E. rhusiopathiae* morphologically and biochemically. It has been recovered from water and the tonsils of normal swine and is not considered pathogenic. They can be differentiated by deoxyribonucleic acid (DNA) homology and biochemically.

ERYSIPELOTHRIX RHUSIOPATHIAE

Formerly *Erysipelothrix insidiosa*.

Habitat

Erysipelothrix rhusiopathiae is found on the mucous membranes of normal swine and some other animals. It may also be present in slime on bodies of freshwater and saltwater fish and crustacea. The organism lives and multiplies during the warm months in alkaline soil throughout the world. Carrier pigs are the primary reservoir of the organism.

Mode of Infection and Transmission

Erysipelas is worldwide in distribution and is acquired by direct contact with infected pigs and fomites. The mode of infection is mainly by ingestion. The organism occurs in the surface slime of freshwater and saltwater fish and consequently may be transmitted in fishmeal.

Pathogenesis and Pathogenicity

Toxins have not been demonstrated. Hyaluronidase, coagulase, and neuraminidase are produced by some strains and may be related to virulence. Neuraminidase cleaves alpha-glycosidic linkages in neuraminic acid, a mucopolysaccharide on the surface of the host's cells.

The organisms regularly invade the bloodstream, and the type of disease that develops probably depends to a considerable extent on the immune status of the individual.

SWINE. Erysipelas is **enzootic** and of considerable economic significance in certain regions. Pigs are most susceptible in the 3–18-month age range. The forms of disease include the acute form, the skin or urticarial form, the arthritic form, and the cardiac form (endocarditis). These various forms may occur separately, in a sequence, or together.

In the acute septicemic form, the course is short and the mortality is high. Reddish or purple rhomboidal blotches, scabs, and sloughing are seen in the skin form. Lesions are probably the result of thrombus formation following Arthus-type reactions (immune complexes). The arthritic form is usually seen in older pigs; it is characterized by a marked periarticular fibrosis resulting in part from an allergic reaction to the bacteria and their fragments that may persist in joints. Valvular endocarditis is seen in the cardiac form.

SHEEP. Postdipping lameness is a laminitis resulting from an extension of a focal cutaneous infection in the region of the hoof. Nonsuppurative polyarthritis is seen in lambs. The organisms gain entry via the unhealed navel and wounds. This form of the disease also may be seen in calves.

FOWL. Turkeys, chickens, ducks, geese, and many game and wild birds are susceptible. Erysipelas is an important economic disease of growing turkeys. The acute disease is characterized by septicemia, and the organism may be recovered from all tissues.

DOGS. A number of cases of valvular endocarditis have been reported in dogs. The organism may be recovered in blood cultures.

CATTLE. Infrequent occurrences of polyserositis, septicemia, and arthritis have been reported.

MARINE MAMMALS.   Serious and fatal infections are encountered in cetaceans (dolphins, porpoises) and pinnipeds (sea lions, walruses).

Specimens

ACUTE OR SEPTICEMIC FORM.   Blood and blood smears from live animals and liver, spleen, and coronary blood of necropsied animals.

CHRONIC FORM.   Affected tissues, such as heart, skin, and joint fluid. The organism may be difficult to obtain from advanced skin and joint lesions.

Isolation and Cultivation

Erysipelothrix rhusiopathiae grows readily on media enriched with serum or blood. Five percent to 10% CO_2 stimulates growth. Selective media are available to aid in the isolation of *E. rhusiopathiae* from contaminated specimens.

Two kinds of colonies are seen. Smooth colonies are small and round; rough colonies are larger, with irregular borders. Rough colonies are obtained more frequently from chronic infections. Growth is slight after 24 hours incubation but is readily apparent after 48 hours. Alpha hemolysis (greenish) is usually seen around young colonies. Gram-stained smears from smooth colonies reveal slender gram-positive rods resembling those of *Listeria* species. Smears from rough colonies disclose highly pleomorphic and filamentous forms.

Characteristic organisms can be demonstrated from the blood and tissues of infected animals.

Identification

Erysipelothrix rhusiopathiae and *E. tonsillarum* most closely resemble *Listeria* species. In contrast to *Listeria* spp., *Erysipelothrix* species are catalase and indole negative and nonmotile. Evidence of H_2S near the stab line in **TSI agar medium** is highly characteristic of *E. rhusiopathiae*. Unlike *E. rhusiopathiae*, *E. tonsillarum* is sucrose positive.

With regard to experimental animals, mice are susceptible to infection and usually die within 4 days after intraperitoneal inoculation. Guinea pigs are resistant to infection. Pigs can be infected by applying virulent organisms to scarified skin.

Antigenic Nature and Serology

Based on heat-stable somatic antigens, at least 22 different serotypes (designated 1 to 22) have been recognized using an agglutination procedure. The various serologic varieties are closely related immunologically. Serotypes 1 and 2 were recovered most frequently from tonsils and acute disease of swine. Serovar 7 is identical to *E. tonsillarum*. Serologic tests are of little value in diagnosis.

Resistance

The organism is remarkably resistant for a non-spore-former. It survives drying at room temperature for several months. Moist organisms survive for years; a broth culture remained viable for 17 years. The organism survived boiling for 2 hours in pork 6 in thick. It survives for long periods in smoked and unsmoked meats and in cadavers. Disinfectants, except for phenolic compounds, are quite effective.

Immunity

Immunity is mainly humoral. The formation of immune complexes and the occurrence of hypersensitivity reactions are responsible in part for some of the lesions seen.

Hyperimmune antierysipelas serum is no longer widely used. It is prepared in horses and cattle. It may be used therapeutically during an outbreak and to protect in-contact pigs. Protection is of short duration.

Avirulent living vaccines are widely employed. One of these is administered orally. Bacterins, usually prepared from serotype 2 and consisting of formalin-killed cultures adsorbed on alumina gels (adjuvant–slow release), are widely employed and generally protect pigs until market age. They are also of value in preventing the disease in turkeys.

Treatment

Penicillin is the drug of choice for swine and turkeys; it may be given with antiserum. The treatment of the chronic disease is ineffective, and affected animals are culled.

Public Health Significance

Erysipeloid is the name given to *E. rhusiopathiae* infection in humans. It is an occupational disease of veterinarians, packinghouse workers, butchers, and fish handlers. Cooks are occasionally infected from fish and contaminated meat and poultry. The organism usually enters via the skin (intact or broken), and after 1–5 days of incubation, a painful erythematous swelling develops at the site of entry. Infection is usually localized and most frequently involves the hand or fingers. The course is usually about 3 weeks; occasionally, severe systemic complications follow. Several cases of septicemia, valvular endocarditis, and septic arthritis have been reported. *Erysipelothrix tonsillarum* has not been recovered from humans.

Erysipeloid responds well to penicillin, erythromycin, and cephalosporins, and clindamycin is used in human patients who are allergic to penicillin.

BACILLUS

Species of the genus *Bacillus* are large, spore-forming, gram-positive rods (Fig. 23.1). They are aerobic or facultatively anaerobic, most are motile and catalase-positive, and fermentative or respiratory or both. The many species (at least 73) occur widely in the soil, air, dust, and water. They are among the most common laboratory contaminants. *Bacillus anthracis* is the only important pathogen of the genus in animals and humans. Infrequent infections

Young Culture   Older Culture

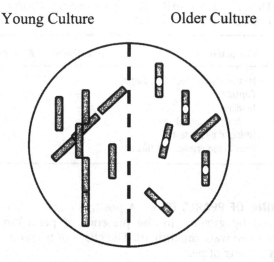

FIGURE 23.1 Morphology of *Bacillus anthracis.* The left side of the figure depicts a young culture where large bacilli can be seen, often in chains. The right side shows an older culture, with vegetative cells containing central endospores.

in animals have been attributed to *Bacillus cereus*, but animal disease caused by other species is rare.

BACILLUS ANTHRACIS

Distribution

Bacillus anthracis, in the spore form, is found worldwide. Anthrax organisms sporulate with greater frequency in low-lying marshy areas with a soil pH higher than 6. Apparently vegetative forms grow poorly, if at all, in the soil. Some regions of the Mississippi and Missouri River valleys harbor spores, and flooding disseminates them. States within the United States with regions where anthrax occurs are South Dakota, Nebraska, Arkansas, Texas, Mississippi, and California. Outbreaks and sporadic cases have occurred, however, in other locations in the United States.

Animals may become infected from contaminated soil, water, bone meal, oil cake, tankage, offal, carrion birds, and wild animals.

Pathogenesis

Typical sources of *B. anthracis* spores include contaminated soil, water, dust, hides, hair, wool, tankage, oil cake, bone meal, offal, excrement, and infected animals. In animals, the most common mode of infection is by ingestion. Infection also takes place via wounds, minor scratches and abrasions of the skin, and inhalation. Mechanical transmission of *B. anthracis* by blood-feeding insects has been reported in humans. Anthrax is not transmitted from animal to animal or from human to human.

For many years, death was attributed to the plugging of capillaries by large numbers of anthrax bacilli. Neither endotoxin nor exotoxin had been demonstrated, al-

though it was apparent that animals died of toxemia. Exotoxin subsequently was found in the plasma of dead or dying animals.

The anthrax toxin is complex, consisting of three protein components, I, II, and III. Component I is the edema factor (EF), component II the protective antigen (PA), and component III the lethal factor (LF). Each component is a thermolabile protein. Components I and II cause edema with low mortality; however, when component III is included, there is maximum lethality. Only encapsulated, toxigenic strains are virulent. The unique capsular polypeptide (poly-D-glutamic acid) is antiphagocytic, but does not elicit protective antibodies. The edema factor is an inherent adenylate cyclase, similar to the adenylate cyclase toxin of *Bordetella pertussis*.

The three components, EF, PA, and LF act synergistically to produce the toxic effects seen in anthrax.

When virulent strains are grown in media containing serum or bicarbonate or both, they produce capsules, and the colonies are smooth to mucoid. In the absence of serum or bicarbonate, they fail to produce capsules, and the colonies are rough. Virulent strains harbor two large plasmids: pX02 codes for the capsule and pX01 codes for the exotoxin.

The spores usually enter through the skin or mucous membranes and germinate at the site of entry. The vegetative cells multiply and there follows a gelatinous edema, a papule in 12–36 hours, a vesicle, then a pustule, and finally a necrotic ulcer. From this lesion there is dissemination to lymph nodes and finally the blood stream, resulting in septicemia.

Death is attributed to respiratory failure and anoxia caused by the toxin. In the more localized form, as seen in swine, the infection may principally involve the lymph nodes of the head and neck.

Large numbers of bacilli are shed from the orifices of animals during the terminal stage.

Pathogenicity

The organism is generally classed as an obligate pathogen. Acute, septicemic infections occur in cattle, sheep, goats, horses, and mules.

SWINE. The disease is usually subacute and may result in pharyngitis with extensive swelling and hemorrhages of the mouth and throat. An intestinal form with gastroenteritis also occurs. Chronic infection with localization in the tonsils and lymph nodes of the cervical region is frequent.

DOGS AND CATS. A rare infection resembling that seen in swine.

HUMANS. Depending on the portal of entry, the forms seen in humans are pulmonary or inhalation anthrax; cutaneous anthrax (malignant carbuncle or pustule), for greater than 90% of cases; and intestinal anthrax, which is analogous to the cutaneous form. The site of infection in the human cutaneous form is most often the face, neck, hands, or arms.

Specimens

To prevent sporulation, animals thought to have anthrax should not be opened. Great care should be taken when working with suspected *B. anthracis* material.

CUTANEOUS FORM. This form is frequently overlooked in animals and leads to the septicemic form; swabs, biopsies from lesions.

SEPTICEMIC FORM. Occurs in cattle, sheep, goats, horses, and possibly other species; swabs from exuded blood or blood taken by syringe. Blood smears may also be submitted.

LOCALIZED FORM. Occurs in swine; swabs from the cut surface of hemorrhagic lymph nodes or fluid aspirated from affected lymph nodes are preferred.

Direct Examination

Smears from tissues or blood are made and stained by the Gram method. If unstained central areas are seen in rods, it is advisable to do a spore stain. The finding of large, square-ended, gram-positive rods suggests the possibility of anthrax. In areas where anthrax appears periodically, M'Fadyean's polychrome methylene blue stain has been a useful rapid, presumptive diagnostic procedure. With this stain, rods appear blue surrounded by pink capsular material.

It should be kept in mind that clostridial organisms are frequently found in the blood and tissues shortly after death. They are not square-ended, lack capsules, and do not grow aerobically.

Isolation and Cultivation

If tissues are submitted, a composite suspension is prepared with a tissue grinder or mortar and pestle using sterile physiologic saline or broth as a diluent. Blood agar plates are inoculated from the suspension, blood, swabs and biopsies and incubated at 37°C.

Colonies appear in 24 hours. They look rough, flat, and grey and usually are nonhemolytic. Some are called "**Medusa-head**"–type or "judge's wig"–type colonies because the wavy edge of the colony resembles a tangled mass of curly hair. Colonies are smooth to rough. The organisms from smooth colonies possess the most capsular material. When the plasmid associated with capsule production is transferred to nonencapsulated organisms by transduction, the encapsulated phenotype is expressed.

Smears from *Bacillus* colonies disclose large, gram-positive rods, singly, in pairs, or in long chains. Unstained central areas representing spores may be seen in individual rods.

Identification

Bacillus anthracis must be distinguished from other *Bacillus* species. It resembles most closely *B. cereus*, which is found in soil worldwide. The differential characteristics listed in Table 23.1 distinguish *B. anthracis* from most strains of *B. cereus*.

Table 23.1   Differential Characteristics of *Bacillus anthracis* and *Bacillus cereus*

Characteristic	B. anthracis	B. cereus
Hemolysis on sheep blood agar	–	+
Capsule	+	–
Motility	–	+
Lysis by gamma phage	+	–
String of pearls test	+	–
Growth requirement for thiamin	+	–

STRING OF PEARLS TEST. A positive reaction is characterized by growth, in the presence of penicillin, that shows cell wall impairment. The chain of bacteria resembles a string of pearls.

BACTERIOPHAGE. A preparation of specific phage (gamma phage) is added to a diffusely inoculated plate of suspected *B. anthracis* culture. Only *B. anthracis* is lysed.

ANIMAL TESTS. These can be used for confirmation. *Bacillus anthracis* is much more pathogenic for guinea pigs and mice than *B. cereus* and other *Bacillus* species. Guinea pigs and mice are inoculated with tissue suspensions or blood. If virulent *B. anthracis* is present, the animals usually die within 24 hours; large, capsulated rods can be demonstrated in smears from the spleen and blood.

Test strips and other identification systems, available commercially, can be used to identify many of the *Bacillus* species encountered in clinical specimens.

Bacillus anthracis Genetics

As a result of recent terrorist activities, the genes of *B. anthracis* have become an area of heated investigation. Of particular importance has been the sequencing of plasmids pXO1 and pXO2, as these plasmids possess the virulence genes of the species. The virulence genes of interest have been the gene products associated with capsule production and the major exotoxins PA, LF, and EF. The remaining genes associated with these plasmids have yet to be determined.

The genes associated with capsule production are *capA*, *capB*, and *capC*. All of these genes are necessary for the production of capsule.

From the cloning and subsequent analysis of the exotoxins, it has been found that PA binds to the cell surface receptor where it ultimately facilitates the import of LF and EF into the cell. The receptor for PA is known as the anthrax toxin receptor, and the human form of the receptor has been cloned. Studies are examining the efficacy of producing a soluble form of the anthrax toxin receptor as a vaccine to inhibit the amount of exotoxins that enter cells.

Genetic analysis of the *B. anthracis* genome has led to means whereby particular strains of the bacterium could be identified. These procedures are important in the investigation of the source of anthrax-tainted materials. A procedure known as amplified fragment length polymorphism (AFLP) analysis has been used to analyze a variety of anthrax samples. AFLP is a process that begins with restriction enzyme digestion of the anthrax DNA, cutting it into smaller fragments. The cut fragments are then used in polymerase chain reaction, which amplifies particular regions of specific fragments. These amplified fragments are then separated by size by gel electrophoresis and the DNA bands visualized. This "picture" is then the "fingerprint" for that particular anthrax strain. The fingerprints of many different strains can be compared, often indicating relatedness amongst the strains.

A more recent technique used in the analysis of the anthrax genome is multiple locus variable number tandem repeat analysis (MLVA). MLVA is an improvement over AFLP in that it provides a very detailed genetic fingerprint. MLVA recognizes repeated DNA sequences next to each other in the genome. For example, ACTTACCAG ACTTACCAG ACTTACCAG ACTTACCAG ACTTACCAG has five tandem repeats of the sequence ACTTACCAG that could be recognized. These regions are identified using a set of markers that occur on either side of the repeat. This could be illustrated as (M = marker)

M1 − ACTTACCAG ACTTACCAG ACTTACCAG
ACTTACCAG ACTTACCAG − M2

Originally, the markers used in the analysis came from what was known from AFLP data. Subsequently, other markers have been identified. If two strains of anthrax look identical by AFLP, they can be further examined by MLVA to see whether there are any differences not detected by AFLP. The combination of these two genetic procedures is very powerful and yields a very specific fingerprint. All of the fingerprints collected to date are kept in a large database for reference.

Immunity

Recovered animals have permanent immunity.

Strains are considered to be antigenically identical. The polypeptide capsule is antiphagocytic but does not stimulate protective antibodies. Protective immunity is thought to be largely antitoxic.

Enzyme-linked immune assays (such as ELISA) for PA, LF, and EF are used to confirm anthrax infection and monitor antibody responses in epidemiological and other studies.

Treatment

Sick animals should be treated, and uninfected animals should be immunized. The organism is susceptible to many antibiotics; penicillin and tetracyclines are most frequently used to treat animals. Treatment in humans is effective in the cutaneous infection but not usually in the pulmonary form. Ciprofloxacin, doxycycline, and penicillin are the drugs most commonly used to treat human anthrax. Natural strains appear to be uniformly susceptible to the aforementioned drugs. Early treatment is essential.

Prevention and Control

In most states and countries, all suspected cases of anthrax must be reported to government veterinary officials.

IMMUNIZATION. Sterne's live, noncapsulated, avirulent spore vaccine gives good protection and is widely used to protect animals.

A vaccine consisting of protective antigen from a culture filtrate of an avirulent, nonencapsulated strain has been used to protect U.S. military personnel and others at risk. Multiple doses are given, and an annual booster is required.

RESISTANCE. The endospores of *B. anthracis* are highly resistant to physical influences and chemical disinfectants. They may survive at least two to three decades in dried cultures. They remain viable in soil for many years, and freezing temperatures have little, if any, effect on them. They are destroyed, however, by boiling for 30 minutes and by exposure to dry heat at 140°C for 3 hours.

When used, most chemical disinfectants must be employed in high concentrations over long periods of time. Spores are destroyed by lye in 8 hours; by 5% phenol in 2 days; by 10%–20% formalin in 10 minutes; and by autoclaving at 121°C for 15 minutes. Mercuric chloride 1:1000 added to heat-fixed smears kills in 5 minutes. Wool, hides, and horsehair from areas where anthrax occurs should be gas (e.g., chlorine dioxide, formaldehyde) sterilized. Spores are killed by a 0.05% sodium hypochlorite solution.

Cremation or deep burial (at least 6 ft) in lime (calcium oxide) is recommended for disposal of animal carcasses.

Public Health Significance

Some sources of spores for humans are soil, hair, hides, wool (wool sorter's disease), feces, milk, meat (inadequately cooked), and blood products. The disease is seen most frequently in farmers, herdsmen, butchers, and veterinarians and in wool, tannery, and slaughterhouse workers.

Necropsies on animals should be performed with particular care if anthrax is suspected. Human infections most often result from spores entering injuries to the skin. Cutaneous anthrax (malignant pustule) accounts for more than 95% of the human disease. The skin lesion is usually solitary, painless, seropurulent, necrotizing and hemorrhagic, and ulcerous. It leaves a black eschar, which accounts for the name malignant pustule. Pulmonary anthrax resulting from the inhalation of spores is almost always fatal. Following germination of the spores there is pulmonary necrosis, septicemia, and meningitis.

Failure to diagnose human anthrax correctly and treat it adequately can result in death.

ADDITIONAL *BACILLUS* SPECIES

Bacillus cereus has been incriminated as a cause of gangrenous bovine mastitis and abortion in cows and ewes. In humans, it has been implicated in food poisoning. Spores germinate in various foods, including fried rice, meats, desserts, sauces, and soups, where an enterotoxin or emetic toxin may be produced. Two syndromes, the emetic and the diarrheal, are seen. The emetic type is caused by a heat-stable toxin, and the diarrheal form by a heat-labile toxin. *Bacillus cereus* has also been implicated in a number of human infections, usually in immune compromised patients.

Bacillus subtilis is claimed to cause occasional conjunctivitis, **iridocyclitis**, septicemia, endocarditis, respiratory infections, and food poisoning in humans.

Bacillus licheniformis has been implicated as an infrequent cause of bovine, ovine, and porcine abortions. It occasionally causes septicemia, peritonitis, and food poisoning in humans.

Bacillus stearothermophilus spores are used to test the efficacy of autoclaving and other sterilizing procedures.

Bacillus thuringiensis contains a crystalline toxin and is thus pathogenic for *Leptidoptera* larvae. It is currently being investigated for potential use in insecticide development.

GLOSSARY

enzootic Present in a district or region at all times.
iridocyclitis Inflammation of the iris and ciliary body.
Medusa-head From Greek mythology: one of the Gorgons with snakes for hair.
TSI agar medium Bacteriological medium, triple sugar iron agar, used mainly for preliminary screening of enterobacteria.

24 *Streptococcus*

The streptococci are a large (at least 68 species), heterogeneous group that occurs widely in nature and also as members of the normal flora of man and animals. They are gram-positive, nonmotile, non-spore-forming cocci that occur singly, in pairs, or in chains. A relatively small number of species cause important diseases in animals and humans. They are facultatively anaerobic, fermentative, and catalase- and oxidase-negative. Potentially pathogenic and nonpathogenic species may be present on the skin and on the mucous membranes of the genital, upper respiratory, and digestive tracts.

STRUCTURE AND COMPOSITION

Freshly isolated group A and C strains of streptococci have a hyaluronic acid capsule that, although nonantigenic, interferes with phagocytosis (see Fig. 24.1). Under the capsule is the cell wall, consisting of a mosaic of proteins, peptidoglycan, and the group-specific carbohydrate.

The most important protein is the M protein, which is responsible for virulence. The more than 70 types of *Streptococcus pyogenes* are based on serological differences in the M protein. This important protein is responsible for type-specific immunity, inhibits phagocytosis, and has an immunotoxic effect on polymorphs and platelets. The peptidoglycan group–specific carbohydrate complex makes up the remainder of the cell wall.

Another component of the cell wall is lipoteichoic acid. The hairlike fimbrae that extend through the cell wall and hyaluronic acid to the outside of the cell are composed of lipoteichoic acid and M protein. The fimbrae are involved in the attachment of streptococci to epithelial cells.

EXTRACELLULAR PRODUCTS

Group A streptococci produce more than 20 extracellular products. No doubt many of these are produced by pyogenic animal streptococci. Some of the better known products follow.

Hemolysins

Streptolysins O and S are responsible for beta-hemolysis; each is produced under certain conditions. Antibody to

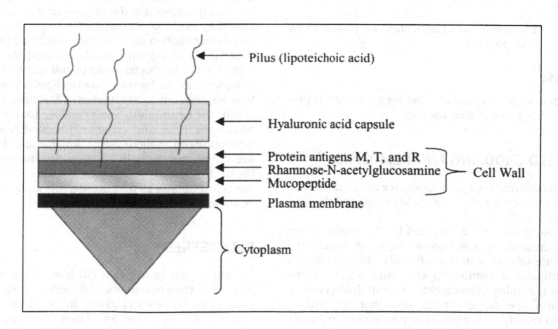

FIGURE 24.1   Structure of a typical group A *Streptococcus* cell.

streptolysin O is a good indicator of present or past infection. Streptolysin O is oxygen sensitive, but streptolysin S is not; both are toxic for neutrophils and macrophages. Streptolysin O, a protein, elicits neutralizing antibodies, whereas streptolysin S, a peptide, is nonantigenic.

Streptokinase (Fibrinolysin)

This enzyme activates plasminogens to become plasmin (protease), thus leading to the digestion of fibrin clots. This process prevents the buildup of fibrin clots that may contain and protect organisms. Several antigenically distinct forms exist. It elicits neutralizing antibodies in many streptococcal infections.

DNases A, B, C, and D (Streptodornase)

These extracellular enzymes assist in the production of substrates for growth. Antibody to DNase B is used in the serodiagnosis of group A human infections. These enzymes reduce the viscosity of fluid containing DNA. Streptococcal pus may be thin because of this enzyme. In addition, DNases B and D are ribonucleases.

Hyaluronidase

A correlation probably exists between the production of this enzyme and virulence, as seen in streptococcal cellulitis. Hyaluronidase promotes the spread of infection in tissues. Convalescent serum is rich in neutralizing antibodies.

Erythrogenic Toxins (Types A, B, and C)

These are low–molecular weight proteins. One of the group A erythrogenic toxins is responsible for the rash in scarlet fever.

NADases

These enzymes, which kill phagocytes, are produced by some group A streptococci.

Proteinase

This enzyme, which has broad substrate specificity, is produced by some group A streptococci.

LANCEFIELD GROUPING AND HEMOLYSIS

Two characteristics of major importance in the identification of streptococci are the Lancefield groups and the kind of hemolysis produced.

Lancefield groups are designated by the capital letters A–U. This grouping is based on serologic differences in a carbohydrate substance in the cell wall called component C. The antigenic determinants are amino sugars. A precipitin test is employed using extracts containing component C and specific grouping sera that are usually prepared in rabbits. Other serologic procedures, including latex agglutination, coagglutination, and fluorescent antibody tests are also used to identify Lancefield groups.

Some of the Lancefield groups may be further divided into serotypes by means of the agglutination test. These serotypes are based on serologic differences in the M protein, which are responsible for type-specific immunity. There are at least 60 serotypes of group A *Streptococcus pyogenes*; in contrast there is only one serotype of *Streptococcus equi*. Serotypes are designated by Arabic numbers.

The type of hemolysis is also of importance in identification:

- Alpha-hemolysis: Partial hemolysis, often revealed as a zone of green discoloration around the colony; hemolysis with an inner zone of unhemolyzed cells.
- Beta-hemolysis: Clear, colorless zone caused by complete hemolysis.
- Gamma-hemolysis: No detectable hemolysis.
- Alpha-prime-hemolysis: A small zone of partially lysed red blood cells (RBCs) lying adjacent to the colony, followed by a zone of completely lysed RBCs extending farther into the medium. It can be confused easily with beta hemolysis.

MODE OF INFECTION AND TRANSMISSION

Infections may be endogenous or exogenous. Exogenous infections are usually acquired by inhalation or ingestion. Aerosol, direct contact, or fomites are the most common modes of spread. Carriers and infected subjects are the important reservoirs of *S. equi* and *S. pyogenes*.

PYOGENIC INFECTIONS IN GENERAL

Some species of staphylococci and streptococci, for example, *S. equi*, are termed pyogenic because they elicit a response characterized by pus. When pyogenic bacteria invade a tissue, such as the mucous membrane of the pharynx, they evoke an inflammatory response characterized by vascular dilation and a marked exudation of plasma and neutrophils. In response to chemotaxis, the neutrophils move toward the bacteria and engulf many of them. After phagocytosis, the bacteria may be digested, but some bacteria are resistant to the lysosomal enzymes and multiply within the neutrophils. Some produce toxins that kill the phagocytic cells, and enzymes liberated from the dead neutrophils bring about partial liquefaction of the dead tissue and phagocytic cells. The liquefied mass becomes visible as thick, usually yellow, pus. The viscous consistency of pus is attributable to the considerable amount of deoxyribonucleoprotein from the nuclei of dead cells.

PATHOGENESIS

Various disease processes result from streptococcal infections, and their development depends on various factors, such as portal of entry, tissue involved, animal species, and streptococcal species. Three diseases, illustrating somewhat different pathogeneses, are strangles of horses, jowl abscesses of swine, and streptococcal arthritis. Although usually localized, streptococcal infections may become bacteremic or septicemic, resulting in foci of infection in various locations or death. As in many microbial diseases, the severity of the infection depends on the immune status of the animal.

Surface M protein and, to a lesser degree, surface hyaluronic acid are considered to be major virulence factors in streptococci. The capacity of streptococci to spread within tissue and cause damage results at least partially from DNase, hyaluronidase, streptolysins O and S, NADase, M protein, leukotoxins, and cell wall mucopeptide complex.

Protein X, a surface protein of *Streptococcus agalactiae*, is frequently associated with strains recovered from cases of bovine mastitis. This protein behaves as a target of opsonins and, therefore, is possibly an important protective antigen against *S. agalactiae* mastitis. Bovine complement S (vitronectin) is thought to be important in the adherence of *S. agalactiae* to bovine epithelial cells.

PATHOGENICITY

Streptococcus pyogenes

This strain of group A, with more than 80 serotypes, is the principal cause of streptococcal disease in humans, including pharyngitis, scarlet fever (pharyngitis with skin rash), puerperal fever, rheumatic fever, glomerulonephritis, and toxic shock syndrome. It rarely causes bovine mastitis, but when it does, there is the potential of spread to humans via milk. It occasionally causes lymphangitis in foals and various infections in dogs and cats.

Streptococcus agalactiae

This strain of group B, with five serotypes, and *Staphylococcus aureus* are the most important and frequent causes of bovine mastitis. *Streptococcus agalactiae* is an obligate pathogen that can be eliminated from herds. Infection is spread by the milker's hands or by contaminated teat cups. *Streptococcus agalactiae* also causes mastitis in sheep and goats.

A different variety of *S. agalactiae* causes septicemia, meningitis, and pneumonia that can be fatal in newborn infants. This streptococcus is carried by about one-third of pregnant women as part of the flora of the intestine or the vagina. This variety of *S. agalactiae* has been associated with several canine neonatal deaths and kidney and uterine infections in cats.

Streptococcus dysgalactiae

This variety of group C, with three serotypes, is an important cause of bovine mastitis and polyarthritis of lambs.

Streptococcus equisimilis (Proposed Name, S. dysgalactiae subsp. equisimilis)

A member of group C, with eight serotypes, it is occasionally recovered with *S. equi* from strangles, wound infec-

tions, genital infections, and mastitis in the mare; it is also the cause of various infections in swine, cattle, dog, and fowl and a rare cause of human infections.

Streptococcus equi (Proposed Name, S. equi, subsp. equi)

A variety of group C, with one serotype, it is the cause of strangles and other infections of the horse and of genital and udder infections in the mare. Strangles is an acute contagious disease of young equidae. It begins as a rhinitis and pharyngitis and progresses to abscesses, particularly in the intermandibular and parapharyngeal lymph nodes. Rarely the disease becomes generalized terminating in death. Bastard srangles is a very severe chronic form with disseminated abscesses.

Streptococcus zooepidemicus (Proposed Name, S. equi subsp. zooepidemicus)

Belonging to group C, with 15 serotypes, it is the primary cause of genital infections in the mare, epididymitis in stallions, and navel infections in foals. It causes cervicitis, metritis, and mastitis in cattle; arthritis, abortion, and septicemia in swine; fibrinous pleuritis, pericarditis, and pneumonia in lambs; mastitis in goats; and fatal septicemia in chickens.

Streptococcus canis

This member of group G causes miscellaneous pyogenic infections in dogs and cats. Canine streptococcal shock syndrome is considered to be caused by the toxins of *S. canis*. It is thought to be initiated by minor trauma followed by local cellulitis, then progressing to shock and necrotizing fasciculitis.

Streptococcus bovis

It occurs in the alimentary tract of ruminants. A member of group D, it has been recognized as a probable cause of lactic acidosis and other gastric disorders in ruminants and infrequent bovine mastitis. In humans *S. bovis* causes endocarditis and meningitis and is recovered from the blood of patients with colon cancer. The human strains of *S. bovis* can be distinguished from the animal isolates.

Streptococcus equines

This group D strain occurs in the alimentary tract of horses.

Group E

This group has a number of serotypes that cause cervical lymphadenitis (jowl abscesses) in swine. This disease, mainly of feeder swine, is characterized by the development of one or more heavily encapsulated abscesses involving the cervical lymph nodes. Infrequent human pyogenic wound infections have been attributed to group E streptococci.

Streptococcus suis

These are strains of groups S (type 1), R (type 2), T, and ungroupable strains. Type 1 causes polyarthritis and meningitis in suckling pigs. Type 2 strains cause acute and often fatal meningitis, polyarthritis, endocarditis, myocarditis, genital infections, and abortion in sows and meningitis, arthritis, septicemia, diarrhea, and deafness in humans.

Streptococcus uberis

Serologically heterogeneous, *S. uberis* causes bovine mastitis and is found in the vagina and tonsils of cattle.

Streptococcus porcinus

It causes abscesses of mandibular, pharyngeal, and other lymph nodes in pigs and infrequent human infections. *Streptococcus porcinus* is serologically heterogeneous (some strains belong to Group E), resistant to bacitracin, and CAMP positive.

Streptococcus iniae

A pathogen of fish that occasionally causes endocarditis, cellulitis, menigintis, and bacteremia in fish handlers; its strains are not groupable.

Streptococcus pneumoniae

Formerly known as *Diplococcus pneumoniae*, this species is not groupable but resembles the other streptococci, except that it occurs principally as pairs of cocci rather than as chains. It includes more than 80 serotypes that are identified on the basis of serologic differences in the polysaccharide capsular antigen. It is found as a commensal in the upper respiratory tract of humans and, less commonly, of animals.

Most of the human infections are caused by fewer than 10 different serotypes. Lobar pneumonia, empyema, sinusitis, and conjunctivitis are among the important diseases caused by *S. pneumoniae* in humans. Unless eradicated, it is an important cause of pneumonia in guinea pig colonies. It has been implicated infrequently in respiratory infections in calves, horses, dogs, goats, monkeys, rabbits, and rats. There are several reports of bovine mastitis caused by pneumococci; septicemia and septic arthritis have been reported in the domestic cat.

Viridans Streptococci

Usually not groupable, these are frequent commensals of the oropharynx and female genital tract that are often isolated from clinical specimens from animals and humans. Although not often pathogenic in animals, they are a significant cause of endocarditis, abscesses, and opportunistic infections in humans. A number of species have been described.

Enterococcus faecalis, Enterococcus faecium, and Enterococcus durans

Formerly known as *Streptococcus faecalis, Streptococcus faecium,* and *Streptococcus durans*, these *Enterococcus* spp. are common inhabitants of the intestinal tract of animals and humans. *Enterococcus faecalis* may cause urinary infections in various animals and endocarditis in chickens.

Lactococcus lactis

Formerly known as *Streptococcus lactis*, *L. lactis* is present in milk and dairy products.

Former Streptococci

The bacteria formerly referred to as "anaerobic streptococci" and those referred to formerly as "nutritionally variant streptococci" are no longer included in the *Streptococcus* genus. They are now included in the genus *Abiotrophia*.

IMMUNITY

Animals infected with streptococci often develop a hypersensitivity of the delayed type. The role of this reaction in streptococcal disease is not known. It has been suggested that immune complexes may be responsible for **purpura hemorrhagica** in the horse after *S. equi* infection. Immunity to streptococcal infections is considered to be primarily humoral. Protection is type specific and considered to depend upon antibodies to M protein.

GENERAL

Specimens

These vary with the disease. Among the infectious materials submitted are pus (strangles, abscesses), joint fluid (arthritis), milk (mastitis), organs and blood (septicemia), and meningeal swabs and cerebral spinal fluid (meningitis).

Laboratory Diagnosis

Gram-positive cocci, singly or in chains, can be demonstrated in smears from clinical specimens. The pathogenic strains grow best on serum or blood-enriched media; blood agar is preferred. Colonies vary from large to small in size and are round, smooth, and glistening, looking somewhat like dewdrops. Hemolysis may or may not be present. Colony varieties are mucoid (hyaluronic acid), matt (much M protein, virulent), and glossy (little M protein, low virulence).

Many, but by no means all, streptococci that cause infections are beta-hemolytic. To save time, susceptibility tests may be conducted while identification is pending. It is not always feasible to make a definitive identification.

Identification is based on some of the following criteria:

- Hemolysis.
- Lancefield group: Several methods are used including the original Extraction Method, the Latex Agglutination Test, and the Slide Coagglutination Test. The latter two are available as commercial kits.
- Discs containing bacitracin inhibit the growth of *S. pyogenes* on blood agar. The test is not totally reliable.
- Edward's medium containing esculin, crystal violet, and thallium acetate is used for the rapid presumptive identification of the important mastitis streptococci. It inhibits gram-negative bacteria and staphylococci.
- The CAMP test may be used for the presumptive identification of *S. agalactiae*. It involves the completion of the partial hemolysis (beta toxin zone) of *S. aureus* when *S. agalactiae* is streaked at right angles to the *Staphylococcus* streak on blood agar (Fig. 24.2).
- *Streptococcus porcinus* and *S. iniae* give positive CAMP reactions.
- The CAMP test may be conducted in a medium that contains beta toxin of *S. aureus* to screen for *S. agalactiae*. The incorporation of esculin into the medium makes possible the presumptive recognition of *S. agalactiae*, *S. dysgalactiae*, and *S. uberis*.
- Group B streptococci hydrolyse sodium hippurate.
- Nucleic acid–based probes are available for the identification of isolates of group A and B isolates.

Streptococcus pneumoniae grows well on blood agar. It appears as small round colonies with elevated edges and is alpha-hemolytic. It is gram-positive, and paired cocci are seen in stained smears. It is bile soluble and inhibited by **optochin**. Nucleic acid probes are available for the identification of pneumococcal isolates.

The identification of many streptococcal species is described in detail in Murray et al. (Murray PR et al., *Manual of Clinical Microbiology*, 7th ed. ASM Press, Washington, D.C., 1999).

Treatment

Penicillin is the drug of choice for the treatment of most streptococcal infections. Alternative agents are erythromycin, cephalosporins, lincomycin, and vancomycin. Penicillin resistance occurs with viridans streptococci and enterococci. The latter are usually susceptible to ampicillin or a trimethoprim-sulfonamide. Penicillin is recommended for pneumococcal infections, although resistance has been reported.

The incidence of cervical lymphadenitis is swine has been markedly reduced by the addition of tetracyclines to feed. Penicillin is the preferred drug for the treatment of strangles in horses; alternative drugs are trimethoprim-sulfonamide and ceftiofur. Treatment should be started early and continued past the febrile stage. Bastard strangles (disseminated with abscesses) has been attributed to inadequate treatment. Penicillin has been effective in the treatment of streptococcal mastitis.

Prevention and Control

An *S. equi* bacterin is available to prevent strangles, although it must be used with care because severe local reactions sometimes occur. A vaccine consisting of predominantly M protein has been developed to reduce undesirable reactions. A modified-live intranasal vaccine is also available.

A live attenuated strain of group E *Streptococcus* is used to vaccinate pigs against jowl abscesses. Group E bacterins are reported to be effective.

None of the pathogenic streptococci is particularly resistant to the usual chemical disinfectants. Many species survive for weeks in soil, clothing, bedding, food, stalls, milking machines, and milk containers.

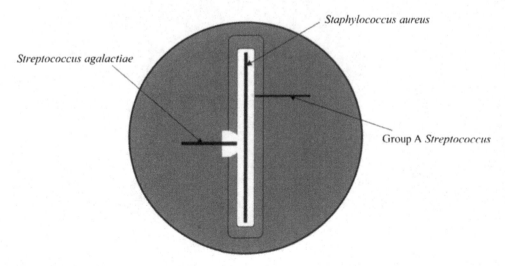

Staphylococcus aureus

Streptococcus agalactiae

Group A *Streptococcus*

FIGURE 24.2 CAMP test. The large central streak of *Staphylococcus aureus* is surrounded by a narrow zone of hydrolysis (clear zone). Around this zone is a region of partial hemolysis, where the integrity of the red blood cells within the agar is compromised (indicated by the region with small dots). Perpendicular to this, a streak of *Streptococcus agalactiae* is to the left and a group A *Streptococcus* streak is to the right. As *S. agalactiae* produces the CAMP factor, a characteristic arrowhead indicates complete lysis of the red blood cells in this area (clear zone). In contrast, the group A *Streptococcus* does not produce a zone of hydrolysis and is therefore negative for the CAMP factor.

Public Health Significance

Streptococcus pyogenes (group A) may infect the bovine udder and be spread to humans via milk. As was stated previously under Pathogenicity, a number of pathogenic animal streptococci may cause infrequent humans human infections.

GLOSSARY

optochin Ethylhydrocuprein that strongly inhibits the growth of *S. pneumoniae* but not certain streptococci whose colonies resemble the pneumococcus.

purpura hemorrhagica Condition in horses, as a sequella of strangles, mediated by immune complexes of antibody and streptococcal antigen in vascular basement membranes.

25   *Listeria*

The genus *Listeria* (eight species) is placed taxonomically between streptococcus/enterococcus and staphylococcus. They are small, motile (at 25°C), gram-positive rods that are catalase positive, oxidase negative, facultatively anaerobic, fermentative, and non-spore-forming. *Listeria* spp. occur widely in the environment. They are found in soil and are saprophytes in decaying vegetable matter. Their optimum temperature for growth is in the range of 20°–45°C.

For decades after its discovery, *Listeria monocytogenes* was the only species recognized. At present, two lines of descent are recognized. One includes the following species:

- *Listeria monocytogenes:* This is the principal pathogen of the genus for animals and humans.
- *Listeria ivanovii:* This is the only species other than *L. monocytogenes* that is naturally pathogenic for animals. It can cause abortion in sheep and cattle. Little is known at present about the extent of infections caused by this species. There is a carrier state in normal animals. A subspecies of *L. ivanovii, londoniensis,* has been described.
- *Listeria innocua, Listeria welshimeri,* and *Listeria seeligeri:* These species have been recovered from soil, decaying vegetation, and animal feces.

The other line of descent includes only one species, *Listeria grayi* (identical to *Listeria murrayi*). This species is nonpathogenic and rarely isolated.

LISTERIA MONOCYTOGENES

Habitat

As indicated above, *Listeria* spp. are widely distributed in the environment. *Listeria monocytogenes* has been recovered from feces (many enteric carriers), genital secretions, and nasal mucus of apparently healthy animals. Its presence in silage is particularly important. Organisms multiply when the pH of silage rises above 5.5.

Of particular importance to human disease is the occurrence of *L. monocytogenes* in poultry, meats, dairy products, and fresh and frozen foods.

Mode of Infection

The modes of infection of the neural and visceral forms are different. In the neural form, infection is via branches of the trigeminal nerve and the eye, nose, and oropharynx. In the visceral form, ingestion is the mode of infection. Most infections are thought to be exogenous.

Pathogenicity

The disease is called listeriosis, and the neural form is sometimes called "circling disease." The neural form of the disease is most common in ruminants. It is seen in cattle and sheep, particularly in winter and early spring; all ages are susceptible. Outbreaks occur in feedlots. The occurrence of the disease has been associated with feeding of silage that may contain large numbers of *L. monocytogenes*. An increase in iron consumption resulting from eating silage is thought to contribute to listeriosis. Central nervous system signs include unilateral ataxia and meningitis. Microabscesses are found, principally involving the brain stem.

Keratoconjunctivitis and ophthalmitis have been described in cattle and sheep.

Abortions occur in cows and ewes, but without the neural manifestations of the disease. The organism can be recovered from the aborted fetus and uterus. Equine abortion caused by *L. monocytogenes* has been reported.

The neural form of the disease occurs in the horse but is infrequent. Both the neural and abortion forms have been reported in llamas.

In chickens and turkeys, listeriosis usually takes a septicemic form. Necrotic foci of the liver and myocardium are seen. The neural form of listeriosis has been reported in broiler chickens.

A visceral or septicemic form of the disease with liver necrosis is seen in the rabbit, guinea pig, chinchilla, reindeer, antelope, and other species. Several cases of neural listeriosis have been encountered in the dog.

Pathogenesis

Listeria monocytogenes is a facultative intracellular parasite. The following is a brief summary of processes relating to its intracellular survival.

- The cell wall surface protein internalin interacts with the protein E-cadherin, a receptor on epithelial cells, facilitating phagocytosis into phagocytic and nonphagocytic cells.
- After phagocytosis, the bacterium is enclosed in a phagosome, where it produces the hemolysin listeriolysin O (a thiol-activated cytolysin that can

lyse the cholesterol-containing membranes of eukaryotic cells), which lyses the membrane of the phagosome and allows the bacteria to escape into the cytoplasm of the host cell.

- Bacteria proliferate and induce polymerization of host cell actin (a component of the host cell cytoskeleton on the bacterial surface), which moves them to the cell membrane (actin-based motility), where they push against the cell membrane and form protrusions called filopods.
- The filopods are ingested by adjacent macrophages and other cells. The listeria are released, and the cycle takes place again.

The use of host cell actin to spread infection is also applied by some other bacteria and rickettsia.

Listeriolysin O, referred to above, is considered a major virulence factor, although a similar hemolysin is produced by the nonpathogenic species *L. seeligeri* and the infrequent pathogen *L. ivanovii*.

The neural form of the disease is seen most frequently in ruminants. The visceral form is seen most often in monogastric animals, and spread appears to be hematogenous after ingestion. Organisms are intracellular (macro-phages and other cells) in both forms. As with some intracellular bacteria, a granulomatous reaction occurs, which in the visceral disease leads to focal areas of necrosis in the liver.

Specimens

For the neural form, specimens should be the pons and medulla; for the visceral form, portions of affected organs and particularly the liver; and for abortion, the fetus and fetal membranes.

Isolation and Cultivation

The organism is frequently difficult to recover from the brain in neural listeriosis, presumably because the organisms are intracellular and present in small numbers. If no growth is obtained initially, ground brain stored at refrigerator temperature ("cold enrichment") should be recultured weekly for as many as 12 weeks before it is discarded as negative. The organism is able to grow at refrigerator temperatures; thus the value of cold enrichment. *Listeria monocytogenes* is more difficult to recover from the bovine brain, where the number of organisms is fewer than in the sheep and goat brain. Cultural procedures may be indicated by the finding of microscopic lesions characteristic of listeriosis in the brain or brain stem.

The organism grows well on ordinary media but is routinely isolated on blood agar. Primary growth is stimulated by 5%–10% carbon dioxide. Smooth colonies are approximately 2 mm in diameter, round, entire, glistening, and bluish by transmitted light; narrow zones of beta-hemolysis are evident. Small, gram-positive rods occurring singly, in pairs, or in short chains are seen in stained smears. Morphologically, they may resemble some diphtheroids and streptococci.

Identification

Listeria monocytogenes is motile at room temperature, catalase positive, and oxidase negative. Motility can be seen in wet mounts (tumbling motility) and in subsurface growth (umbrella-shaped growth) in semisolid motility medium. *Listeria monocytogenes*, *L. ivanovii*, and *L. seeligeri* are beta-hemolytic. Fermentation of several carbohydrates is used with other characteristics in the differentiation of species (Table 25.1)

Listeria monocytogenes monoclonal antibodies have made possible an effective fluorescent conjugate for use with food specimens and cultures. It is not suitable for clinical specimens. Several DNA probes have been developed to detect *L. monocytogenes* in enrichment cultures of foods. Identification of *L. monocytogenes* is particularly important, as all species can contaminate foods.

The CAMP test (see Chapter 24, *Streptococcus*) is helpful in the differentiation of *Listeria* spp.; however, there are occasional variations in reactions. The usual results with the CAMP tests are as follows:

Table 25.1   Differentiation of Some *Listeria* Species

Biochemical Characteristic	L. monocytogenes	L. ivanovii	L. grayi	L. innocua	L. seeligeri	L. welshimeri
Beta-hemolysis	+	+	−	−	+	−
CAMP reaction						
Staphylococcus aureus	+	−	−	−	+	−
Rhodococcus equi	V	+	−	−	−	−
Acid produced from						
Mannitol	−	−	+	−	−	−
Rhamnose	+	−	V	V	−	V
Xylose	−	+	−	−	+	+
Ribose	−	+	V	−	−	−
Hippurate hydrolysis	+	+	−	+	ND	ND
Reduction of nitrate	−	−	V	−	ND	ND

Note: +, ~90% positive; −, ~90% negative; V, variable; ND, no data.

- With *Staphylococcus aureus* streak. Negative: *L. innocua*, *L. ivanovii*, *L. welshimeri*, and *L. grayi*. Positive: *L. monocytogenes* and *L. seeligeri*.
- With *Rhodococcus equi* streak. Negative: *L. grayi* and *L. welshimeri*. Positive: *L. ivanovii*.

Commercial kits consisting of miniaturized biochemical tests are available for the identification of *Listeria* spp.

Listeria monocytogenes and *L. ivanovii* are pathogenic for mice and other experimental animals, but animal inoculations are not routinely used in diagnosis.

Antigenic Nature and Serology

Sixteen serotypes of *Listeria* have been identified on the basis of somatic (O) and flagellar (H) antigens. They bear no relation to the host species, except for serovar 5 (*L. ivanovii*). Serotype 4b is the predominant strain in Canada and the United States. Most infections are caused by three serotypes: 1/2a, 1/2b, and 4b. Numbers indicate O antigens, and letters indicate H antigens. Serologic tests are carried out in reference laboratories.

Resistance

Pasteurization (62°C for 30 minutes; 71.6°C for 15–30 seconds) destroys *L. monocytogenes*. It is remarkably resistant to drying; it can survive for months in food, straw, soil, and shavings; and is susceptible to common disinfectants.

Immunity

For the most part, immunity depends on the T-cell-mediated activation of macrophages by lymphokines, particularly gamma-delta T cells. The role of the humoral response is not clear. However, limited studies in mice report a predominance of IgA and IgG1 antibodies in response to gut infections. Immunization has not been widely practiced.

Autogenous bacterins have given inconclusive results. As the immunity in listeriosis is mainly cellular, live attenuated vaccines may be of value. A live attenuated vaccine has been used successfully to prevent listeriosis in sheep.

Public Health Significance

The possible sources for human infections are soil (contaminated dust), contaminated dairy products, meat, fruits, vegetables, and animal and human (genital and enteric) carriers.

Infections in humans frequently involve immunocompromised and immunologically immature individuals (infants); thus, contributing factors may be other underlying diseases, for example, HIV infection, the use of corticosteroids, and radiation therapy.

Listeria monocytogenes causes bacteremia, meningitis and encephalitis, and occasionally valvular endocarditis. Perinatal infections include uterine infections with abortion, stillbirths, and a neonatal septicemic form called granulomatosis infantiseptica.

Several cases of bovine mastitis caused by this organism have been reported. Unpasteurized cow's milk yielding the organism is a potential source of human infections.

Treatment

Treatment is usually of little value, particularly in sheep and goats, after neurologic signs are seen. The drugs of choice are chloramphenicol and the tetracycline antibiotics, given at maximum dosage. Cephalosporins are not recommended because of their limited penetration of the meninges. Treatment may be of some value in cattle, but relapses may occur. Sulfonamides, penicillin, and tetracyclines may be used prophylactically.

Erythromycin and ampicillin have been the drugs of choice in the human disease. The cure rate is low in the immunocompromised host.

26 *Staphylococcus*

The staphylococci are placed in the same Order as *Listeria* spp. and *Streptococcus* spp. They are gram-positive cocci occurring in pairs, short chains, and clusters. They are facultatively anaerobic, nonmotile, catalase positive, oxidase negative, and fermentative. There are more than 47 species in the genus *Staphylococcus*. The species of greatest veterinary significance are *Staphylococcus aureus*, *Staphylococcus intermedius*, *Staphylococcus hyicus*, and *Staphylococcus schleiferi* subsp. *coagulans*. They and other staphylococci occur frequently as commensals on the skin and mucous membranes of animals and humans.

The species of major veterinary significance are discussed below.

STAPHYLOCOCCUS AUREUS

Habitat

Staphylococcus aureus is a frequent commensal of the skin and mucous membranes, especially of the upper respiratory and digestive tracts.

Structure

Peptidoglycan, a polysaccharide polymer, together with teichoic acid, provides rigidity for the cell wall. Peptidoglycan in the host elicits the production of interleukin-1 (IL-1) by phagocytes. IL-1 in the bloodstream will eventually reach the hypothalamus. Here, the IL-1 will stimulate neurons to produce prostaglandins that elevate the body temperature, resulting in fever. In addition, the IL-1 will aid in the production of a local inflammatory response and participate in generation of a specific immune response.

Teichoic acids are linked to peptidoglycan and are antigenically species specific.

Protein A is present as a surface component on most strains of virulent *S. aureus*. It is antiphagocytic and has the unique ability to bind to the Fc region of IgG. This coating of the bacterial cell by antibody serves as a disguise and is thus protective.

The useful serologic procedure coagglutination depends on protein A. When specific IgG antibody is added to staphylococci possessing protein A and then followed by homologous antigen, coagglutination is produced.

The polysaccharide microcapsule of some strains of *S. aureus* is also antiphagocytic. The ability to produce capsule, however, does not appear to be a prerequisite for virulence.

The cell wall of all *S. aureus* strains contains a species-specific polysaccharide A. The antigenic component of this polysaccharide is the *N*-acetyl glucosaminyl ribitol unit.

Carotenoid pigments impart an orange or yellow color to strains of *S. aureus*.

Important structural components of the staphylococcal cell are shown diagrammatically in Fig. 26.1.

Extracellular Products

CATALASE. This enzyme converts hydrogen peroxide to oxygen and water. It is produced by staphylococci but not by streptococci.

COAGULASE. Two kinds of coagulase are produced: free coagulase and bound coagulase (clumping factor). Free

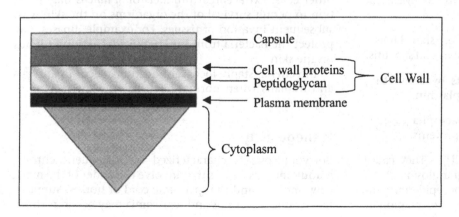

FIGURE 26.1 Structure of a typical *Staphylococcus* cell.

coagulase is released into the growth medium and is detected in a tube test. Bound coagulase is cell associated and tested for by a slide procedure. The clotting of plasma by both coagulases involves the conversion of prothrombin to thrombin, which converts fibrinogen to fibrin (clot). Strains of *S. aureus*, *S. intermedius*, and *S. hyicus* produce coagulase. More strains are positive to the tube test than to the slide test. Coagulase may contribute to infection by coating the surface of staphylococci with fibrin and thus protecting them from phagocytosis and from killing within phagocytes.

ENTEROTOXINS. At least six enterotoxins (A–F) have been identified. They are heat-resistant (100°C/30 minutes), extracellular proteins composed of single polypeptide chains of about 30 kd. Approximately 50% of *S. aureus* strains produce one or more enterotoxins. Other *Staphylococcus* species occasionally produce enterotoxins. These toxins are classed as **superantigens**, and their action may involve cytokines. A favorable milieu, such as unrefrigerated custards, raw milk, cream, ice cream, meat gravy, fish, cheese, or oysters, is required for their production. Clinical signs of this human food poisoning are nausea, vomiting, and diarrhea within 1–6 hours. In contrast, *Salmonella* food poisoning takes effect in 24–48 hours. Enterotoxins in the food can be detected by an agar gel precipitin test.

HEMOLYSINS α, β, γ, AND δ (hemotoxins, cytolysins). All are antigenically distinct. Erythrocytes from various species differ in susceptibility to these toxins. The alpha and beta toxins are potent hemolysins. The alpha toxin is most active against rabbit erythrocytes and is responsible for the inner clear zone of hemolysis. It causes spasms of smooth muscle and is dermonecrotizing and lethal. The beta toxin is sphingomyelinase C and is responsible for the outer partial zone of hemolysis. It is most active against sheep erythrocytes. The gamma toxin has a narrow hemolytic spectrum and is inhibited by agar and cholesterol. The delta toxin has a broad hemolytic spectrum and is inhibited by phospholipids. The mode of action of gamma and delta toxins and their roles in pathogenesis are not well understood.

HEAT-STABLE NUCLEASE. This enzyme cleaves both deoxyribonucleic acid (DNA) and ribonucleic acid (RNA). It is produced by most strains of *S. aureus*, *S. hyicus*, *S. schleiferi* subsp. *coagulans*, and *S. intermedius*.

LIPASE. Degrades protective fatty acids on skin. Lipase-positive strains tend to cause abscesses of skin and subcutis.

STAPHYLOKINASE. Degrades fibrin clots by converting plasminogen to the fibrinolytic enzyme plasmin.

LEUKOCIDIN. Kills granulocytes and macrophages; it is composed of two heat-labile interacting proteins.

EXFOLIATIVE TOXINS A AND B (EXFOLIATIN). They cause cleavage of **desmosomes** in the stratum granulosum of the epidermis. The toxins are specific for the epidermis; intraperitoneal inoculation results in epidermal exfoliation in mice. The toxins are potent **mitogens** that act on T- and B-lymphocytes. These toxins produced by *S. aureus* and *S. hyicus* cause staphylococcal scalded skin syndrome in infants and may be involved in porcine exudative epidermitis.

TOXIC SHOCK SYNDROME TOXIN-1. This toxin, which is identical to enterotoxin F and pyrogenic exotoxin C, causes human toxic shock syndrome. This serious disease is characterized by fever, shock, skin rash, and multisystem involvement. Approximately 15% of *S. aureus* strains produce this toxin.

HYALURONIDASE. This enzyme is referred to as the "spreading factor." It degrades hyaluronic acid, the ground substance of connective tissues, and thus is thought to facilitate spread of the organism through tissues.

LYSOSTAPHIN. This lytic enzyme is produced by *S. simulans* and is active against staphylococci but not micrococci. It is used in a test to distinguish these genera.

Pathogenesis

Staphylococcus aureus cells express proteins on their surface that attach to host proteins laminin and fibronectin. The latter is present in blood clots and on endothelial and epithelial surfaces.

Endogenous infections are probably most frequent, but exogenous infections also occur. Transmission is usually by direct contact or by fomites.

Strains of this widespread commensal have the capacity to invade tissues, producing abscesses, pustules, various other pyogenic infections, and on occasion, bacteremia and septicemia.

The inflammatory response to infection mobilizes neutrophils to the site of infection, which leads to the pyogenic response. Then abscess formation, and eventually rupture of skin and drainage of pus at the surface, follow. Some of the extracellular products of *S. aureus*, referred to earlier, are involved in the development of these infections. Both capsules and protein A of staphylococci are thought to be strongly antiphagocytic. Delayed hypersensitivity is considered to play a role in local tissue damage in staphylococcal infections. As stated earlier, leukocidin, hemolysins, and other enzymes and toxins of *S. aureus* damage blood cells, macrophages, and epithelial and other cells. Extracellular products of *S. aureus* may function to permit survival of the organisms on the skin with subsequent invasion of tissues. For example, lipases may protect the bacteria from the bactericidal action of lipids on the skin.

In general, staphylococcal infections occur in animals and humans when normal host defenses are lacking or impaired.

Pathogenicity

Botryomycosis is characterized by infrequent chronic granulomatous lesions that involve the udder of the mare, cow, and sow and the spermatic cord of horses. Suppurative wound infections and septicemia may occur in all animals. Pyoderma is seen in dogs (more commonly caused by *S. intermedius*) and horses; pyemia, especially from tick-bite wounds; lameness; and bacteremia are seen in lambs.

Staphylococcus aureus is an important cause of mastitis in the cow, goat, sow, and ewe. Staphylococcal bovine mastitis can be acute, but most frequently, it is chronic and subclinical. It is common and of great economic importance. Gangrenous mastitis caused by alpha-toxin is seen in postparturient cows.

There are various pyogenic infections of the skin of many animals, including subcutaneous abscesses with cellulitis in horses and various suppurative infections in rabbits.

Staphylococcal arthritis and septicemia occur in turkeys.

Staphylococcus aureus is an important cause of urinary tract infections in animals and humans.

Staphylococcal enterocolitis is seen principally in humans after prolonged antibiotic therapy; for example, after intestinal surgery.

Impetigo involving the sow's udder is initiated by the bites of piglets.

Many infections in humans, including osteomyelitis, sinusitis, mastitis, **furuncles**, **carbuncles**, endocarditis, toxic shock syndrome, pneumonia, tonsillitis, impetigo, nosocomial infections, and food poisoning are caused by *S. aureus*.

Specimens

Pus, usually provided on swabs; affected tissue; and milk samples are the usual specimens.

Direct Examination

Gram stain of clinical material shows singles, pairs, chains, and small clusters of gram-positive cocci and usually numerous polymorphonuclear leukocytes.

Laboratory Diagnosis

Staphylococcus aureus and other staphylococci grow well on common laboratory media. Selective media are available for *S. aureus*; for example, mannitol salt agar. Blood agar is preferred for primary isolation. Colonies appear in 24 hours and are up to 4 mm in diameter, round, smooth, and glistening; they range in color from white to deep yellow or orange (gold). Double-zone hemolysis is especially characteristic. Bovine red cells are best for demonstrating

the hemolysis of *S. aureus*. Smears disclose clumps of gram-positive cocci.

Presumptive identification is made on the basis of the double zone of hemolysis and cultural and morphologic features. Definitive identification is based on coagulase production and the other characteristics listed in Table 26.1. Although staphylococci are sensitive to lysostaphin, micrococci are not.

Rapid miniaturized commercial systems are available for identifying most staphylococci encountered in clinical specimens. A latex agglutination test is available for the rapid identification of *S. aureus*.

Some strains of *S. aureus* can be identified by their susceptibility to one or several staphylococcal phages; for example, strain 80/81 (penicillin resistant) is susceptible to lysis by phages 80 and 81. This variety has been important in human nosocomial infection. Phage typing is of value in the study of the epidemiology of staphylococcal infections. There are many phage types, and animal staphylococcal types are usually different from human types.

A number of phage culture lysates are used in the typing procedure. A single drop of each lysate is added to a plate confluently inoculated with the organism to be tested; it is incubated overnight at 30°C and then is observed for zones of lysis. The pattern of lysis indicates the type.

Resistance

Staphylococci are susceptible to common disinfectants. Pus is protective, and organisms remain viable in dried pus for weeks, an important consideration in clinics. Unlike many other vegetative bacterial forms, some staphylococci can survive a temperature of 60°C for 30 minutes. Their resistance to high salt concentration (as high as 15%) is taken advantage of in the selective medium mannitol salt agar.

Immunity

Strains of *S. aureus* possessing capsular and certain surface antigens are most immunogenic. **Bacterins** and toxoids are employed in active immunization. They are considered to be of questionable value in the prevention of bovine mastitis. A vaccine based on the fibronectin binding protein has been reported to elicit protective immunity against staphylococcal mastitis in cattle. **Autogenous bacterins** have given variable results. Hypersensitivity to staphylococci probably plays a role in aggravating infections; thus, dogs with pyoderma should

Table 26.1 Some Differential Characteristics of Important Staphylococci

Characteristic	S.aureus	S. hyicus	S. intermedius	S. epidermidis	S. schleiferi subsp. coagulans
Coagulase	+	V	+	+	+
Clumping factor	+	−	V	−	−
β-hemolysis	+	−	+	−	+
Pigment	+	−	−	−	−

Note: +, positive; −, negative; V, variable.

be desensitized with small doses when using an autogenous bacterin. The delayed hypersensitivity reaction, however, may have a beneficial effect on the host in that the reaction tends to localize the infection and thus to prevent systemic spread.

Immunity is both cell mediated and humoral; the latter is antibacterial as well as antitoxic. Humoral antibodies are thought to be important for protection. Opsonization may play a key role in humoral immunity by promoting phagocytosis by neutrophils.

There is little to no immunity to reinfection.

Treatment

Antimicrobial susceptibility tests should be conducted on all staphylococci considered clinically significant. Penicillin is the drug of choice if strains are susceptible; however, many strains of *S. aureus* are penicillin resistant. Most resistance is attributable to penicillinase (β-lactamase), an enzyme that hydrolyzes the β-lactam ring of penicillin (see Chapter 8). Plasmid-based penicillin resistance may be transferred by transduction. The synthetic (penicillinase-resistant) penicillins are of value, including methicillin, oxacillin, and nafcillin. Methicillin resistance is common in human strains, but infrequent thus far in animal isolates.

Other effective drugs are lincosamide, macrolides, amoxicillin-clavulanate, chloramphenicol, clindamycin, and sulfonamide-trimethoprim. Vancomycin, sometimes referred to as the drug of last resort for *S. aureus*, is the most widely effective antibiotic.

Treatment may be ineffective because of abscessation. Surgical drainage may be indicated.

Public Health Significance

Human beings may become infected with *S. aureus*, *S. schleiferi* subsp. *coagulans*, *S. hyicus*, and possibly other staphylococci of animal origin.

OTHER STAPHYLOCOCCI

Many of the basic properties described above for *S. aureus* also apply to the less studied but important staphylococci referred to below. Their isolation and cultivation is the same as for *S. aureus*, and the same principles of treatment apply. Their identification is based on the criteria listed in Table 26.1.

A considerable number of species of no veterinary significance cause a variety of infections in humans; for example, *Staphylococcus saprophyticus* is an important cause of urinary tract infections in young women.

For discussion and identification of the numerous species of staphylococci, readers are referred to Murray et al., 1999 (Murray PR et al., *Manual of Clinical Microbiology*, 7th ed. ASM Press, Washington, D.C., 1999).

Staphylococcus intermedius

Staphylococcus intermedius is similar to *S. aureus* in many respects. Colonies are grey-white, smooth, nonpigmented, glistening, and beta hemolytic on blood agar. *Staphylococcus intermedius* possesses two different teichoic acid antigens in its cell wall, poly (C) and poly (P). Dog strains possess poly (P); pigeon strains possess poly (C). Protein A is not present in this species. *Staphylococcus intermedius* produces coagulase and hemolysins (alpha, beta, and delta). Important differential characteristics are listed in Table 26.1.

This species is a normal inhabitant of the nasopharynx and skin of dogs, raccoons, foxes, and mink. It causes a variety of infections in dogs, including pyoderma, otitis extema, mastitis, eye infections, urinary tract infections, folliculitis, and furunculosis. It is has also been recovered from infections in other animals, including cats, cattle, horses, and pigeons.

Staphylococcus hyicus

Staphylococcus hyicus is the cause of exudative epidermitis or "greasy pig disease" of swine.

Colonies are creamy white, glistening, nonpigmented, nonhemolytic, convex, and circular on blood agar. It produces a heat-stable nuclease. Coagulase and fibrinolysin are produced by some strains. Protein A and enterotoxins are produced by some strains, but the latter are not identical to those of *S. aureus*. It does not produce alpha-, beta-, or delta-hemolysins. A cytotoxin produced by *S. hyicus*, however, has some properties similar to the delta-hemolysin of *S. aureus*. In addition, *S. hyicus* produces an exfoliative toxin that causes exfoliation in chickens, some laboratory animals, dogs, and cats.

Staphylococcus hyicus, which is closely related to *Staphylococcus epidermidis* antigenically, occurs frequently on the skin of pigs and on the skin and nares of healthy poultry. In addition, it can be found less frequently on the skin and in the milk of cattle, in various animal products, and in slaughterhouse effluents. Exudative epidermitis is highly contagious and varies in severity from one group of pigs to another. It also has been implicated in septic arthritis of pigs, abortion in sows, seborrheic dermatitis of a pygmy goat, dermatitis of donkeys and horses, and skin and udder infections of cattle.

Staphylococcus hyicus is susceptible to many antibiotics. High dosage is recommended for 7–10 days. Antiseptics are applied to the whole body.

Staphylococcus epidermidis

This species is found commonly on the skin of humans and, to a lesser extent, as a commensal on the skin and hair of many animals. It is an occasional opportunist of low pathogenicity. Among the infections attributed to *S. epidermidis* are low-grade bovine mastitis, suture abscesses, and abscesses in various sites, including wounds.

Staphylococcus epidermidis is coagulase negative. Colonies are nonhemolytic and unpigmented but otherwise resemble those of *S. aureus*.

Staphylococcus schleiferi subsp. coagulans

This organism is recovered from dogs with otitis externa, from animal bites in humans, and from joint and wound infections in humans.

Colonies are smaller (3–5 mm) than those of *S. aureus* and are unpigmented, smooth, and glossy.

Staphylococcus xylosus and S. sciuri

Staphylococcus xylosus and *S. sciuri* have been reported to cause bovine mastitis. The former species is of human origin and the latter is a resident of rodents.

MICROCOCCI

The micrococci (genus *Micrococcus*) consist of two species, *Micrococcus luteus* and *Micrococcus lylae*, which occur on the skin of humans and animals. The former is the most common in nature and in clinical specimens. They resemble the staphylococci morphologically but differ biochemically. They are nonpathogenic and mainly important because they resemble staphylococci and are frequently recovered from clinical specimens.

They split sugars by oxidation, in contrast to staphylococci, which ferment sugars. Staphylococci can be distinguished readily from micrococci in the laboratory because staphylococci are resistant to bacitracin and susceptible to furazolidone.

GLOSSARY

autogenous bacterin Bacterin prepared from bacteria isolated from infected animals in a herd, flock, and so forth.
bacterin Killed suspension of bacteria.
carbuncle Local purulent, necrotic, inflammatory process involving the skin and deeper tissues with multiple openings from which pus is discharged.
desmosomes One of the types of cell junctions by which cells join or communicate with each other. The desmosome of one cell adheres to the desmosome of another. This system of joining cells is designed to resist mechanical separation. Desmosomes are important in the structure of the epithelium, for example.
furuncle Localized inflammatory process of the skin and subcutis that discharges pus and is caused by an infection.
impetigo Acute, contagious staphylococcal or streptococcal skin disease characterized by vesicles, pustules, and crusts.
mitogen Any agent that causes a cell to divide.
superantigen Antigens (mostly from bacterial toxins) that interact with a particular subset of T cells resulting in direct activation of large numbers of T cells.

27

Actinobaculum, Actinomyces, and Arcanobacterium

The genera *Actinobaculum*, *Actinomyces*, and *Arcanobacterium* belong to the lineage of gram-positive bacteria with a high guanine-plus-cytosine content. They are non-spore-forming, non-partially acid-fast, gram-positive rods. Species differ in their oxygen requirements and cellular morphology and are referred to generally as the actinomycetes. They are sometimes called "higher bacteria" because they have some of the cultural and morphologic characteristics of the fungi.

ACTINOBACULUM: ACTINOBACULUM SUIS

This species, formerly called *Eubacterium suis*, causes ureteritis, cystitis, and pyelonephritis in sows. Boars carry *A. suis* in the preputial diverticulum and serve as the source of infection. Transmission takes place during breeding. The disease is ascending and limited to females. Among the signs are anorexia, weight loss, purulent discharge, infertility, increased urination, purulent and bloody urine, and sudden death. Sows may die without clinical signs being observed.

The disease is most often diagnosed at slaughter. Definitive diagnosis is based on culture of urine or clinical materials from affected tissues and identification of *A. suis*. In stained smears, the gram-positive rods have coryneform morphology. The organism only grows anaerobically and has the following biochemical characteristics: indole, nitrate, and catalase negative; fermentation: glucose, lactose, mannitol, and sucrose negative, maltose positive; acetic and formic acid from peptone-yeast-glucose (gas chromatography).

Penicillin may be effective if given early, but treatment of chronic cases is unsuccessful.

ACTINOMYCES

Actinomyces are gram-positive, non-acid-fast rods that may show branching. They are nonmotile and non-spore-forming; microaerophilic or anaerobic except for *Actinomyces viscosus* and *Actinomyces naeslundii*, which are facultatively anaerobic. They are catalase negative (except for *A. viscosus*) and fermentative. All of the actinomyces causing disease in animals and humans occur as commensals in the oropharynx.

Significant species, of the 20 in the genus, are as follows:

- *Actinomyces bovis*: Actinomycosis in cattle.
- *A. viscosus*: Pneumonia, pyothorax, and subcutaneous infections in dogs.
- *Actinomyces hordeovulnaris*: Pleuritis, peritonitis, pyothorax, and septic arthritis in dogs.
- *A. naeslundii*: Infrequent infections in animals; recovered from aborted porcine fetuses.
- *Actinomyces suis*: Pyogranulomatous mastitis in sows.
- *Actinomyces israelii*: Actinomycosis in humans; lesions may involve the jaw, thorax, or abdomen.

ACTINOMYCES BOVIS

Actinomyces bovis is a commensal in the oropharynx of cattle and probably of some other animals.

Infections are usually initiated in wounds of the oral mucous membrane.

Pathogenesis

Exotoxins have not been demonstrated. Organisms grow in the anaerobically damaged tissue, usually as the result of trauma to the oral mucous membrane. A suppurative process develops, and infectious material may be aspirated into the lungs, producing pulmonary actinomycosis, or swallowed, producing visceral or abdominal actinomycosis.

Pathogenicity

Actinomyces bovis causes a subacute or chronic progressive disease, principally of cattle, characterized by the development of indurated, granulomatous, suppurative lesions involving bone and soft tissue, principally involving the jaw. Abscesses develop and discharge through fistulas; tortuous sinuses result from the burrowing process.

CATTLE.   The disease involves the mandible or other bony tissue of the head ("lumpy jaw"). Seen less often are orchitis, mastitis, and lesions of the liver and other internal organs. Actinomycosis is rare in sheep.

PIGS.   See *Actinomyces suis* below.

DOGS AND CATS.   *Actinomyces bovis* infection is rare.

Actinomyces bovis and *Actinobacillus lignieresii* (the cause of actinobacillosis) are occasionally found together in lesions.

Direct Examination

A small amount of pus is placed in a Petri dish and washed to expose the small 1–3-mm sulfur granules associated with the disease. The actinomycotic granules are larger than the grey-white granules seen in actinobacillosis. A granule is transferred to a slide, and a drop of 10% sodium hydroxide is added. A cover slip is placed on the granule, which is crushed by gentle pressure. In actinomycosis, the characteristic "ray fungi" with club-shaped margins can be seen under low-power microscopy. The "clubs" are caused by a gelatinous sheath and the deposition of calcium phosphate around the terminal filaments. The granule is held together by a polysaccharide–protein complex. The cover slip is removed and the material spread to make a smear. It is dried, fixed, and stained by the Gram method. If the granules are from an actinomycotic lesion, delicate, intertwined, branching, gram-positive filaments are seen.

Isolation and Identification

The organism grows well on blood agar and brain heart infusion agar and in thioglycolate broth. An anaerobic atmosphere containing 5%–10% CO_2 is preferred. Colonies are white, rough, nodular, and difficult to remove. The radiating mycelia can be seen under a dissecting microscope. Small cottony colonies may be seen suspended discretely in thioglycolate broth.

Gram-stained smears from growth on solid or fluid media reveal masses of gram-positive, coryneform rods and slightly branched, slender filaments. Some filaments fragment into bacillary and coccal forms (Fig. 27.1).

A strongly presumptive identification is usually made on the basis of the gross pathology, characteristic sulfur granules, and demonstration of the gram-positive branching filaments. Cultivation of an organism from characteristic lesions and granules in animals possessing the morphologic characteristics of *A. bovis* is usually considered sufficient for identification. Definitive differentiation of *A. bovis* from other *Actinomyces* and from anaerobic **diphtheroids** is accomplished by various biochemical tests.

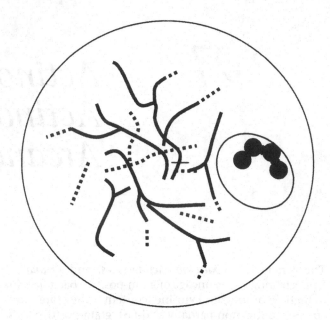

FIGURE 27.1   Branching filaments of *Actinomyces bovis* in pus.

Treatment

Establish and maintain drainage of abscesses. Penicillin or clindamycin are effective if treatment is begun early. Iodides given orally or intravenously are also useful. Treatment is of no avail in advanced cases.

ACTINOMYCES VISCOSUS

This organism differs from *A. bovis* and some other actinomyces in that it grows aerobically and is catalase positive. It has been isolated from the human and canine oral cavity, from periodontal disease in humans and animals, and from actinomycosis in dogs. It is occasionally recovered from infections in other animals.

Actinomycosis in the dog is characterized by the presence of actinomycotic granules containing gram-positive, non-acid-fast, filamentous organisms that resemble *A. bovis* morphologically.

Two forms of actinomycosis are usually seen in the dog. The more common is the localized granulomatous abscess involving mainly the skin and subcutis (actinomycotic mycetoma). This form, resulting from a cutaneous wound, responds well to treatment.

The other form principally involves the thorax, with or without extension to the abdominal cavity. Pneumonia and pyothorax with granulomatous lesions of thoracic tissues and accumulation of pleural and pericardial fluid containing soft grey-white granules are characteristic of this deep form.

Skin pustules and nodules in a horse, attributed to *A. viscosus*, have been reported.

Actinomyces viscosus grows at 37°C on blood and brain heart infusion agar (and broth) but not on Sabouraud agar. Colonies are readily apparent in 3–7 days. Final identification is based on a number of biochemical tests.

Prolonged antimicrobial therapy, as with penicillin, amoxacillin, chloramphenicol or tetracycline, and surgical drainage are effective if begun sufficiently early.

OTHER *ACTINOMYCES* SPECIES

Actinomyces hordeovulnaris

This species has been isolated from dogs with localized abscesses and systemic infections characterized by one or more of the following: pleuritis, peritonitis, pyothorax, and septic arthritis. The infections were initially reported from California and were associated with injuries to the skin by the foxtails of the grass of *Hordeum* spp.

The organism, which is pleomorphic with branching filaments, grows well on blood agar in an anaerobic or microaerophilic atmosphere; a candle jar is satisfactory. White colonies, somewhat adherent, achieve a diameter of 2 mm in 72 hours. Biochemical tests are required for final identification.

Treatment is essentially the same as for *A. viscosus.*

Actinomyces suis

This name has been proposed for strains of *Actinomyces* recovered from a pyogranulomatous mastitis (actinomycosis) of sows. Although these strains resemble *A. bovis,* they have minor biochemical and antigenic differences.

Actinomyces israelii

This species, which closely resembles *A. bovis,* is the principal cause of actinomycosis in humans. On rare occasions, *A. israelii* has been recovered from pyogranulomatous lesions in cattle and pigs.

Actinomyces spp.

Unspeciated *Actinomyces* are occasionally associated with supra-atlantal bursitis (poll evil) and supraspinous bursitis (fistulous withers) in horses and various infections of other animals including the dog. These infections are usually initiated by various injuries.

ARCANOBACTERIUM

This genus is closely related to *Corynebacterium* and *Actinomyces.* It differs from *Actinomyces* in the diamino acid of the cell wall, the **menaquinones,** and the cellular fatty acid content. Like the corynebacteria, the cells are pleomorphic, and except for one species, are catalase negative. They are nonmotile and fermentative and only one

species, *Arcabobacterium pyogenes,* of the four recognized, is pathogenic for animals.

ARCHANOBACTERIUM PYOGENES

Formerly *Actinomyces pyogenes.*

Pathogenicity and Pathogenesis

Archanobacterium pyogenes is a very important pyogenic organism of cattle, sheep, and swine. Among the frequent infections it causes, mainly in these species, are chronic abscessing mastitis, particularly in cows; chronic suppurative pneumonia, frequently with mycoplasmas and species of *Pasteurella* and *Mannheimia*; septic arthritis; vegetative endocarditis (cattle); endometritis and pyometra; umbilical infections; infections of wounds and surgical incisions; and seminal vesiculitis (bulls and boars). It is frequently found in mixed infections, such as with *Fusobacterium necrophorum* in bovine liver abscesses. Infections may affect single or multiple animals.

This species is a common commensal on the mucous membranes of the nasopharynx of cattle, sheep, and swine. It may be shed from apparently normal udders and is frequently recovered from tonsils and retropharyngeal lymph nodes. Infections arise when the organisms gain entrance to tissue as a result of various injuries and other infections, including those caused by viruses, mycoplasmas, and other bacteria. Dissemination to lungs and other tissues may be hematogenous.

Archanobacterium pyogenes produces a relatively weak hemolytic, protein exotoxin, which kills mice when given intravenously and produces skin necrosis. This 58-kDa cytolysin is thought to be an important virulence factor. It resembles the thio-activated cytolysins produced by listeria and clostridia. Antitoxin can be demonstrated in naturally infected animals, but its correlation with protection is questionable. A protease, which may be identical to the gelatinase produced by the organism, has been suggested as a possible virulence factor.

Abscesses are variable in size, with usually a substantial fibrous capsule. The character and odor of the pus depends on whether the infection is pure or mixed. *Fusobacterium necrophorum, Bacteroides* spp., and other anaerobes may be responsible for a foul odor.

Isolation and Identification

Gram-stained smears of pus disclose small, slender gram-positive, pleomorphic rods that may be somewhat curved and clubbed at the ends. The organism grows readily on blood agar, producing pinpoint, glistening streplike beta-hemolytic colonies in 48 hours. With age, colonies become opaque and dry. *Archanobacterium pyogenes* is nonmotile, nitrate reduction negative, catalase negative, and gelatinase positive. Most strains peptonize litmus milk and are CAMP positive (see Chapter 24, *Streptococcus*).

Immunity

The immune response to *A. pyogenes* has received little attention. Serum antibodies, including those against exotoxin are detectable, but they confer little or no protection. The organism and its products have been included in vaccines and bacterins, but their value is questionable.

Treatment

Archanobacterium pyogenes is susceptible to penicillin, ampicillin, tetracyclines, trimethoprim-sulfonamides, and other antimicrobial drugs. Resistant strains have been reported but are uncommon. Because of the nature of infections—abscesses with thick fibrous capsules—the response to antimicrobial treatment is poor. Prophylactic treatment of heifers and dry cows with long-acting penicillin is effective in preventing mastitis caused by *A. pyogenes*. Cattle, sheep, and swine with pulmonary abscessation respond poorly to antimicrobial treatment and are usually culled.

GLOSSARY

diphtheroid Synonym of coryneform (*Corynebacterium*-like). Usually refers to nonpathogenic corynebacteria.

habronemiasis Cutaneous habronemiasis is a granulomatous skin disease of horses caused in part by the larvae of spirurid stomach worms.

inspissated Thickening in consistency of, frequently, pus.

menaquinones Family of compounds that are structurally similar to vitamin K2.

28

Dermatophilus and *Cornyebacterium*

Dermatophilus and *Corynebacterium* are included in the Order Actinomycetales, but they are in different suborders in that they have marked distinguishing features. There are two species of *Dermatophilus*, *Dermatophilus congolensis* and *Dermatophilus chelonae*, but only the former is a significant pathogen. In contrast, there are 67 recognized species of *Corynebacterium*, only a small number of which are pathogenic for animals. Some are harmless commensals of animals and many occur in soil and vegetation.

DERMATOPHILUS CONGOLENSIS

This species is a gram-positive, branching, filamentous, segmenting rod. It is aerobic, non-spore-forming, and not acid-fast; motile zoospores are produced.

Dermatophilus congolensis causes dermatophilosis or streptothricosis, which is worldwide in distribution. Although it may affect many animal species, it is seen most frequently in cattle, sheep, goats, and horses.

A recently described species, *D. chelonae*, was recovered from two turtles and one tortoise.

Habitat and Transmission

As far as is known, *D. congolensis* is an obligate parasite living only on animals.

Infection is spread by contact, fomites, and biting insects. Moist conditions probably promote its dissemination.

Pathogenicity

Streptothricosis or dermatophilosis has been encountered in horses, cattle, sheep, goats, dogs, cats, deer, squirrels, and humans. Recent studies indicate that the disease is widely prevalent, especially in cattle. It is an infection involving the superficial layers of the skin and is characterized by the formation of crusts or scabs varying in size from quite small to about 2.5 cm. In advanced cases, large areas of the skin may be involved as a result of coalescence of smaller lesions. Removal of the scab leaves a moist, depressed area.

A severe form of the disease has been responsible, on occasion, for deaths of calves, sheep, and goats.

In sheep, the disease is referred to as mycotic dermatitis and is generally seen in three forms:

- Dermatitis of the wool-covered areas, or "lumpy wool."
- Dermatitis of the face and scrotum.
- Dermatitis of the lower leg and foot, which may result in a severe ulcerative dermatitis, referred to as "strawberry foot rot."

Several cases, acquired from animals, have been described in humans. Infections can be produced experimentally in the rabbit.

The disease in cats is probably initiated by puncture wounds. Abscesses develop involving the subcutis, muscles, and lymph nodes; chronic draining fistulas may result.

Immune Response

Animals with dermatophilosis develop an antibody response, but the relative importance in protection of the humoral and cell-mediated responses is not clear.

Direct Examination

Smears are made from scabs softened with distilled water and then stained by the Giemsa or Gram method. Segmenting (longitudinal and transverse) filaments and coccoid spores stain deep purple. The spores are seen in packets (Fig. 28.1).

Isolation and Identification

The organism grows well on blood agar, tryptose agar, and other media. Small, rough, greyish-white colonies appear in 24–48 hours; they have fimbriated, lacelike borders; they enlarge to 4 mm in diameter on further incubation; and they become yellowish to yellow-orange. The organism can usually be recovered in the conventional manner on blood agar.

Motile zoospores approximately 1 μm in diameter are formed as a result of the septation of hyphal elements; they possess polar flagella and can be seen in wet mounts from colonies. Gram-positive, branching hyphal elements in various stages of segmentation are seen in stained smears. The hyphal elements are larger and more irregular in shape than the filaments of *Streptomyces* and *Nocardia*.

Identification is usually based on the finding of the characteristic morphologic elements in Giemsa or Gram-stained crusts and scabs and on the growth of organisms

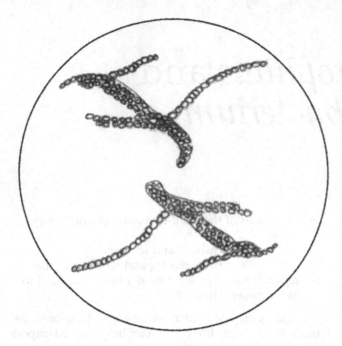

FIGURE 28.1 Characteristic segmenting forms of *Dermatophilus congolensis.*

with the cultural features of *D. congolensis.* Immunofluorescent staining has been used to identify the organism in clinical specimens.

Treatment and Control

The disease has been effectively treated in some animals by a single large dose of combined penicillin and streptomycin. It is important that both drugs be used. Tetracyclines and chloramphenicol are also effective. Removal of scabs with a brush and mild soap is recommended before topical application of iodine compounds, copper sulfate, or other disinfectant solutions. Control measures against ectoparasites and biting insects are recommended. Mild cases usually respond to regular grooming and isolation in dry quarters.

Animals can remain infected for long periods; however, when they are cleared of infection, reinfection does not occur. Vaccines have not proved effective in field trials.

CORYNEBACTERIUM

They are small, pleomorphic rods, some of which have club-shaped swellings at one or both ends. Organisms from fluid media appear as single cells, pairs, palisades, V forms, and clusters that resemble Chinese letters. The cell wall contains meso-diaminopimelic acid, an arabanogalactan polymer, and certain short-chain mycolic acids (most species). They are catalase positive, fermentative or nonfermentative, nonmotile (except for some plant pathogens), and non-spore-forming. Many corynebacteria possess metachromatic granules that are thought to be reserves of phosphate; they are readily stained with methylene blue.

Some corynebacteria are commensals of animals. The nonpathogenic species, which are often referred to as "diphtheroids," are frequently recovered from clinical specimens.

Corynebacterium diphtheriae, the cause of human diphtheria, has been studied extensively. It produces a potent exotoxin that is encoded by a bacteriophage carrying the *tox* gene.

CORYNEBACTERIUM RENALE GROUP

Three immunologic types of *Corynebacterium renale*, I, II, and III, are now recognized. On the basis of taxonomic studies, each type has been given a species name: type I, *C. renale*; type II, *Corynebacterium pilosum*; and type III, *Corynebacterium cystitidis*. They can be distinguished by biochemical characteristics (Table 28.1).

Habitat

All three species have been recovered from the normal bovine female and male genital tracts, where they may reside as harmless commensals.

Mode of Infection

With all species, infection is transmitted venereally and indirectly by contaminated urine. Infections may also be endogenous. The adherence of all three species to the mucous membrane of the urogenital tract is mediated by pili.

Pathogenicity and Pathogenesis

Ulcerative posthitis and vulvitis, mainly a disease of sheep, is caused by either *C. renale* or *C. pilosum*. Male castrated sheep are mainly affected, but it is also seen occasionally in goats and cattle. The disease is considered to result from the inflammation caused by the ammonia released by the hydrolysis of urea by urease produced by the causal bacteria. As a result, the disease is seen most frequently in animals on a high-protein diet.

Each of the three species causes cystitis, ureteritis, and pyelonephritis in cows and occasionally in sheep. Cystitis may occur without pyelonephritis; the latter may develop after parturition and is more common in individuals on a high protein diet. Bovine pyelonephritis is sporadic and global in distribution.

The infection is ascending and involves the bladder, ureter(s), and one or both kidneys in a severe pyogenic inflammatory process. The bladder wall, ureters, and kidney are greatly thickened and enlarged. Hemorrhage, necrosis, and ulceration are extensive, and abscesses may be found throughout the kidney. The urine is purulent and blood stained.

Direct Examination

Gram-stained smears from purulent urine disclose clumps of short, pleomorphic, gram-positive rods. Definitive diagnosis depends on isolation and identification.

Isolation and Identification

Carefully collected urine samples are usually plated on blood agar. Young colonies are initially small, and the colony characteristics of each species vary somewhat. Those of *C. renale* become opaque and ivory colored as they enlarge. The colonies of *C. pilosum* resemble those of *C. renale*, but tend to be cream colored to yellow. Those of *C. cystitidis* tend to be semitransparent to white. All three species produce urease. Criteria for the identification of the three species of the *C. renale* group are given in Table 28.1.

Antigenic Nature and Immunity

The classification of *C. renale* into type I (*C. renale*), type II (*C. pilosum*), and type III. (*C. cystitidis*) was based on the recognition of different surface antigens by agar diffusion precipitin tests. The protein of the pilus is antigenic and distinct for each species. Although various serologic procedures have been used to detect antibodies in these infections, none has been found to be of diagnostic value. As in other urinary tract infections, corynebacteria in cows with upper urinary tract involvement are coated with antibody (IgG). The immune response in pyelonephritis is not sufficient to effectuate recovery.

Treatment

There are reports of successful treatment of *C. renale* group infections with large doses of penicillin, although remissions were frequent. Treatment is most satisfactory if it is begun early. Effectiveness of treatment should be monitored by urine culture.

Ulcerative posthitis in sheep is dealt with by clipping and cleaning of hair around the prepuce, by application of antiseptics, and by changes in diet. Administration of

Table 28.1 Differentiation of *Corynebacterium renale*, *Corynebacterium pilosum*, and *Corynebacterium cystitidis*

Characteristic	C. renale	C. pilosum	C. cystitidis
Colony color	yellow	yellow	whitish
Growth in broth at pH 5.4	+	−	−
Acid from			
Xylose	−	−	+
Starch	−	+	+
Nitrate reduction	−	+	−
Casein digestion	+	−	−
Hydrolysis of Tween 80	−	−	+

Note: +, positive; −, negative.

testosterone every 3 months reduces the occurrence; castrated animals are more susceptible.

CORYNEBACTERIUM PSEUDOTUBERCULOSIS

Corynebacterium pseudotuberculosis resembles *C. diphtheriae* somewhat. When lysogenized with the tox+ phage, *C. pseudotuberculosis* synthesizes diphtheria toxin.

Habitat

It may occur on the normal skin and mucous membranes of sheep and goats. The organism can survive in pus for long periods.

Mode of Infection

The organisms in pus most commonly enter via abrasions resulting from shearing (contaminated shears) and injuries to the skin. Infection by inhalation or ingestion is considered infrequent.

Pathogenicity

Corynebacterium pseudotuberculosis causes caseous lymphadenitis, an important economic disease of sheep and goats. The disease progresses with time, and eventually 40% of the flock may be infected. *Corynebacterium pseudotuberculosis* also causes abscesses and chronic lymphadenitis in wild ruminants, camels, and rarely, in cattle and humans.

In horses and mules, mainly in warm climates, it causes a frequently occurring ulcerative lymphangitis. Pectoral abscesses in horses and purulent arthritis in lambs are also caused by this species.

Pathogenesis

Corynebacterium pseudotuberculosis is a facultative intracellular parasite. When infection spreads, it does so via the lymphatics. The pus is greenish yellow or white, frequently caseous, and may be inspissated and arranged in onion-like concentric layers in lymph nodes.

A relatively weak exotoxin, phospholipase D (PLD) is considered an important virulence factor. It is leukotoxic and produces hemolysis, dermal necrosis in rabbits, and death in some laboratory animals. Antibodies to it are protective. A lipid of the cell wall has been observed to protect the organisms from phagocytosis and contribute to their intracellular survival.

Superficial caseous lymphadenitis affects mainly the prescapular and prefemoral lymph nodes, and animals show no ill effects. However, in some animals, mainly sheep, the disease spreads, and visceral disease results, with abscesses developing in various locations such as lung, liver, and kidney. Animals with the visceral form do poorly, and the term "lean ewe syndrome" has been applied to some.

Ulcerative lymphangitis in horses and mules, and rarely in cattle, appears as nodules, most often involving the superficial lymphatics around the fetlocks. The organism enters via injuries, and the disease is frequently chronic and long lasting.

Slowly developing abscesses of the pectoral, lower abdominal, and inguinal regions of horses have frequently yielded *C. pseudotuberculosis*. These infections, which have been reported mainly from California, may be complications of habronemiasis and dermatitis caused by the horn fly.

Isolation and Identification

This gram-positive, pleomorphic rod, which can readily be isolated from pus, grows well on blood agar aerobically. Colonies are initially small, but after several days of incubation, they enlarge to 3–4 mm in diameter, become dry and crumbly, and turn cream to orange in color. Complete hemolysis is usually seen on blood agar.

Definitive identification is based on the differential biochemical characteristics. Strains produce catalase and urease, and casein is digested. Cultures from horses and cattle have been reported to reduce nitrate, whereas those from sheep and goats seldom do. On blood agar, *C. pseudotuberculosis* inhibits the staphylococcal beta-toxin but results in a synergistic hemolysis with *Rhodococcus equi*. When a streak of *C. pseudotuberculosis* crosses at right angles to a streak of *R. equi*, there is enhancement of hemolysis.

Antigenic Nature and Immunity

Two serotypes, 1 and 2, have been identified. The first is recovered most frequently from sheep and goats, whereas serotype 2 has been mainly found in cattle and buffaloes. Differences in restriction endonuclease analysis and nitrate reduction have been noted between equine strains and those from sheep and goats.

Corynebacterium pseudotuberculosis is a facultative, intracellular parasite, and consequently, the cellular immune response is particularly important. Some protective immunity is elicited by the exotoxin phospholipase D.

Autogenous (flock) bacterins have been used in an attempt to control outbreaks of caseous lymphadenitis, but their value is questionable. Commercial vaccines containing PLD toxoid reduce the severity and incidence of the disease but do not prevent it.

An enzyme-linked immunosorbent assay, employing phospholipase D as antigen, and other serological procedures have been used effectively to detect infected or carrier animals.

Treatment and Control

Although *C. pseudotuberculosis* is susceptible to many antimicrobial agents, including penicillin, tetracyclines, erythromycin, and chloramphenicol, the nature of the lesion precludes their effectiveness. Exposure to the causal agent must be prevented. Culling and segregation, avoiding infection associated with shearing, and prevention of spread via dipping and feeding equipment are effective.

As mentioned above, commercial vaccines are of value, and serological screening with segregation of positive animals is useful. Through a combination of preventive measures, the disease in a flock can be greatly reduced and even eliminated.

Public Health Significance

Human infections from contact with infected animals are rare. They are characterized by a mild lymphadenitis.

OTHER SPECIES

Corynebacterium bovis

This organism is a commensal found in the reproductive tract of some cows and bulls and on the squamous epithelium of the teat duct of as many as 20% of the quarters of cows. Although it is not considered a cause of mastitis, the slight inflammation it causes is thought to aid in protecting the udder from infection. *Corynebacterium bovis* is a lipophilic organism that grows best in the presence of unsaturated long-chain fatty acids. Although it grows well on enriched media, colonies are more prevalent on the fatty areas of plates inoculated with milk. The morphology is characteristic of the genus, and identification is based on biochemical criteria.

Corynebacterium kutscheri (C. murium)

This organism culturally resembles *C. pseudotuberculosis*. It causes an important, although infrequent, disease of mice and rats characterized by caseous tuberculosis-like focal lesions in the skin, liver, lungs, and other organs.

Corynebacterium kutscheri is morphologically indistinguishable from other corynebacteria. Identification is based on the differential biochemical characteristics.

Corynebacterium minutissimum

This organism has been recovered from docking wounds in lambs, inflammation of interdigital spaces ("scald"), and scabs on the brisket of sheep. In humans it causes a chronic, contagious dermatitis of the axillary and pubic regions called erythrasma (scaly plaques) and infrequent bacteremia and endocarditis.

Corynebacterium parvum (now renamed Propionibacterium acnes)

This is a nonpathogenic anaerobe used as an immunological adjuvant in tumor therapy. It has immunopotentiating effects, mainly by activating macrophages.

Corynebacterium ulcerans

This organism, which resembles *C. diphtheriae* in some respects, has been recovered from bovine mastitis. Like *C. pseudotuberculosis*, it produces phospholipase D, and some strains produce small quantities of diphtheria toxin.

29 *Mycobacterium*

The mycobacteria most closely resemble the other mycolic acid–producing bacteria, *Corynebacterium*, *Nocardia*, and *Rhodococcus*. They comprise two major groups, the slow growers and the more rapidly growing species. The slow growers require a number of weeks to produce observable colonies, whereas most of the more rapid growers produce colonies in 3–21 days. The slow growers consist of the *Mycobacterium tuberculosis* Complex, which includes *M. tuberculosis*, *Mycobacterium bovis*, *Mycobacterium microti*, and *Mycobacterium africanum*. The more rapidly growing groups consist of the *Mycobacterium avium* Complex and at least 80 "environmental" species sometimes referred to as the atypical mycobacteria or nontubercular mycobacteria. A small number of these may take longer than 3 weeks to produce colonies.

The principal species of *Mycobacterium* from a veterinary and medical standpoint and the main diseases and hosts with which they are associated are as follows:

- *M. bovis:* Bovine tuberculosis.
- *M. tuberculosis:* Human tuberculosis.
- *M. microti:* Tuberculosis in voles.
- *M. africanum:* Closely related, if not identical, to *M. tuberculosis*; causes tuberculosis in humans in Africa.
- *M. avium:* Avian tuberculosis. The term "tubercle bacilli" refers to *M. bovis*, *M. tuberculosis*, and *M. avium*.
- *M. avium* subsp. *paratuberculosis* (formerly *Mycobacterium paratuberculosis*): Johne's disease (paratuberculosis) of cattle, sheep, and goats.
- *Mycobacterium lepraemurium:* Feline leprosy and rodent infections.
- *Mycobacterium leprae:* Human leprosy.
- *M. avium* Complex (MAC): Includes *M. avium* and *M. intracellulare*, each of which causes animal and human infections. They are distinguishable serologically and by probes, but not phenotypically.

The species listed above, except for the MAC species, are obligate parasites. The MAC species and many other mycobacteria are free-living in soil and water. Some of them cause rare to infrequent infections in animals. They have been placed in four groups based mainly on the basis of rate of growth, colony morphology, and pigment production. These groups are discussed below, along with the pathogenicity of the more important species.

Mycobacteria are gram-positive, acid-fast, small, slightly curved to straight rods. They are aerobic, nonmotile, non-spore-forming bacilli with occasional branching and sometimes a mycelium-like growth that fragments into coccoid and rod forms. The cell walls have a high lipid content, accounting for the acid-fastness discussed below. Colonies vary from smooth to rough, and some are pigmented.

The environmental or free-living mycobacteria were placed in categories by Runyon (1959). He established the following four groups based mainly on rate of growth, colony morphology, and pigment production:

Group I. Photochromogenic, producing pigmented (yellow) colonies only after exposure to light; slow-growing in that it requires 7 days or more for visible growth; for example, *Mycobacterium kansasii*, *Mycobacterium marinum*, *Mycobacterium asiaticum*, *Mycobacterium simiae*.

Group II. Scotochromogenic, producing yellow or orange pigment in the absence of light; slow-growing; for example, *Mycobacterium gordonae*, *Mycobacterium scrofulaceum*, *Mycobacterium szulgai*, *Mycobacterium xenopi*.

Group III. Nonphotochromogenic, producing no or slight pigment with exposure to light; slow-growing; for example, *M. avium*, *M. intracellulare*, *Mycobacterium terrae*, and *Mycobacterium ulcerans*.

Group IV. Variable pigmentation; grow rapidly in that there is visible growth in less than 7 days (Rapid Growers); for example, *Mycobacterium phlei*, *Mycobacterium smegmatis*, *Mycobacterium fortuitum*, *Mycobacterium chelonei*.

Additional organisms within each of these groups have now been speciated on the basis of cultural and biochemical characteristics, and thus, the groups introduced by Runyon have been expanded and more precisely defined.

Given the presence of mycobacteria in soil and water, isolation alone does not necessarily indicate pathogenic significance. Some mycobacteria can be recovered from feces. Those that are infective can sensitize animals to tuberculin.

TUBERCULOSIS

This disease is caused by the tubercle bacilli: *M. bovis*, *M. avium*, and *M. tuberculosis*.

Cell Constituents of Mycobacteria

None of the mycobacteria has yet been shown to produce exotoxins. The way in which they produce disease is not clearly understood. The chemistry of the tubercle bacilli is quite complex. They have a high concentration of lipids, 20%–40% dry weight, which is thought to be in part responsible for their resistance to humoral defense mechanisms and to disinfectants, acids, and alkalis.

The thick cell wall of mycobacteria is rich in mycolic acid and other complex lipids, making it hydrophobic and impermeable to aqueous stains without heat. Heat is applied in the Ziehl–Neelsen stain. The cell wall of mycobacteria contains N-glycolyl-muramic acid rather than N-acetyl-muramic acid.

Some of the specific lipids are the following:

- Mycolic acids: These are 13-hydroxy fatty acids that vary in size with species and are responsible for acid-fastness, the property of retaining carbol fuchsin after application of the decolorizer, acid alcohol, in the Ziehl–Neelsen stain.
- Mycosides: They are responsible for control of cellular permeability (resistance to water-soluble enzymes, antibiotics, and disinfectants). They are associated with cord factor and wax D, a mycoside that enhances the immune response. Wax D and various proteins induce delayed-type hypersensitivity. Cord factor inactivates the mitochondrial membranes within the phagocyte and also inhibits chemotaxis. If present systemically, cord factor is lethal. Recent evidence supports the hypothesis that factors responsible for virulence reside in mycosides, certain sulfolipids, and sulfatides.
- Glycolipids: They are toxic, contribute to a granulomatous response, and enhance survival of phagocytosed mycobacteria. Cord factor, a glycolipid, is responsible for the characteristic colonial growth (long palisade-like growth resembling serpentine cords) of virulent mycobacteria. Chemically, the cord factor is made up of trehalose-6-6′-dimycolate. Phenolic glycolipids associated with the cell wall act to scavenge and detoxify the toxigenic oxygen radicals that are produced by the macrophage oxidative burst. The cell wall glycolipid, lipoarabinomannan, suppresses T-cell proliferation by blocking transcription of those genes activated by interferon-γ within the macrophage, thereby interfering with the activation of additional macrophages.
- Sulfolipids: Associated with the organism's cell wall, sulfolipids are thought to inhibit phagosome–lysosome fusion within macrophages. They may also potentiate the toxic effect of cord factor on the mitochondrial membranes of the infected macrophage. In addition, they inhibit mitochondrial oxidative phosphorylation.

The release of lysosomal components by macrophages, as the result of the presence mycobacterial cell wall components (Fig. 29.1), induces the release of tumor necrosis factor α, which is associated with local lung damage in the case of *M. tuberculosis*.

Some Factors Contributing to Tuberculosis

First, crowding is important because it increases exposure to organisms from carriers. Thus, the infection rate is higher in stabled cattle as opposed to range cattle.

Second, genetic factors play a role in susceptibility; some races are more susceptible, including American Indians and Eskimos. Genetic differences in susceptibility among different domestic animal species do not appear to have been recognized.

Third, there is both natural and acquired resistance to tuberculosis; the latter is a result of previous exposure.

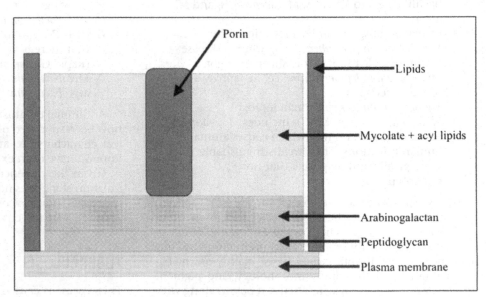

FIGURE 29.1   The mycobacterial cell wall. Starting with the plasma membrane, the mycobacterial cell wall comprises a thin layer of peptidoglycan, arabinogalactan, and the layer of mycolate and acyl lipids. Within these layers are various lipids and porins, as indicated.

Fourth, human immunodeficiency virus in humans and possibly some immunosuppressive infections in animals predispose an individual to tuberculosis.

Mode of Infection

MYCOBACTERIUM BOVIS. Organisms leave the host in respiratory discharges, feces, milk, urine, semen, and genital discharges. Infection is by inhalation. Localized lesions of lymph nodes of head and nodes of lungs and parenchyma of lungs are produced. In calves, the mode of infection is probably by ingestion. Lesions are seen in intestinal wall, mesenteric nodes, liver, and spleen and, secondarily, in lungs.

MYCOBACTERIUM AVIUM. Organisms are shed in feces and are acquired mainly by ingestion of contaminated food, water, and soil. Lesions may be found anywhere but usually involve intestines, liver, spleen, and bone marrow. Lung lesions are infrequent.

***MYCOBACTERIUM TUBERCULOSIS* (HUMAN).** Organisms are shed in the sputum and respiratory discharges. Direct spread is by droplet infection and fomites. Lesions are found in the lungs and lymph nodes principally.

Pathogenesis

The local manifestations depend on the route of invasion. In inhalation, the route is via the lungs and tracheobronchial lymph nodes. In ingestion, it is usually through the mesenteric nodes and intestinal wall and to the liver via the portal system. Organisms from lymph nodes may reach the thoracic duct with general dissemination. Animals develop delayed hypersensitivity and cell-mediated immunity, usually with a lessening of multiplication and dissemination. It is thought that delayed hypersensitivity of an exaggerated level attributable to large amounts of tubercular antigen may have a destructive effect on tissues. Most foci are microscopic, and most disappear. Some, however, may persist for years and in some instances may progress to form the characteristic tubercle. A tubercle consists of a centralized aggregation of enlarged macrophages (epithelioid cells), multinucleated giant cells (fused macrophages) containing tubercle bacilli, macrophages, lymphocytes, and fibroblasts. The center of the tubercle undergoes caseous necrosis.

Miliary tuberculosis is an acute form of the disease, with general dissemination and production of large numbers of small tubercles.

Pathogenicity

MYCOBACTERIUM BOVIS. Cattle are a natural host; swine are readily and severely infected. Rare infections occur in dogs, horses, and sheep. Cats are susceptible and may perpetuate the bovine disease. In cattle, there is pulmonary tuberculosis with involvement of associated lymph nodes. Infection of viscera and bones occurs in humans, especially from milk. Chickens are resistant, but

rabbits, mice, and guinea pigs are very susceptible (generalized infections).

MYCOBACTERIUM AVIUM. Chickens are most susceptible, but other birds can be infected; not all infected chickens have gross lesions. Crowding is an important factor. Waterfowl are quite resistant, but house birds are susceptible. In swine, disease usually occurs in lymph nodes of the head. Cattle are refractory but can be sensitized. Mink fed infected chickens will become infected. Infections in humans are of little consequence. Guinea pigs are slightly susceptible; rabbits are quite susceptible. Sporadic cases have been reported in horses, dogs, and cats. Psittacine birds are resistant to *M. avium* but susceptible to *M. tuberculosis*.

MYCOBACTERIUM TUBERCULOSIS. It occurs in humans and primates; the latter acquire the disease from humans. Cattle are sensitized by the human organism. In swine, disease usually occurs in lymph nodes of the head, and organisms are acquired by the eating of uncooked garbage. Parrots are susceptible, chickens are rarely infected, dogs can be infected, and cats are very resistant. Guinea pigs and mice are very susceptible, and rabbits are slightly susceptible. The pulmonary form occurs in elephants.

Laboratory Diagnosis

Great care should be exercised in handling suspected clinical materials. The organism can be demonstrated in smears from lesions by employing acid-fast stains. The organisms are small, straight, or slightly curved, and they occur singly or in clumps. They stain red by the Ziehl–Neelsen acid-fast stain.

An alternative, sensitive staining procedure uses fluorescein dyes. Acid-fast organisms examined by this procedure stain yellow. A negative smear does not mean that the specimen is negative for acid-fast organisms.

Frequently, a preliminary diagnosis of tuberculosis is made on the basis of the demonstration of typical acid-fast organisms in characteristic lesions. Definitive diagnosis of tuberculosis requires isolation and identification. Isolation should be attempted only if the laboratory is equipped with proper biocontainment facilities.

One procedure for isolation and cultivation from clinical material, such as nodules, is, briefly, as follows:

1. Trim fat off tissues and add 4% NaOH to digest tissue and kill contaminating bacteria.
2. Grind tissue in a sterile mortar with sterile sand, centifuge, then add HCl to neutralize sediment.
3. Inoculate sediment onto Lowenstein–Jensen slants and egg yolk agar slants and incubate at 37°C for up to 8 weeks.
4. Stain smears from growth if the latter is characteristic of mycobacteria; identify if organisms are acid-fast.

Cultural characteristics of the "classic" species of mycobacteria are given in Table 29.1.

Identification is based principally on cultural, morphologic, and biochemical characteristics. This phenotypic

Table 29.1 Cultural Characteristics of Classic Species of Mycobacteria

Mycobacterium bovis	*Mycobacterium avium*	*Mycobacterium tuberculosis*
Dry, sparse, delicate nonluxuriant; growth on solid media incubated at 37°C usually appears within 3–6 weeks.	Moist, slimy, glistening, luxuriant, frequently yellow or gray; growth on solid media incubated at 40°–42°C usually appears within 2–3 weeks.	Dry, crumbly, luxuriant; colonies are usually yellowish with roughened surfaces; growth on solid media incubated at 37°C usually appears within 2 weeks.

approach is complex and time-consuming and is being replaced by the use of specific probes. Definitive identification is usually carried out in a reference laboratory. Identification based on phenotypic characteristics can take more than a week for rapid growers and several weeks to months for slow growers.

To identify mycobacteria from clinical specimens in a relatively shorter period of time, commercially available, species-specific isotopic and nonisotopic deoxyribonucleic acid (DNA) probes are available. Genetically, identification is based on specific amplification of the 16S rRNA sequences of *Mycobacterium* species. Probes are used to detect **IS6110** that are common to all *M. tuberculosis* strains.

Antigenic Nature and Serology

Mycobacterium bovis and *M. tuberculosis* are antigenically closely related. Monoclonal antibodies appear to be helpful in recognizing the antigenic variations between these two species. DNA homology between *M. bovis* and *M. tuberculosis* is nearly 100%. *Mycobacterium avium* can be readily differentiated serologically from *M. bovis* and *M. tuberculosis*.

Mycobacterium avium resembles *M. intracellulare* antigenically; each possesses different serotypes. Both were referred to as the *M. avium-intracellulare* complex, but *M. avium* complex is now preferred. Species-specific DNA probes have been constructed and used for the rapid identification of *M. avium* and *M. intracellulare*.

The serological diagnosis of mycobacterial infections (except for paratuberculosis) in animals and humans is not reliable. Sufficiently sensitive, specific, and standardized testing procedures are not available.

Resistance

In general, mycobacteria are rather resistant to various physical influences and chemical disinfectants. Their considerable resistance is partly the result of the presence of lipid in the cell wall. Species causing tuberculosis retain their viability in putrefying carcasses and in moist soil for 1–4 years and survive for at least 150 days in dry bovine feces. Freezing temperatures have little, if any, effect. Drying is only effective when the organisms are also exposed to direct sunlight. They are fairly resistant to acids and alkalis; phenolic disinfectants are effective. In addition, sodium hypochlorite at 1:200 or 1:1000 concentration and phenol–soap mixtures or other phenol derivatives are suitable for laboratory use.

Treatment

Treatment is usually not feasible or desirable in animals. One of the most useful drugs in the treatment of tuberculosis is isoniazid. It has been employed prophylactically to control tuberculosis in zoos and animal parks. Isoniazid and ethionamide both work by inhibiting the synthesis of mycolic acids.

The 6-month regimen recommended for human tuberculosis is isoniazid, rifampin, and pyrazinamide for the first 2 months, followed by isonizid and pyrazinamide for 4 months. A four-drug regimen that includes ethambutol and streptomycin is also used. Regimens are altered if there is evidence of drug resistance. Treatment may be continued for up to 18 months. Because of possible side effects, streptomycin is only given for several months. The new fluoroquinolones, such as spafloxacillin, have been used with some success; however, resistant strains have been observed.

Immunity

Although antibodies are produced in tuberculosis, immunity is primarily cell-mediated. *Mycobacterium tuberculosis* produces a fibronectin binding protein, which potentially interferes with stimulation of T cells and activation of additional macrophages. However, those T cells that secrete interferon-γ stimulate the endothelial cells to bond T cells and allow their movement to the infected area. In addition to activated macrophages, cytotoxic T cells are activated to kill those macrophages infected with *M. tuberculosis*. If this process is elicited early in the infection, no clinical signs are observed. However, the individual will test positive to exposure to the bacteria. Unfortunately, some of the bacteria may escape the sequestration as described above and pass to the regional lymph nodes. From there, they can disseminate via the blood stream to other locations within the body. In addition, if the infection is not cleared, the characteristic tubercle is formed, which may become calcified.

The only vaccine used to any extent is the BCG vaccine (bacille Calmette Guerin). It is a live bovine strain that has been attenuated by growth in potato–glycerin bile medium through several hundred transfers. It is used for the prevention of tuberculosis in children and calves, in which the disease is prevalent. It has not been used in the United States because it has no place in an eradication program; it sensitizes animals to tuberculin.

Hypersensitivity to tuberculin indicates some resistance to tuberculosis. The tuberculin reactions are sometimes negative (**anergy**) if the infection is overwhelming or if there is a deficiency in cell-mediated immunity.

Field Diagnosis and Control

In the field, diagnosis is carried out by means of the tuberculin test, which depends on a reaction of the delayed hypersensitivity type. Several tuberculins are used; all contain mycobacterial proteins, to which infected animals may be hypersensitive. Koch's "Old Tuberculin," which has been used widely in the standardization of tuberculins, is a filtrate of an 8-week-old culture of *M. tuberculosis*. The tuberculin used for the routine testing of cattle in the United States is prepared from strains of *M. bovis*. Avian tuberculin is used in the comparative test (double intradermal) in cattle as well as in swine and poultry. PPD (purified protein derivative) is a relatively pure tuberculin.

The tuberculin tests commonly used are

- Intradermal: Read at 72 hours; firm swelling indicates a positive reaction. This is the most widely used test. The sites of inoculation in cattle are the caudal fold, the vulvar lips, or the sides of the neck.
- Comparative cervical: Intradermal inoculation of regular and avian tuberculin at two different sites in the neck. Read at 72 hours by measuring swelling.
- Ophthalmic: Mostly used on primates; dilution of regular "bovine" tuberculin is inoculated intradermally into the upper eyelid.

The tuberculosis eradication program is based on the detection and slaughter of infected animals as determined by the tuberculin test. The eradication program began in 1917 when the infection rate was ~5%; it is now near 0%. At present, most of the reactors do not have gross lesions characteristic of bovine tuberculosis. Their tuberculin sensitivity is mostly attributed to other mycobacteria, and it was for this reason that the comparative cervical test was introduced.

The absence of infected cattle and the pasteurization of milk have all but eliminated human infection with *M. bovis*.

FREE-LIVING MYCOBACTERIA

This includes many species, only a small number of which are pathogenic (see Runyon groups discussed earlier). They are worldwide in distribution, occurring and living in soil and water. The species distribution varies with the kind of soil and various climatic and environmental factors. They can sometimes be isolated from animal feces. Generally speaking, severe infections caused by some species of these mycobacteria occur in humans and animals only after impairment of the body's immune system.

Pathogenicity

The pathogenicity of some of the many free-living mycobacteria is referred to briefly below.

***MYCOBACTERIUM AVIUM* COMPLEX.** This includes the species *M. avium* and *M. intracellulare* of which there are a number of serotypes. The pathogenicity of *M. avium* was discussed above. Various serotypes of this complex cause opportunistic infections in domestic animals and humans. Some strains formerly called the Battey bacilli cause serious human infections.

***MYCOBACTERIUM FORTUITUM*.** Causes skin infections in dogs and cats, lymph node infections in cattle and pigs, mastitis in cattle, joint and respiratory infections in pigs, and pneumonia in dogs. Highly resistant to a number of commonly used antimicrobial drugs.

***MYCOBACTERIUM CHELONII*.** Causes injection and wound infections.

***MYCOBACTERIUM KANSASII*.** Has been recovered from lymph nodes of cattle, pigs, and other animals.

***MYCOBACTERIUM MARINUM*.** Causes infections in fish and other cold-blooded animals. Causes swimming pool granuloma in humans.

***MYCOBACTERIUM SCROFULACEUM*.** Infects cervical lymph nodes of cattle and pigs.

***MYCOBACTERIUM XENOPI*.** Isolated from amphibians and seafowl.

***MYCOBACTERIUM ULCERANS*.** Rats, mice, rabbits, and guinea pigs are susceptible. Causes skin ulcers in humans.

***MYCOBACTERIUM GENAVEUSE*.** Causes infections in pet birds.

***MYCOBACTERIUM SMEGMATIS*.** Soil and smegma; mastitis in cattle.

***MYCOBACTERIUM PHLEI*.** Soil; nonpathogenic. An extract of this organism (mycobactin) is used in a medium for the isolation and growth of the cause of paratuberculosis.

***MYCOBACTERIUM SENEGALENSE* AND *MYCOBACTERIUM FARCINOGENES*.** These closely related species cause bovine farcy (cutaneous infection) in Africa.

Laboratory Diagnosis

These mycobacteria grow well on Lowenstein–Jensen medium and other culture media used for mycobacteria. The procedures used for isolation are similar to those referred to earlier for the tubercle bacilli. DNA probes may be available for the identification of some species. Identification based on phenotypic characteristics is beyond the scope of most diagnostic laboratories.

Among the tests used for the identification of potentially pathogenic free-living mycobacteria (nonphotochromogens, photochromogens, scotochromogens, and rapid growers referred to above) are the following: time required for growth, urease production, deamination of pyrazinamide, pigment production, NaCl tolerance, growth on MacConkey agar, niacin production, tween 80 hydrolysis, inhibition by glycerol, nitrate reduction, iron uptake, arylsulfatase (time required), catalase production, and optimum growth temperature. The various species of mycobacteria can be identified in reference labs using HPLC (high performance liquid chromatography) analysis of mycolic acids.

SKIN TUBERCULOSIS OF CATTLE

Mycobacteria have been demonstrated from skin lesions consisting of cold, firm, rounded swellings and fluctuant thick-walled abscesses. They occur most commonly in the skin of the legs and ventral abdomen; they may soften and ulcerate. Because of the lymphatic distribution of lesions, the term ulcerative lymphangitis has been used. The organisms, which have not been cultivated, may sensitize cattle to tuberculin.

MYCOBACTERIUM LEPRAE

Mycobacterium leprae causes leprosy (Hansen's disease), a chronic disease affecting the skin and peripheral nerve trunks of humans. The incubation period may be up to 20 years. It occurs worldwide but is most prevalent in tropical countries and is infrequent in countries in temperate regions. It has not been cultivated in vitro, but experimental infections have been produced in the armadillo, mice, hamsters, rats, ground squirrels, hedgehogs, and monkeys. Mice and the nine-banded armadillo are the most susceptible. Armadillos in Texas and Louisiana have been found naturally infected with a disease identical to leprosy.

A combination of three drugs, dapsone, rifampicin, and clofazimine, is curative and overcomes drug resistance.

FELINE LEPROSY

Feline leprosy, which occurs widely, is presumed to be caused by an organism identical to *M. lepraemurium*, the cause of a leprosy-like disease of rats.

The feline disease is characterized by the formation of single and multiple granulomas or nodules of the skin 1–3 cm in diameter. They are painless and move freely. Some may be ulcerous and discharge a slight, serosanguineous exudate. Affected cats are usually in good health, and only in rare cases does the disease become generalized. It is thought that cats acquire the infection via rat bites.

Long, slender, acid-fast rods can be demonstrated in smears from the nodules. The slow-growing feline and rat organisms have been cultivated on a special medium containing cytochrome C and α-ketoglutarate.

Treatment involves the surgical removal of nodules, which do not usually recur. Variable results have been obtained with the antileprosy (human) drug dapsone. Streptomycin and isoniazid are toxic for the cat.

MYCOBACTERIUM AVIUM SUBSP. PARATUBERCULOSIS

Mycobacterium avium subsp. *paratuberculosis* was formerly known as *M. paratuberculosis*.

This organism, the cause of Johne's disease or paratuberculosis, is found worldwide. Cattle, sheep, goats and other wild and domestic ruminants are affected, including deer, camels, and llamas. Because there is no national eradication plan for this disease in the United States, it is difficult to determine its precise incidence. It may be sufficiently prevalent in some dairy herds to constitute a real problem. Annual death losses within an infected herd may reach 10%.

Animals are infected by ingestion of food and water contaminated by feces. The incidence of subclinical cases shedding organisms intermittently may be as high as 15%. The organism may be present in colostrum and milk and thus infect calves, and intrauterine infection has been reported.

Pathogenesis and Pathogenicity

The ingested bacteria of paratuberculosis are taken up by macrophages that are found in the intestinal lymph nodes mainly in the ileocecal region. If the infection progresses, there is an immune-mediated granulomatous reaction in the submucosa with the accumulation of large numbers of macrophages and lymphocytes. The migration of macrophages and lymphocytes is mediated by cytokines such as IL-12 and γ-interferon. These are aided by T-helper-cells secreting cytokines associated with a cell-mediated immune response. As infected macrophages do not respond well to these cytokine signals, they accumulate in the submucosa and are eventually sloughed off.

Iron appears to play an important role in the pathogenesis. Presence of a large quantity of intracellular iron correlates well with the severity of lesions. High levels of iron and iron-containing compounds are also positively correlated with fecal shedding of organisms from infected cattle. Experimental infections can be established orally or intravenously. Dosage of organisms is probably important in establishing infections. Toxic substances have not been demonstrated.

In cattle there is chronic enteritis, often with severe diarrhea. The diarrhea in sheep, goats, and other ruminants is usually less severe or absent. The incubation period may be a year or more. Calves are susceptible but do not show signs until adulthood. The disease is usually progressive, leading to emaciation and death. Mortality is caused in large part by the malabsorption of amino acids and the loss of protein into the intestine (protein-losing enteropathy). The ileum and colon are usually involved, and the infection may extend to the rectum in advanced cases. The mucous membrane becomes corrugated and thickened because of epithelioid and giant cells, both of which contain many organisms. Large numbers of organisms may be shed in the feces.

The organism has been isolated from the udder and from the reproductive tracts of both male and female cattle. Disseminated paratuberculosis of both kidneys of a cow has been reported. Bovine fetal infection with the organism has also been reported. Mice, hamsters, pigs, and horses have been infected experimentally.

Laboratory Diagnosis

The organisms are often difficult to demonstrate in smears, and failure to demonstrate organisms does not exclude Johne's disease. A number of smears may have to be examined. Thin smears are made from feces, intestinal mucosa (terminal ileum preferred) in the dead animal, and rectal mucosa in the live animal. The rectal smears may only be positive in advanced cases. On average, the rectal smear will only detect about 25% of infected animals. A small piece of the rectum is pinched out, washed, and then squeezed between two slides. The resulting smear and other smears are stained by the Ziehl–Neelsen method. Johne's bacilli occur singly and in characteristic clumps and stain a pinkish red. Bovine feces frequently yield saprophytic acid-fast organisms that can be mistaken for Johne's bacilli.

A reliable but complicated procedure requiring laparotomy is to examine smears of biopsies of mesenteric lymph nodes taken in the region of the terminal ileum for acid-fast organisms.

The organism grows very slowly, and cultivation and identification may take months. The feces or tissue is treated for contaminants. A medium containing mycobactin (extract of *M. phlei*) is used. Colonies appear in 4–12 weeks.

In smears, organisms appear as short, thick, small, acid-fast rods similar to the avian tubercle bacillus. Identification is based on cultural (including growth rate and mycobactin dependency), morphologic, and staining characteristics and seroagglutination.

DNA probes with polymerase chain reaction amplification have been used for rapid identification of the organism in bovine feces.

Serologic tests used for the diagnosis of paratuberculosis include the enzyme-linked immunosorbent assay (ELISA), a complement-fixation test, and an agar gel immunodiffusion test. The ELISA is more sensitive and specific than the complement-fixation and immunodiffusion tests.

Resistance

Mycobacterium paratuberculosis resembles other mycobacteria in its resistance to physical and chemical influences; it will survive in contaminated stables for months.

Control

The intravenous johnin test will detect about 80% of cases found to be infected by cultural methods. A positive reaction is indicated by a temperature rise of 1.5°F or more. The complement-fixation test is used as a screening procedure, but it is not as reliable as culture of feces. The agar gel immunodiffusion test is widely used but lacks sensitivity. An ELISA has been developed that is sensitive and specific.

Among steps taken to control paratuberculosis are the following:

- Animals with persistent diarrhea or chronic weight loss should be isolated or sent to slaughter.
- Culture the feces from all animals 2 years old or older every 6 months and remove and slaughter animals (and their offspring) whose cultures are positive.
- Adults from the herd should be sold only for slaughter or to quarantined feedlots.
- Clean and disinfect the premises after the removal of infected animals.
- Calf-rearing quarters should have separate cleaning and feeding equipment; calves are easily infected.
- Continue surveillance until there have been four consecutive negative fecal cultures of all animals 2 years of age or older.
- Purchase only animals with johnin-negative tests from herds with no history of the disease.
- If artificial insemination is used, semen should come from culturally negative bulls.

Immunity

The antigenic relationship between this organism and the avian tubercle bacillus is indicated by the fact that animals with Johne's disease often react to avian tuberculin.

Bacterins have been used in sheep and calves with some success, but immunization has not been widely practiced and is not permitted in cattle in some countries. Vaccinated animals may be johnin- and tuberculin-positive.

As in tuberculosis, immunity in Johne's disease is considered to be predominantly cell-mediated.

Public Health Significance

Mycobacterium avium subsp. *paratuberculosis* has been isolated from the tissues of several human patients with **Crohn's disease.** Micro- and macroscopically, Crohn's disease (Crohn's ileitis) is very similar to Johne's disease. Whether or not this organism has a role in the etiology of Crohn's disease remains to be determined.

GLOSSARY

anergy Failure to react immunologically to the injection of an allergen or antigen.

Crohn's disease Disease mainly affecting the small intestine (regional ileitis) and characterized by cramps, diarrhea, local abscesses, weight loss, and inappetence. The cause is not known.

IS6110 Insertion sequences typically associated with transposons.

30

Nocardia and *Rhodococcus*

The genera *Nocardia* (14 species) and *Rhodococcus* (12 species) are in the family Nocardiaceae and are related taxonomically to the corynebacteria and mycobacteria. These gram-positive, aerobic rods occur worldwide as saprophytes in soil and water. *Mycobacterium*, *Gordona*, *Nocardia*, and *Rhodococcus* all possess mycolic acid as a constituent of their cell wall. Differences are based on chain length and number of double bonds. In the case of *Nocardia*, the mycolic acids are called nocardomycolic (44–60 carbons) acids. Only one species of *Rhodococcus* and several species of *Nocardia* are of veterinary significance.

NOCARDIA

Nocardia are nonmotile, non-spore-forming, gram-positive rods that usually show branching and aerial hyphae. They are aerobic, split sugars by oxidation and are usually partially acid-fast. There is considerable confusion in the taxonomy of *Nocardia*. Several species, all soilborne, have been described. The following are important pathogens:

- "*Nocardia asteroides* complex" infects domestic animals and humans.
- *Nocardia otitidiscaviarum* (formerly *Nocardia caviae*) infects the guinea pig and humans and causes bovine mastitis.
- *Nocardia brasiliensis* is one of the causes of nocardiosis in humans.

NOCARDIA ASTEROIDES

What has been referred to as *N. asteroides* is now considered a complex made up of *N. asteroides*, *Nocardia farcinica* and *Nocardia nova*. As the animal hosts of these species are not yet clearly defined, we will consider *N. asteroides* to be the principal pathogen of domestic animals.

Nocardia asteroides is found widely distributed in the soil as a saprophyte. Infection is by inhalation or wounds. It is exogenous and not considered contagious.

Pathogenesis

The pathogenesis of nocardiosis is somewhat like that of actinomycosis. Infection begins as a nodule or pustule that ruptures. There is suppuration with subsequent induration. A localized form (skin) and thoracic and systemic forms are seen.

Toxins have not been demonstrated. The cell wall of nocardiae possesses mycolic acids that contribute to virulence by resisting killing by macrophages.

In vitro, virulent *N. asteroides* can grow within and destroy macrophages. The resistance of this species to oxidative killing by neutrophils and monocytes has been attributed to nocardial catalase and superoxide dismutase. Some human strains of *N. asteroides* display an as yet unexplained neurotropism.

Pathogenicity

Nocardiosis is usually a chronic progressive disease characterized by suppurating, granulomatous lesions. Sporadic infections occur in many animal species.

CATTLE.   It causes an acute or chronic mastitis with granulomatous lesions and draining fistulous tracts.

The tropical disease bovine farcy was initially attributed to *N. farcinica*; however, its precise cause is in question. The diseases is a suppurative infection mainly involving the neck and limbs. It begins in the skin and may involve the superficial lymph vessels and nodes. A similar disease occurring in Africa has been attributed to *Mycobacterium senegalense* and *Mycobacterium farcinogenes*.

DOGS AND CATS.   There is a localized form of the disease, with subcutaneous lesions (mycetomas) or lymph node involvement or both. In the dog, there is a thoracic form with occasional extension to the abdominal cavity. Like actinomycosis in the dog caused by *Actinomyces viscosus*, there is a suppurative pleuritis or peritonitis or both, with the accumulation of pleural, pericardial, and peritoneal fluid. Abscesses may be found in the heart, brain, liver, and kidneys as well. Severe halitosis, gingivitis, and ulceration of the oral cavity are common in dogs with nocardial stomatitis.

HORSES.   Nocardiosis is infrequent in the horse; however, respiratory and disseminated nocardiosis have been reported in immunosuppressed horses.

Unlike actinomycosis, granules are not found in infections caused by *N. asteroides*. Because the treatments of nocardiosis and actinomycosis may be different, it is very important that a correct diagnosis be made.

HUMANS.   The most common forms in humans are pulmonary nocardiosis and a subcutaneous form (hands and feet of agricultural laborers). Because of central nervous system involvement proceeding from the pulmonary form, the case–fatality rate is high.

Nocardiosis is not considered a zoonotic disease.

Direct Examination

Gram-stained smears of pus reveal some rods to coccoid forms and gram-positive branching filaments. The acid-fast stain of most strains shows retention of some of the carbolfuchsin.

Isolation and Identification

The organism grows on unenriched media, on blood agar, and Sabouraud agar, at 25°or 37°C. Growth is evident in 4 or 5 days, and colonies are irregularly folded, raised and smooth, or granular. The color varies from white through yellow to deep orange. Gram-positive, partially acid-fast, branching mycelial filaments, which break up into bacillary and coccoid forms, are evident under oil immersion. The presence of mycelial elements distinguishes *Nocardia* from saprophytic and atypical mycobacteria. The mycelial forms of *Nocardia* can be readily seen in slide cultures on Sabouraud dextrose agar. The mycelial elements may give regular cultures a powdery appearance. The branching filaments of *N. asteroides* resemble those of *Actinomyces bovis*.

A presumptive identification is based on pathology and demonstration of typical organisms in clinical material and on colonial, cultural, morphologic, and staining characteristics. Although pathogenic nocardiae are usually partially acid-fast, some strains are not. Nocardiae reduce nitrate and are catalase positive.

Nocardia species are definitively identified by a number of biochemical and growth tests and resistance to some antibiotics. These procedures are beyond the scope of most diagnostic laboratories.

Streptomyces spp. and *Actinomadura* spp. have aerial hyphae, are not acid-fast, and are not pathogenic for mice and guinea pigs. They are occasionally isolated from mycetomas in animals in the tropics.

Rapidly growing *Mycobacterium* spp., which occur widely, can be distinguished by their occurrence as rods rather than as fragmenting hyphae and by their strong acid-fastness.

Treatment

Treatment consists of surgical debridement and drainage of lesions. Antimicrobial susceptibility tests should be performed, as there are differences in susceptibility among the species of the *N. asteroides* complex. Trimethoprim-sulfonamides are effective. Antimicrobial treatment may have to be continued for as long as 12 weeks.

There is no effective treatment for nocardial mastitis.

STREPTOMYCES AND ACTINOMADURA

These non-acid-fast actinomycetes are rarely causes of infections in animals. *Streptomyces griseous* and *Actinomadura madurae* have been isolated infrequently from mycetomas in cats and goats, respectively.

RHODOCOCCUS

The genus *Rhodococcus* is a diverse group, with 12 species that differ considerably in morphology, growth characteristics, biochemical activity, and capacity to produce disease. They are soilborne, and all produce pigments of various colors. They possess mycolic acids but are not acid-fast. They are gram-positive, aerobic, nonfermentative, and catalase and urease positive. Many have the ability to metabolize unusual substrates and are therefore of interest in bioremediation (use of microorganisms in environmental clean up) studies.

Only one species, *Rhodococcus equi*, is an important animal pathogen.

RHODOCOCCUS EQUI

Rhodococcus equi was formerly known as *Corynebacterium equi*.

Habitat

Rhodococcus equi is soilborne and often is present in manure. It is present in the intestine of many horses and persists for long periods in the manure and litter of stables.

Mode of Infection

Infection may result from direct contact with, or inhalation of, contaminated soil (dust), manure, infectious secretions, or feces. Infection can also be by ingestion and congenitally via umbilical exposure.

Pathogenesis and Pathogenicity

The principal disease is suppurative bronchopneumonia in foals 1–6 months old, characterized by suppurative abscesses of varying size in the lungs and in associated lymph nodes. On occasion, there may be infection of the skin, joints, and spleen. Ulcerative intestinal lesions and infections of the mesenteric lymph nodes are occasionally observed. Foals 1–2 months old are the most severely affected, and the overall case–fatality may exceed 50%. Sporadic cases are seen, and also a number of foals may be affected on the same premises. It is thought that recurring cases on so-called problem farms is attributable to a build up of *R. equi* in the environment.

Clinical signs of the respiratory disease include coughing, mucopurulent nasal discharge, fever, and difficulty breathing. Chest radiographs indicate the extent of the pulmonary disease.

Aside from the respiratory form, various infections have been noted in adult horses and foals, including abortion, uterine infections, and in foals necrotizing enterocolitis and subcutaneous abscesses.

It is a common cause of submandibular and cervical lymphadenitis of swine. The lesions resemble those of tuberculosis. *Rhodococcus equi* is an infrequent cause of abscesses of the lungs and lymph nodes of various animals. Abscesses probably initiated via wounds have been reported in cats. In some instances, these various abscesses may lead to a bacteremia or septicemia.

Rhodococcus equi is a facultative intracellular parasite that survives in macrophages. The large polysaccharide capsule and cell wall constituents probably contribute to its virulence and pathogenesis. The *R. equi* factors, phospholipase C and cholesterol oxidase, are also considered to have a role in disease development.

After an initial granulomatous response in the foal disease, there is suppuration and development of abscesses.

Both virulent and avirulent strains are encountered. Several different plasmids have been isolated from *R. equi*. A virulence plasmid (85–90 kb) has been associated with virulence. It is correlated with a cell surface protein called Vap (virulence associated protein), the role of which is not known. The genetic map of this plasmid is available (*Can. J. Vet. Res.* 1995. Vol 59(3), pp. 229–231). Many additional putative genes have been identified on the plasmid but have yet to be characterized.

Isolation and Identification

Gram-positive, usually coccoid, occasionally rod-shaped organisms are seen in pus.

The organism grows well on blood agar aerobically at 37°C. In 48 hours, colonies are smooth, mucoid, translucent, and 3–5 mm in diameter. On some media, a pink pigment is produced.

Identification is based on the characteristic cellular and colonial morphology and some biochemical characteristics, including positive tests for catalase and urease.

A phenomenon resembling the CAMP reaction can be used to identify *R. equi*. Partial hemolysins from *R. equi* enhance the hemolysis of the phospholipase D of *Corynebacterium pseudotuberculosis* or the beta-hemolysin of *Staphylococcus aureus*.

Antigenic Nature and Immunity

Rhodococcus equi possesses a large polysaccharide capsule that is antigenically diverse. More than 25 different capsular types have been identified from different animal and geographic sources. Although antibody to *R. equi* is found in the sera of normal horses and can be elicited by inoculation of killed organisms, most protection is attributed to cell-mediated immunity. Autogenous bacterins have not been effective in preventing the disease. Adult horses are generally immune to infection.

Treatment

A combination of erythromycin and rifampin for 4–10 weeks is the preferred treatment. Because of the suppurative nature of the lesions, treatment is only effective if started early.

Public Health Significance

Human infections caused by *R. equi* are infrequent and are not considered to be animal related. Infections occur most commonly in immunocompromised individuals—for example, those with HIV infection. The disease is usually a subacute necrotizing pneumonia, although abscesses may occur in the central nervous system, subcutaneous tissue, pelvis, and lymph nodes.

31 *Chlamydia*

We will use *Chlamydia* and chlamydiae to refer to organisms in the genera *Chlamydia* and *Chlamydophila*. These genera are placed in Phylum IX "Wall-less Forms," and the Family Chlamydiaceae, in which they are the only genera. In contrast, the *Rickettsia* are in Phylum VII, Proteobacteria. Until recently, there was only one genus, *Chlamydia*, in the family. From studies employing 16S and 23S rRNA genes of a number of organisms within *Chlamydia*, another genus, *Chlamydophila*, was designated.

Chlamydiae are nonmotile, gram-negative, pleomorphic, obligate intracellular bacteria. They replicate within host cells and have a unique developmental cycle.

The following species are recognized:

- *Chlamydophila psittaci*: Causes avian chlamydiosis and bovine abortion and, in humans, psittacosis.
- *Chlamydophila pecorum*: It has been recovered from cattle and sheep with various diseases including sporadic bovine encephalitis, infectious polyarthritis, pneumonia, and diarrhea.
- *Chlamydophila abortus*: Enzootic abortion of sheep and goats; chlamydial abortion in cattle, pigs, and goats.
- *Chlamydophila suis*: Intestinal infections in pigs.
- *Chlamydophila caviae*: Inclusion conjunctivitis in guinea pigs.
- *Chlamydophila pneumoniae*: One serovar; cause of a variety of respiratory infections in humans. Similar organisms have been recovered from horses and koalas with respiratory infections and conjunctivitis, respectively.
- *Chlamydia felis*: Conjunctivitis (feline pneumonitis).
- *Chlamydia trachomatis*: Many serovars; causes trachoma, inclusion conjunctivitis in infants, lymphogranuloma venereum, other genital tract infections, and proctitis in humans. Organisms similar to this species have been isolated from swine and ferrets.
- *Chlamydia muridarum*: Respiratory infections in mice.

Chlamydia have both ribonucleic acid (RNA), deoxyribonucleic acid (DNA), and cell walls like gram-negative bacteria. They possess some bacterial enzymes, but their metabolism is restricted. As a result, they are very dependent on the host cell. Metabolically, they are capable of hydrolyzing glucose, pyruvate, and glutamate. They are susceptible to many broad-spectrum antibiotics. They exist in two stages: infectious forms called elementary bodies, and intracytoplasmic forms called reticulate bodies. Their developmental cycle follows.

Developmental Cycle

There are four phases of the chlamydial life cycle. The chlamydiae begin their life cycle as highly infectious elementary bodies, capable of entering host epithelial, mucosal, or phagocytic cells via phagocytosis. The elementary bodies are spherical and approximately 0.25 μm in diameter.

Phase 1, known as the dormant phase, refers to elementary bodies before uptake by a target cell. This is the case during initial infection or release of infectious particles from a lysed host cell. The elementary bodies have very little metabolic activity during this time.

Phase 2 is the induction of metabolic activities with the elementary bodies. This activity is stimulated by the uptake of an elementary body by a host cell. Once phagocytosized, they form intracytoplasmic, membrane-limited inclusions within the phagocytic vacuole.

Phase 3 is characterized by the transformation of the elementary bodies into noninfectious reticulate bodies. This transformation is the result of nucleoid dispersion. The reticulate body enlarges in diameter to 0.5–0.6 μm. Ten to 15 hours later, the reticulate bodies divide by binary fission.

Phase 4 is characterized by the reversion of the mature reticulate bodies back into elementary bodies. This occurs within 20–30 hours following replication. Forty to 60 hours following replication, the host cell lyses and releases the new elementary bodies, which are capable of infecting more host cells (Fig. 31.1).

Antigenic Nature

All chlamydiae share a group (genus)-specific antigen. This antigen, also known as complement fixation antigen, is lipopolysaccharide in nature, with ketodeoxyoctanoic acid as the reactive moiety. In addition, chlamydiae possess species-specific and serovar (serotype)-specific antigens. For example, more than 15 serovars of *C. trachomatis* have been described.

Toxins have not been demonstrated from *Chlamydia*. However, as with other gram-negative bacteria, the lipid A

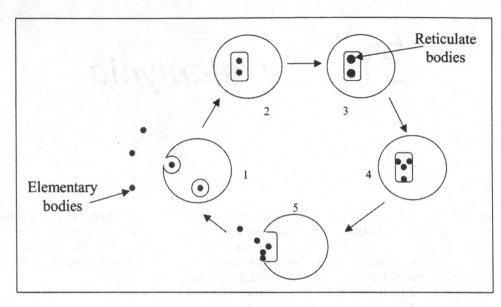

FIGURE 31.1 Developmental cycle of *Chlamydia*. **(1)** Elementary bodies are taken up by host cells and reside within intracellular vacuoles. **(2)** The elementary bodies then undergo metabolic activity. **(3)** The elementary bodies have developed into reticulate bodies. **(4)** The reticulate bodies divide by binary fission to form elementary bodies. **(5)** The new elementary bodies are then released and the cycle continues.

portion of the lipopolysaccharide (LPS) does have endotoxic properties. The elementary bodies produce hemagglutinin, whereas the reticulate bodies do not.

Habitat and Mode of Infection

Chlamydiae infect the mucous membranes of the respiratory and gastrointestinal tracts of many normal animals, including avian species. The organisms (elementary bodies) are shed in secretions and feces in small numbers from asymptomatic animals. Chlamydiae can survive for long periods in soil and feces.

Animals and humans are infected by the inhalation of infectious dust and droplets. In some chlamydioses, such as enzootic abortion of ewes or enteritis, infection may take place by ingestion. There is evidence suggesting that arthropod-borne infections may occur. In contrast to chlamydiae, the rickettsiae are transmitted by arthropods.

Immunity

Immunity is both cell-mediated and humoral. The serotype-specific antigen stimulates production of protective antibody. The role of cell-mediated immunity is currently unknown.

Pathogenesis

The virulence factors of the chlamydiae are currently an intense area of investigation. The LPS is considered to be a putative virulence factor in that it stimulates inflammatory responses by the host that can result in atherosclerosis and stimulate the production of immune complexes that can result in human stroke.

Another virulence attribute of the chlamydiae is the production of CPAF (chlamydial protease- or proteasome-like activity factor). This factor allows the chlamydiae to escape recognition by T cells, allowing the bacterium to

continue its life cycle repeatedly within the host. CPAF does this by degrading the host transcription factors associated with the production of **MHC** (major histocompatability complex) molecules. Interestingly, CPAF is unique to and highly conserved among the chlamydiae.

Another putative virulence factor is the type III secretion apparatus, as seen in other pathogens, including *Yersinia*. The type III secretion apparatus provides a "pore" in the vacuole membrane and allows the transport of products into the **cytosol** of the host cell. CPAF may be secreted in this manner.

The chlamydiae have a predilection for epithelial cells of the mucous membranes, although other tissues in a variety of locations are regularly infected. Pneumonia may develop from the inhalation of infectious dust and droplets. In enzootic abortion of ewes, the mode of infection is ingestion, and organisms localize in cells of the placenta. Latency is a common feature of chlamydial infections. Latent infections may be activated by various stresses and concurrent infections. Persistent antigenic stimulation provokes chronic inflammation in host tissues. It is thought that chlamydial LPS stimulates the production of interleukin-1, which mediates inflammation and scarring.

Pathogenicity

Chlamydophila psittaci causes avian chlamydiosis, a worldwide disease of poultry, pet birds, wild birds, and other avian species. Psittacosis is the human disease, which is contracted from exposure to avian species shedding the causal agent (see Public Health Significance below). The appellation ornithosis is superfluous and now is rarely used.

Avian chlamydiosis is manifested in a latent (inapparent sublinical), subacute, or chronic form. The respiratory and digestive tracts are affected, and the infection may become systemic. There is considerable variation in the virulence of strains. Outbreaks in poultry flocks are uncommon.

Signs of the avian disease include ocular and nasal discharges, sinusitis, conjunctivitis, weakness, and loss of condition. At necropsy, there may be serofibrinous polyserositis, enlargement of the spleen and liver, and characteristic multifocal necrosis of the spleen and liver. Large, intracytoplasmic basophilic inclusions may be seen in infected tissue.

Laboratory Diagnosis

In the acute disease, a presumptive diagnosis can be made on the basis of clinical signs and gross lesions.

The organism can be demonstrated in impression smears of affected tissues stained by Giemsa and Gimenez procedures.

Enzyme-linked immunosorbent assay (ELISA)-based kits are available for antigen detection in feces. They are sensitive and specific, but false positives are encountered. Paired serum samples from several birds for (rising titers) complement fixation, latex agglutination, and ELISA procedures are used; the last is preferred.

Treatment

Tetracyclines, chloramphenicol, and enrofloxacin are effective. Treatment for 5–6 weeks is recommended for pet birds. Elimination of the organism is not always successful. Avian chlamydiosis in imported birds is controlled by administration of chloramphenicol or tetracycline in the feed or water for 45 days.

Although there may be shedding, outbreaks in poultry flocks are uncommon. To prevent human infections, poultry are sometimes treated with tetracycline in the feed for at least 2 weeks before processing.

ENZOOTIC ABORTION OF SHEEP AND GOATS

This widespread disease is caused by *Chlamyophila abortus* and is manifested by a placentitis leading to premature lambing, stillbirths, and more frequently, abortion in late gestation and retained placentas.

The mode of infection is by ingestion. Infections appear to be latent until conception occurs. Placental infection may follow.

A consistent gross lesion seen in chlamydial abortion is placentitis with multifocal cotyledonary necrosis and a red-brown intercotyledonary exudate.

Laboratory Diagnosis

Fresh placenta(s) and fetus(es) are submitted.

1. Examination of stained cotyledon and fetal tissue smears. Fluorescent antibody–stained smears appear to have no advantage over regularly stained smears (modified Ziehl–Neelsen, Giemsa, or Gimenez).
2. Isolation and cultivation of *C. psittaci* in embryonated chicken eggs or cell cultures.

Characteristic large intracytoplasmic inclusions are seen in cell cultures.

3. A number of serum samples; paired samples are preferred. Complement fixation or ELISA: A number of animals with appreciable titers suggests a chlamydial infection. A fourfold rise in titer between paired serum samples is significant.

Treatment and Prevention

Segregation of infected and aborting ewes is important.

Tetracyclines have been used for infected newborn lambs and for ewes that have aborted. Long-acting tetracyclines are administered to pregnant ewes intramuscularly to prevent abortion.

Bacterins are available.

SPORADIC BOVINE ENCEPHALOMYELITIS (SBE)

This is a widespread but infrequent disease, mainly of young cattle, caused by *Chlamydophila pecorum* and characterized by a neurologic form with meningoencephalitis; a chronic form with fibrinous pericarditis, pleuritis, and peritonitis may be seen. Little is known of the epidemiology of SBE.

When neurologic signs are seen, the disease usually terminates fatally. The course varies from days to weeks, and the morbidity and mortality rates may reach 50%.

Laboratory Diagnosis

1. For smears, culture, and histopathology, brain is used, half fresh and half formalinized; portions of affected pericardium, pleura and lung, and peritoneum.
2. For complement fixation, paired serum samples or samples from affected and nonaffected cattle in the same herd are used.
3. Smears made from brain, pericardium, pleura, lung, and peritoneum are stained and examined for chlamydia. The finding of chlamydia from characteristic lesions is highly presumptive. The characteristic histopathologic changes, which include a purulent inflammation of the meninges and parenchyma of the brain, also support a diagnosis of SBE.
4. A fourfold increase in titer of paired serum samples in the complement fixation test strongly indicates a diagnosis of SBE. A moderate to high titer in a sick or recovered animal with low or negative titers in nonaffected animals supports a diagnosis of SBE.
5. A definitive diagnosis depends on the isolation and identification of *C. pecorum*. This may be beyond the scope of many diagnostic laboratories.

Treatment

Tetracylines or tylosin at high dose levels are effective if administered early in the disease.

FELINE PNEUMONITIS

This is a widespread, frequently occurring contagious disease caused by *Chlamydophilus felis* and characterized mainly by a follicular conjunctivitis with an ocular discharge that may become purulent. The ocular form is seen most commonly in 5–12-week-old kittens. Pneumonitis (interstitial bronchopneumonia) is an infrequent feature of the disease.

Laboratory Diagnosis

The disease is frequently diagnosed clinically based on the persistent conjuctivitis.

Smears from conjunctival scrapings, stained by Giemsa, Gimenez, and fluorescent antibody stains, are examined for forms of *C. felis*. It is not usually feasible to cultivate and identify the agent. Kits employing ELISA are available for antibody detection.

Treatment and Prevention

Tetracycline is administered locally (conjunctivitis) and systemically for 3–4 weeks. Alternative drugs are chloramphenicol and enrofloxacin.

A chicken embryo *C. felis* vaccine is available.

MISCELLANEOUS CHLAMYDIAL INFECTIONS

Specific diseases have been referred to above. Some important miscellaneous infections caused by *Chlamydophilia* species and the animals in which they occur are as follows:

- Cattle: Infertility, abortion, polyarthritis (mainly calves), and metritis.
- Horses: Respiratory infection.
- Sheep: Conjunctivitis, intestinal infection, and polyarthritis (mainly lambs—"stiff lamb disease").
- Pigs: Intestinal infection and abortion.
- Goats: Respiratory infection.
- Koalas: Conjuctivitis and urogenital infection.

Polyarthritis

A sporadic disease primarily of calves, caused by *Chlamydophila pecorum*, polyarthritis can be transmitted through the milk of the dam. It may occur with or be preceded by rhinitis, arthritis, or diarrhea. Affected animals walk with a staggering gait or in circles. It is accompanied by profound depression, fever, anorexia, and weakness.

Conjunctivitis

A rhinitis may be present with a keratoconjunctivitis, resulting in a mucopurulent ocular discharge. It is caused by several species and primarily affects young animals and probably plays a role in the transmission of chlamydial infections.

Various forms of chlamydiosis occur in laboratory animals and in a wide range of wild mammals.

GENERAL

Laboratory Diagnosis

It is likely that many chlamydial infections are not diagnosed. They may be sporadic and mild and resolve without treatment.

The specimens required will depend on the infection. The procedures carried out are similar to those described for the more important chlamydial diseases discussed above. They are

- Demonstration of organisms or elementary bodies in stained smears or sections of lesions. Gimenez and Giemsa stains are used for smears. Fluorescein-labeled antibody may be used for the specific staining of smears. ELISA kits are available for identification of chlamydial genera.
- Isolation and cultivation of organisms is carried out in the yolk sac of chicken embryo or cell cultures. Organisms are detected by staining with fluorescein-labeled antibody. A direct immunofluorescence test kit is available commercially for identification of *C. psittaci* in culture. Isolation, cultivation, and identification is expensive and time-consuming and is rarely carried out in diagnostic laboratories.
- Polymerase chain reaction–based assays for the specific detection of clamydial DNA are currently in development.
- Paired serum samples are tested (provided antigens are available) using complement fixation, immunofluorescence (inhibition test), latex agglutination, and ELISA. A fourfold increase in titer is considered significant.

Treatment

In general, tetracyclines, chloramphenicol, or enrofloxacin are administered for 2–3 weeks.

It is of interest that sulfonamides are effective for *Chlamydia trachomatis*, as these organisms synthesize their own folic acid. In contrast, *Chlamydophila psittaci* requires preformed folic acid from the host cell and, thus, is not inhibited by sulfonamides. Penicillin results in the production of intracellular **spheroplasts** and is therefore not recommended.

Public Health Significance

In humans, 70% of *C. psittaci* infections are caused by exposure to caged pet birds. The disease is often referred to as parrot fever. There is also exposure in breeding aviaries and pet stores and where poultry are processed at dressing plants. Elementary bodies in the environment are infectious for several months. Normal-appearing pet birds may be latently infected and, as a result of various stresses, may shed large numbers of organisms in the feces. The dried feces may produce a dust that is infectious by inhalation or ingestion. The human disease resulting from the inhalation of fecal dust is initially a pneumonitis. The organisms may spread via the blood, producing very serious systemic disease.

Individuals with impaired cell-mediated immunity are particularly susceptible.

Tetracyclines are administered orally for 15–21 days. Mortality may be as high as 20% in untreated individuals.

GLOSSARY

cytosol Fluid portion of the cytoplasm (excludes organelles).

MHC Major histocompatability complex: A group of cell surface proteins that are involved in the immune discretion of "self" versus "nonself" and are important in the generation of specific immune responses.

spheroplasts Refers to a gram-negative bacterium that has had the cell wall removed but in which the cell itself is not ruptured.

Borrelia, Treponema, Brachyspira, and Leptospira

There are three families of spirochetes: Spirochaetaceae contains the genera *Borrelia*, *Spirochaeta*, and *Treponema*. The former and latter genera contain species of veterinary interest. The other important genera of spirochetes, *Brachyspira* (formerly *Serpulina*) and *Leptospira*, are in the families Brachyspiraceae and Leptospiraceae, respectively. These organisms are found in water, soil, and decaying organic materials and in or on the bodies of plants, animals, and humans. The majority are saprophytes, a few are commensals, and some are pathogenic, causing diseases in both animals and humans.

GENERAL FEATURES OF SPIROCHETES

Morphology

Differentiation of the genera is based mainly on morphology. Spirochetes of the significant genera are slender, spiral, actively motile, flexible organisms, 5–200 μm long and 0.1–3 μm wide, that divide by transverse fission. They are helically coiled and round on cross-section and have a varying number of spirals. The three basic cellular elements are the outer sheath, which encompasses the cell; the axial filament or fibril; and the protoplasmic cylinder, which includes the cell wall and cell membrane. The outer sheath, whose function is not known, appears to act as a unit membrane.

All spirochetes have axial filaments that resemble flagella. The axial filaments wind around the protoplasmic cylinder under the outer sheath. It is thought that they may be responsible for motility. Insertion of the axial filament is by a proximal hook and insertion discs. The hook is an extension of the axial filament shaft and bends toward the protoplasmic cylinder. The insertion discs are platelike and are inserted into a depression at the end of the cell. The number of insertion discs varies with the genus: *Borrelia* has two, *Treponema* and *Brachyspira* have one, and *Leptospira* has three to five. Motility involves rapid rotation around the long axis, flexation of cells, and locomotion along a helical path.

Identification

Spirochetes may be anaerobic, aerobic, or microaerophilic. Some groups are **halophilic**, thermophilic, **psychrophilic**, or alkaliphilic. Identification is usually based on morphologic and antigenic properties. Biochemically, some spirochetes metabolize sugars to acetate, H_2, CO_2, ethanol, lactate, or butyrate, depending upon species. Some groups, such as *Leptospira*, do not metabolize carbohydrates but prefer long-chain fatty acids or alcohols. Genetically, some groups have circular chromosomes, whereas others have linear chromosomes. All of these factors aid in the identification of the spirochete.

Although spirochetes are gram-negative, they stain poorly. They may be demonstrated by the following procedures: Giemsa or Wright stain (the larger ones), **negative stains** (India ink or nigrosin), silver impregnation (coating increases their size), dark-field and phase microscopy, and immunofluorescence.

Some distinguishing characteristics of the four genera are given in Table 32.1.

Important morphological features of spirochetes are shown diagrammatically in Figs. 32.1 and 32.2.

BORRELIA

Borreliae are medium to loosely coiled, thin, slow-growing, microaerophilic spirochetes. They are highly motile, with 7–20 flagella at each terminus and attached subterminally at opposite ends of the protoplasmic cylinder. The borreliae require long-chain fatty acids, glucose, amino acids, N-acetylglucosamine, and several vitamins as some of their required organic nutrients. The cell wall contains various lipids, including cholesterol. Borreliae also possess both linear chromosomes and linear plasmids. For the most part, speciation of *Borrelia* is based on the arthropod vector involved.

BORRELIA ANSERINA

This species of *Borrelia* causes a significant disease, fowl spirochetosis (avian borreliosis), in chickens, ducks, turkeys, geese, pheasants, pigeons, canaries, game birds, and some wild birds. Sporadic, infrequent outbreaks have occurred in the southwestern United States.

Transmission

It is transmitted by ticks while feeding (bites). The widespread tick, *Argas persicus*, is the principal vector. The

Table 32.1   Distinguishing Features of *Borrelia*, *Treponema*, *Brachyspira*, and *Leptospira*

Characteristic	Borrelia	Treponema	Brachyspira	Leptospira
Length	3–20 μm	6–15 μm	6–14 μm	6–20 μm
Width	0.2–0.5 μm	0.1–0.2 μm	0.2–0.3 μm	0.1–0.2 μm
Ends	Taper terminally to fine filaments	Pointed, may have terminal filaments	Pointed, may have terminal filaments	One or both ends have a semicircular hook
Spirals				
Number	4–8, loose	6–18, regular, angular	4–6, regular, angular	Many, fine, tight
Amplitude	3 μm	1 μm	1 μm	0.4–0.5 μm
Motility	Lashing, cork-screw-like.	Rotating, undulating, stiffly flexible	Rotating, undulating, stiffly flexible	Spinning, undulating
Cultivation	Anaerobic, microaerophilic	Anaerobic, microaerophilic	Anaerobic	Aerobic
Staining				
Gram	Yes	No	No	Faint
Giemsa	Yes	Poor	Poor	Poor
Silver Impregnation	Not necessary	Yes	Yes	Yes

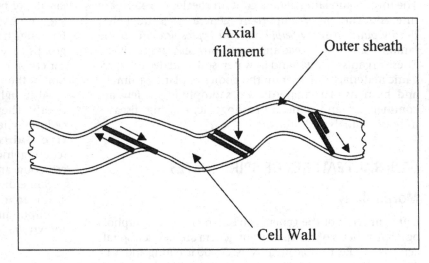

FIGURE 32.1   Basic structure of a portion of a spirochete cell. Beyond the cell wall (inner line designation) is a region known as the outer sheath. Within the sheath reside the axial filaments responsible for spirochete movement. The direction of wrapping of the individual axial filaments is indicated by the arrows.

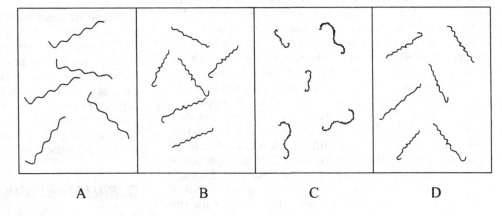

FIGURE 32.2   Features of the four different spirochetes. **(A)** *Borrelia*; **(B)** *Brachyspira*; **(C)** *Leptospira*; **(D)** *Treponema*. For additional detail, see Table 32.1.

organism may be passed in eggs to the next generation of ticks. Other *Argas* ticks, including *Argas sanchezi*, in the United States can transmit the spirochete. The infection is maintained in the tick through the larval, nymphal, and adult stages. The organism may be passed via ova to the next generation of ticks.

Pathogenicity

Although the factors relating to virulence have received little attention for this species, it can be presumed that it possesses some of the virulence features of the much-studied *Borrelia burgdorferi*.

Different serotypes of *B. anserina* occur, and there is no cross-immunity between them.

The disease is characterized by an acute septicemia with accompanying fever, diarrhea, drowsiness, and emaciation. The spleen may be enlarged and mottled, and anemia is usually present. Surviving birds recover after about 2 weeks and have long-lasting immunity against the serotype involved.

Direct Examination

Diagnosis is easily made by demonstration of the organism in carbol fuchsin or Giemsa-stained blood, spleen, and liver smears. It can also be readily demonstrated by dark-field microscopy and immunofluorescence.

Laboratory Diagnosis

Borrelia anserina can be readily cultivated in the turkey or chicken embryo and in enriched media containing rabbit tissue. Diagnosis is based on demonstration of typical *Borrelia* in stained smears from individuals with characteristic lesions and clinical signs.

Treatment, Prevention, and Control

Control requires elimination of the *Argus* ticks, which can be difficult.

Penicillin, chloramphenicol, streptomycin, kanamycin, tylosin, and tetracyclines are effective if treatment is sufficiently early. It is not effective when the number of organisms in blood is large.

A bacterin prepared from chicken embryo cultures is used for prevention. The appropriate serotypes for the region must be included in the bacterin.

BORRELIA BURGDORFERI

Borrelia burgdorferi causes Lyme disease (borreliosis) in humans and animals. The disease was first recognized in 1975 in children from Lyme, Connecticut, and the causal agent was first cultured in 1981 from a tick, *Ixodes dammini*, in New York. The disease, which is tick-borne, occurs in North America, Europe, the former USSR, China, and Japan; in the United States, it is found along the Atlantic coast from Massachusetts to Maryland, in Wisconsin, Minnesota, California and Oregon, and in Ontario and British Columbia in Canada.

Borrelia that cause Lyme disease in Europe and Asia, although closely related to *B. burgdorferi*, are considered genospecies (new varieties) and have been given the names *Borrelia garinii* (Europe), *Borrelia afzelii* (Asia), and *Borrelia japonica* (Asia). It is thought that these genospecies account for some of the differences noted in disease manifestations in humans in different regions. Additional genospecies have been identified and given species names.

The *B. burgdorferi* genome has 855 genes and 430 genes on about a dozen plasmids; some of the genes on the plas-

mids are duplicates of ones on the chromosome. As described for the genus, *B. burgdorferi* possesses both linear chromosomes and linear plasmids.

Transmission

The reservoir hosts are small rodents, including white-footed mice, meadow voles, eastern chipmunks, and white-tailed deer. There is evidence that the dog can also serve as a reservoir host. *Borrelia burgdorferi* is transmitted by *Ixodes scapularis* (formerly *I. dammini*) in the eastern and midwestern United States, by *Ixodes pacificus* in the western United States, by *Ixodes ricinus* in Europe, and by *Ixodes persulcatus* in Asia. The *Ixodes* ticks are three-host ticks, and the larvae and nymphs acquire the organism by feeding on the reservoir hosts. The risk of infection is greatest in the spring and fall.

Pathogenesis and Pathogenicity

Key virulence factors are thought to include antigenic variation of the outer surface proteins and motility. However, *Borrelia* appears to be resistant to nonspecific host defense mechanisms and elicits an inflammatory response consisting primarily of mononuclear cells.

The disease has been reported from both domestic and other animals. Most attention has been given to the disease in humans, horses, cattle, and dogs. Although the disease has diverse manifestations, it is generally similar in each species. Most infections in animals are thought to be subclinical.

Three stages of Lyme disease, which may vary considerably and overlap, are recognized in humans, and an analogous pathogenesis takes place in animals. First, starting a few days to a few weeks after infection, a skin rash appears around the tick bite and in some instances may spread. The infection may be halted at this stage by the body's defenses.

The signs of the second stage appear in several weeks to several months as the infection becomes systemic. They include fever, fatigue, persistence of rash, stiffness of joints and neck, headaches, and lymphadenopathy. Arthritis and central and peripheral nervous systems disorders may be evident.

The third stage may involve chronic arthritis, chronic neurologic symptoms, and cardiac signs caused by infection of heart muscles. The course, severity, and outcome of the disease vary greatly among individuals.

Whether the signs of the chronic disease are the result of persisting live organisms or caused by the immune system, a possible autoimmune reaction, is being actively debated. It is of interest that *B. burgdorferi* has been cultured from human skin lesions 10 years after the initial infection.

HORSES. The first sign seen in horses are a cranky attitude, back soreness, and lameness. Fever, depression, stiffness, arthritis, uveitis, and encephalitis may also be observed. There have been clusters of cases in foals at weaning where the disease is endemic, and in utero infections have lead to the deaths of foals. In areas where the disease is endemic, as many as 10% of horses are seropositive.

DOGS.   That the canine disease is widespread in the United States is suggested by serologic surveys. Cats are resistant to the disease, but serologic surveys suggest that infections occur. Canine infections are generally milder than the human disease, usually with a history of fever, inappetence, lethargy, and sudden onset of lameness associated with pain in two or more joints. The episodes of lameness, which vary from one to several, occur at intervals of roughly 1 month to 1 year. Some infected dogs have developed renal disorders and, rarely, myocarditis and neurologic disease.

CATTLE.   In utero infection has been implicated in the subsequent deaths of calves.

Immune Response

The spirochetes are rapidly killed in vitro by the classical complement pathway. Immunity is primarily humoral, and immune serum passively protects experimental animals from infection. Leukocytes react to the outer surface proteins, heat shock proteins, and other surface molecules. The result of this interaction is the production of interleukin-8 (IL-8), IL-1, and tumor necrosis factor alpha; the interaction is required for the migration of neutrophils to the site. Also produced are IgG antibodies, which are essential to immunity.

Laboratory Diagnosis

1. Specimens include unclotted blood, cerebrospinal fluid, joint fluid, and urine. The organism has been difficult to demonstrate by microscopy in the aforementioned specimens.
2. A fluorescent antibody (monoclonal antibody) procedure is used to detect organisms in tissue.
3. As the borreliae are frequently present in low numbers, a polymerase chain reaction (PCR)-based technique has been used in some laboratories to aid in the detection of organisms.
4. The organism can be grown in modified Kelly medium, but culture and identification are impracticable for the diagnostic laboratory.
5. At present, the indirect immunofluorescence assay and the enzyme-linked immunosorbent assay (ELISA) for antibodies to *B. burgdorferi* are the most useful diagnostic procedures. High titers along with a history of arthritis and intermittent lameness in endemic areas would strongly suggest Lyme disease. However, it must be kept in mind that dogs with subclinical infections may also have appreciable antibody titers.
6. **Western blot** can be used to confirm infection and differentiate antibodies induced by vaccine from those caused by infection.

Treatment and Control

Early, aggressive treatment is important in preventing chronic infections. Doxycycline or amoxicillin for 10–14 days are recommended for acute cases. Clarithromycin and erythromycin are also effective.

Tick control, including avoidance of tick-infested areas, is very important.

Commercial bacterins are used to protect dogs; two doses are given intramuscularly with an interval of 2–3 weeks. Annual revaccination is recommended.

OTHER *BORRELIA*

Borrelia theileri

This spirochete causes a mild febrile anemia in horse, cattle, and sheep in South Africa and Australia. It is transmitted by *Rhipicephalus* spp. and, probably, other ticks. The animal reservoir is horses, cattle, and sheep.

Borrelia coriaceae

This organism is the putative cause of epizootic bovine abortion, a major disease of rangeland cattle in the western United States. It is transmitted by the tick *Ornithodorus coriacens*. The animal reservoir is thought to be deer and cattle.

RELAPSING FEVER (RF)

This spirochetal disease of humans is characterized by alternating febrile and afebrile periods. The untreated disease has a fatality rate ranging from 2% to 10%.

Louse-borne epidemic RF is caused by *Borrelia recurrentis*; humans constitute the reservoir. It occurs worldwide, including the United States.

American tick-borne RF is caused by *Borrelia mazzottii*; the reservoir is rodents. It occurs in the southern United States, Mexico, and Central and South America.

More than a half-dozen additional RFs occur in various regions and countries. The vectors for most are ticks, and the reservoir is rodents.

TREPONEMA

Spirochetes of this genus are of minor veterinary importance. Some of their characteristics were discussed above and referred to in Table 32.1.

Treponema paraluiscuniculi is the cause of a widespread disease: rabbit syphilis, or vent disease. It is a true venereal disease in which lesions consisting of vesicles and scabs are seen mainly involving the prepuce, vagina, and perineal region. Thick, scaly crusts persist in the female for months.

Diagnosis is by the demonstration of organisms in preparations from lesions using stains or dark-field microscopy.

Treponema paraluiscuniculi has not been cultivated in vitro.

Penicillin is an effective treatment.

BRACHYSPIRA (FORMERLY *SERPULINA*)

Species of this genus, whose habitat is the intestine, were once considered treponemes. The genus is now the sole member of the family Brachyspiraceae (formerly Serpulinaceae). Some characteristics that it shares with *Treponema* and that distinguish it from *Leptospira* are given in Table 32.1.

The *Brachyspira* species of veterinary interest are:

- *Brachyspira hyodysenteriae* (formerly *Serpulina hyodysenteriae*): A loosely coiled spirochete; the cause of swine dysentery.
- *Brachyspira pilosicoli*: A loosely coiled spirochete that occurs in the intestine of humans, swine, dogs, mice, rats, and chickens; its pathogenicity is doubtful.
- *Brachyspira innocens*: A small, tightly coiled spirochete; found in the feces of normal pigs and those with swine dysentery; nonpathogenic.
- *Brachyspira intermedius*: Recovered from the feces of pigs; not considered pathogenic.
- *Brachyspira murdochii*: Recovered from the feces of pigs; not considered pathogenic.

BRACHYSPIRA HYODYSENTERIAE

This species is the cause of swine dysentery. Experimentally it produces a dysentery in specific pathogen-free (SPF) pigs but not in germ-free pigs. There is evidence that *Bacteroides fragilis, Fusobacterium necrophorum,* and possibly other bacteria are important secondary agents in swine dysentery. Asymptomatic carriers of *Brachyspira hyodysenteriae* are encountered.

Virulence Factors

Virulence factors of this organism have not been fully characterized. Unique proteins that have been identified as potential virulence factors in the *B. hyodysenteriae* outer membrane include variable surface proteins and lipoproteins. There is indirect evidence to suggest that these may be involved in immune evasion. *Brachyspira hyodysenteriae* also produces a potent beta-hemolysin, which is considered a major virulence attribute. In addition, *B. hyodysenteriae* produces a **NADH** (nicotinamide adenine dinucleotide, reduced form) oxidase, which serves to protect *B. hyodysenteriae* cells against oxygen toxicity, thereby contributing to virulence.

Serotypes and Genetic Variation

Nine serotypes of *B. hyodysenteriae* have been designated based on differences in lipopolysaccharide antigens in an agar gel double immunodiffusion test. Furthermore, examination of individual strains by genetic methods, including deoxyribonucleic acid (DNA) fingerprinting, ribosomal ribonucleic acid homologies, and specific gene variation, has shown that there is great genetic variation within the group. As a result, the reclassification into new species or strains will undoubtedly occur in this group.

Pathogenicity

Pigs of any age may be affected. The disease ranges in severity from very mild to peracute and death. The organism proliferates in the large intestine, causing infection, inflammation, and hypersecretion of the surface mucosa. There are hemorrhagic foci, but the infection is limited to the mucosa. Initially there is a mucoid diarrhea with flecks of blood. In the severe disease, there is a bloody diarrhea that may terminate in death or in a chronic form characterized by a diphtheritic inflammatory process involving the mucosa of the cecum, large intestine, and rectum. Signs in addition to diarrhea and dysentery may include loss of weight, dehydration, and emaciation.

Laboratory Diagnosis

History, clinical signs, and gross lesions suggest a probable diagnosis of swine dysentery. The demonstration of the causal organism in material taken from characteristic lesions provides a strongly presumptive diagnosis of swine dysentery.

The methods used for the demonstration of the organism in the mucosa and feces involve the examination of wet mounts with the phase or dark-field microscope and of Giemsa-, crystal violet–, or Victoria blue–stained smears with the light microscope. It is a large, flexible spirochete that moves rapidly in a snake- or eel-like fashion. Considerable experience is necessary to distinguish *B. hyodysenteriae* from other spirochetes, including the smaller *B. innocens*.

Isolation is not usually practiced. Diagnosis is usually made on the basis of clinical signs and a positive direct examination. *Brachyspira hyodysenteriae* can be isolated from filtered feces or ground colonic mucosa on serum-enriched blood agar containing spectinomycin (400 µg/mL) to prevent the growth of undesirable bacteria. Plates are incubated anaerobically (with 10% CO_2) at 42°C for 48 hours. The small, white translucent colonies have a zone of clear hemolysis. In contrast, *B. innocens* is weakly beta-hemolytic. Stained smears of *B. hyodysenteriae* disclose a loosely coiled organism. It is both oxidase and catalase negative.

Definitive identification is made by biochemical tests, gas chromatographic analysis of volatile fatty acids, DNA probes, and PCR assay. However, these procedures are not carried out in most veterinary diagnostic laboratories.

An ELISA is used to detect antibodies. It is useful as a herd test but not as an individual animal test.

Treatment and Control

Drugs are usually administered in feed or water. The preferred antimicrobials are tiamulin or carbadox; alternatives are tylosin, lincomycin, and dimetridazole. Resistance is encountered to tylosin, lincomycin, and dimetridazole. If feasible, susceptibility tests should be performed.

Immunity is predominantly humoral, in that hyperimmune serum is protective. Bacterins appear to provide considerable protection against *B. hyodysenteriae* infection.

The disease can be eliminated by treatment that eliminates carriers and by moving pigs to quarters and premises that have been thoroughly cleaned and disinfected. Rodent control is important.

LEPTOSPIRA

The family Leptospiraceae contains the two genera, *Leptospira* and *Leptonema*, of which the former contains species of veterinary and medical significance. Leptospirae are aerobic, gram-negative (faintly), right-handed flexible helical rods with more than 18 coils per cell. Each organism is hooked at one or both ends. They are motile by two subterminal periplasmic flagella. They use long-chain fatty acids and alcohols as energy and carbon sources. Some important characteristics of *Leptospira* are given in Table 32.1.

Two taxonomic systems are used for *Leptospira*. The molecular taxonomic approach uses DNA–DNA hybridization. The traditional approach is a serologic system based on antigenic differences. We will use this system, as it is employed in laboratories and clinicians and pathologists are familiar with it.

The basic taxon of the genus *Leptospira* is the serovar (formerly serotype). Two species are recognized, *Leptospira interrogans*, composed of the pathogenic or parasitic serovars, and *Leptospira biflexa*, containing the free-living leptospires. There are more than 218 *L. interrogans* serovars and at least 60 *L. biflexa* serovars. As mentioned, the pathogenic leptospires are included in the species *L. interrogans*. In the serologic system, the former species name, now serovar, is added to *L. interrogans*; for example, *Leptospira canicola* becomes *L. interrogans* serovar *canicola*, and *Leptospira hardjo* becomes *L. interrogans* serovar *hardjo*. Instead of using the species name and serovar, we will only refer to the serovar.

The microscopic agglutination test, which is widely used to detect antibodies, is highly serovar specific. There are both group- and serovar-specific antigens. Serologic procedures are used in the identification of serovars after isolation and cultivation.

Leptospirosis is primarily a disease of animals that, on infrequent occasion, is transmitted to humans directly or indirectly. The natural hosts are rodents, swine, and dogs. Each serovar has certain animal species as natural hosts. Some important serovars, their natural hosts (principally in the United States), and their occurrence in domestic animals are given in Table 32.2. Humans and animals may be infected with a wide variety of serovars, although most infections in domestic animals are caused by only a few serovars.

Mode of Infection and Transmission

The source of the organism is urine from infected or carrier animals. Water, litter, and food may serve as fomites.

Table 32.2   Important *Leptospira* Species or Serovars and Their Hosts

Serovar	Known Host (Natural)	Occurrence in			
		Humans	Dogs	Cattle	Swine
icterohemorrhagiae	Rat, mouse, raccoon, opossum	Common	Occasional	Reported	Reported
canicola	Dog, cattle, swine, skunk, jackal	Common	Common	Rare	Occasional
pomona	Cattle, swine, skunk, raccoon, wildcat, opossum, horse	Occasional	Rare	Common	Common
autumnalis	Opossum, raccoon, mouse	Rare	?	?	?
ballum	Mice, grey fox, rat, opossum, raccoon, wildcat, skunk, rabbit, grey squirrel	?	?	?	?
grippotyphosa	Raccoon, mouse, fox, squirrel, rabbit, bobcat	Rare	Occasional	Occasional	Occasional
bataviae	Rat, mouse	Rare	?	?	?
hardjo	Cattle	Rare	?	Common	?
sejroe	Opossum, raccoon, mouse	?	?	Sporadic	?
hebdomadis	Opossum, raccoon	?	?	?	?
australis	Opossum, raccoon, fox	?	?	?	?
bratislava	Swine	?	Reported	?	Reported

Note: Data principally applicable to the United States; ?, not known.

The organisms can live in alkaline water for days. Direct or indirect infection may be via nasal, oral, or conjunctival mucous membranes and abraded skin. Leptospires are destroyed in the stomach.

Pathogenesis

Although the pathogenic mechanisms are not known, there is considerable damage to vascular endothelium. Virulent strains produce more cytotoxic protein than avirulent strains. The exact role of this protein in the disease is not clear. The hemolysin of *Leptospira* appears to be responsible for intravascular hemolysis. Other virulence factors include the organism's motility, burrowing motility, and production of hyaluronidase.

After epithelial penetration, there is hematogenous dissemination, with localization and proliferation in parenchymatous organs, particularly the kidney and liver. Leptospiral antibody with complement greatly reduces the numbers of leptospira. Kidney infection with multiplication in the convoluted tubules may result in a carrier state or **nephrosis** and sometimes uremia and death. In the carrier state, organisms can be shed in the urine for weeks to months. Among the signs observed are fever, anemia, subserous and submucosal hemorrhages, conjunctivitis, icterus, meningitis, and agalactia. The mechanism of tissue damage may result from the host's immune response. There is damage to the endothelial lining of capillaries, resulting in a reduction of blood flow.

The lesions, signs, and severity vary with different serovars. Death may occur during the febrile stage or later caused by toxemia resulting from liver and kidney damage. Survivors recover from impairment of hepatic and renal function.

The immune response is primarily humoral and servar specific.

Canine Leptospirosis

This disease is primarily caused by serovar *canicola* and less frequently by serovar *icterohemorrhagiae*. The dog is considered an incidental host for serovars *grippotyphosa, autumnalis, australis, pomona,* and *bratislava*. Although the exact incidence is unknown, surveys have shown that up to 38% of dogs in various parts of the United States show serologic evidence of exposure or infection.

Infected dogs and rats sporadically shed leptospirae in their urine and serve as sources of *canicola* and *icterohemorrhagiae* infections. Dogs may shed leptospirae in their urine for 2–6 months; rats usually shed for longer periods. Organisms may survive in nature for approximately 3 weeks if environmental conditions are favorable. The viability of organisms is influenced by the pH of the urine of dogs and rats, and an alkaline pH favors viability.

CLINICAL. Infections may be latent to severe. A chronic progressive nephritis may follow acute *canicola* infection, with death occurring long after initial infection; however, some dogs recover, and their renal function is regained.

These animals may shed organisms in the urine for long periods.

Four principal forms are recognized: (1) the hemorrhagic form, (2) the icteric form, (3) the uremic or subacute form, and (4) the inapparent form. The first two forms are primarily caused by serovar *icterohemorrhagiae*, whereas the latter two forms are usually caused by serovar *canicola*.

In the initial stages of the disease, the first three forms are characterized by depression, anorexia, vomiting, and diarrhea or constipation. Serovar *grippotyphosa* occasionally causes severe leptospirosis in dogs.

DIAGNOSIS. The following procedures are used:

1. Examination of urine by dark-field microscopy. Experience is required to recognize *Leptospira*. They autolyse rapidly, and formalin should be added to preserve them.
2. The microscopic agglutination test (agglutination lysis). This is the preferred serologic procedure. If the titer is 1:100 or higher, it is considered to be of diagnostic significance. It is preferable to have a fourfold increase in paired sera. However, not all cases of leptospirosis produce significant serologic titers.
3. Isolation, cultivation, and identification. Isolation from urine or blood is not usually feasible. Filtration or the addition of 5-fluorouracil may be used to reduce contaminants. Leptospirae are aerobic and may be cultivated in special media at 30°C.
4. Guinea pig or hamster inoculation. Blood, urine, or tissue is used; when bacteremic, the experimental animal's blood is used for isolation and cultivation.
5. Histopathology. Organisms may be demonstrated in kidney sections with special stains.
6. Fluorescent antibody technique can be used to identify *Leptospira* in tissues and urine sediment.

Bovine Leptospirosis

The principal cause is serovar *pomona*. Serovar *hardjo* is also frequent in some regions; it causes fewer abortions than serovar *pomona* but results more often in infertility. On occasion, serovar *grippotyphosa, canicola,* or *icterohemorrhagiae* is involved. Three percent to ~11% of cattle show serologic evidence of infection; 2%–4% are estimated to be actively infected.

SOURCES. Sources of the organisms are cattle and swine with leptospiruria and some wild animals. Cattle may shed for 3 months, but in small numbers and irregularly. Outbreaks of leptospirosis are often associated with heavy rainfall. Leptospirosis is infrequent under dry conditions.

CLINICAL. The infection may be latent in a herd and may be precipitated by stress. Infections are characterized by a variety of clinical signs including fever, diarrhea, anemia, icterus, and hemoglobinuria. Acute infections sometimes result in abortion.

DIAGNOSIS.   Diagnosis of bovine leptospirosis is similar in principle to that of the canine disease; serologic tests are used almost exclusively. An ELISA has been used to detect antibodies (IgM and IgG) to serovars *pomona* and *hardjo* in cattle.

Porcine Leptospirosis

Serovar *pomona* is the principal cause of leptospirosis in pigs. Other serovars including *canicola*, *grippotyphosa*, *icterohemorrhagiae*, and *bratislava* may also be involved in porcine leptospirosis. Serovar *bratislava*, which is extremely difficult to culture, has been one of the predominant serovars in swine in England and Ireland.

Serologic evidence indicates a 3%–22% level of infection; probably 2%–4% are actively infected.

SOURCES.   The organisms occur in swine, cattle, skunks, raccoons, opossums, wildcats, and deer. Organisms may be shed for as long as 3 months; shedding is irregular and not in large numbers.

CLINICAL.   Infections are mostly subclinical or latent. Unthriftiness, abortion, fever, icterus, and anemia are among the signs observed in clinical infections. Metritis and meningoencephalitis are observed occasionally.

DIAGNOSIS.   Diagnosis is similar to that of canine infections; serologic tests are used almost exclusively. *Leptospira* can be recovered from and demonstrated in aborted fetuses.

Equine Leptospirosis

Leptospirosis is an infrequent disease of horses. Most infections are caused by serovar *pomona*; however, rare infections with other serovars have been reported. The disease is usually mild or subacute with fever, depression, and icterus resulting occasionally in abortion and **uveitis**. Recurrent **iridocyclitis** (moon blindness or periodic ophthalmia) may be a sequella. Although leptospirae have been isolated from the eye, it is not clear whether the uveitis is immune-mediated or caused by active infection. Both serovars *pomona* and *grippotyphosa* have been implicated in abortion. Systemic disease is rare, and renal infection has not been confirmed.

IMMUNITY

Immunity appears to be mainly humoral, in that the organisms are not intracellular, and bacterins (killed organisms) elicit considerable protection, although of short duration (less than a year). The levels of antibody resulting from vaccination are low and do not affect serologic testing. There is little cross-immunity between serovars.

Bacterins have not been available for horses.

Dogs

Bacterins usually contain serovars *canicola* and *icterohemorrhagiae*.

Cattle

Bacterins contain serovar *pomona*; some bacterins contain serovars *hardjo*, *grippotyphosa*, *canicola*, and *icterohemorrhagiae* as well. *Leptospira* may be combined with other antigens, including viruses.

Swine

Bacterins contain serovar *pomona*. Some bacterins contain other serovars, including *bratislava*.

TREATMENT AND CONTROL

Ampicillin, penicillin G, streptomycin, tetracyclines, and doxycycline are effective. Early treatment is important. Treatment may be of no avail if renal damage is extensive. Supportive measures including fluid therapy may be indicated in dogs. After dogs have recovered, it may be necessary to further treat them to eliminate the carrier state.

If leptospirosis is a recurring problem, preventive measures such as effective rat control, fencing off of potentially contaminated ponds and streams, and careful screening of replacement stock should be implemented. Although leptospirae will survive for days in alkaline water, they will only live for about 12 hours in sewage, and they are very susceptible to drying and heat.

PUBLIC HEALTH SIGNIFICANCE

Human beings acquire leptospirosis from infected domestic animals, rodents, and contaminated water, particularly water polluted from farm runoff. The disease is referred to by several names, including Weil's disease, Fort Bragg fever, and swineherd's disease. Various serovars of *Leptospira*, including *canicola*, *icterohemorrhagiae*, and *pomona*, can infect humans. Veterinarians, slaughterhouse workers, and farmers are at particular risk. Vacationers can be infected while swimming in water polluted by farm runoff. The disease in humans is not well known and may often not be recognized.

The acute form of the human disease is similar to that seen in some animals and is characterized by fever, jaundice, and nephritis.

The laboratory diagnosis of the human disease is essentially the same as that described earlier for the dog.

It is thought that treatment will only affect the course of the disease if it is initiated within 4 days of onset.

GLOSSARY

halophilic A halophilic organism requires salt (NaCl) for growth.
iridocyclitis Inflammation of the iris and ciliary body.
NADH Acronym for nicotinamide adenine dinucleotide, reduced form. NAD is a coenzyme that carries or releases protons and electrons to and from metabolic reactions. The NADH form is NAD with protons and electrons (thus, reduced).
negative stains Demonstration of the form of bacteria by surrounding them with a stain, for example, India ink, that they

do not take up. They appear as unstained bright bodies against a dark or colored background.

nephrosis A noninflammatory disease of the kidneys that mainly affects function of the nephrons.

psychrophilic A pychrophilic organism is able to grow at low temperatures. Its optimum temperature for growth is less than 15°C.

uveitis Inflammation of the iris, ciliary body, and choroid.

Western blot This is performed in three stages: First, the antigen mixture is electrophoresed on a gel; second, it is blotted onto nitrocellulose paper; and third, the blot is exposed to the antibody of interest (the dark band represents the antigen recognized by the antibody).

33 Non-Spore-Forming Anaerobic Bacteria

The nonsporulating anaerobic bacteria constitute a large group of organisms. Included are anaerobes of the following categories: the gram-negative bacilli, the gram-negative cocci, and the gram-positive bacilli. Some of these are present, often in large numbers, on mucous membranes and in the intestinal tract of animals. The *Actinomyces* and the anaerobic spirochetes and *Campylobacter* are discussed in Chapters 20, 27, and 32.

Many abscesses, and necrotic and suppurative processes in animals, yield non-spore-forming anaerobic bacteria, either alone or more often with aerobic or facultatively anaerobic bacteria.

The taxonomy of the anaerobic gram-negative bacilli has and is undergoing great changes. New species are being described, and old species are being renamed. Phylogenetic analysis using deoxyribonucleic acid (DNA)–DNA hybridization and 16S rRNA sequencing does not always correlate with the phenotypic characteristics used to describe species in the past.

The isolation and identification of the non-spore-forming anaerobic bacteria is time consuming and expensive. A complete examination with identification to species and antimicrobial testing is beyond the capability of many small diagnostic laboratories. However, most diagnostic laboratories can recover anaerobes, place them in major groups, and subject them to antimicrobial tests. Even if the latter is not done, treatment can be empirical. Improved procedures and techniques in recent years have facilitated more work in this neglected area of veterinary bacteriology.

Infectious processes involving these anaerobes may also yield an aerobe or facultative anaerobe. Lower tissue oxidation-reduction potential (**Eh**) favors the growth of these anaerobic bacteria. Normal tissues have an Eh of +120 to +240 mV, whereas necrotic abscesses have an Eh of −250 to −150 mV. Because anaerobes do not survive in an Eh above −100 mV, they are usually restricted to processes in which there is suppuration and necrosis.

As mentioned earlier, many of these anaerobes are commensals on mucous membranes and in the alimentary tracts of animals. The gram-negative anaerobic bacilli make up more than 90% of the bacteria of the intestinal tract, and they are predominant in the large bowel and in the rumen flora, where they have a vital role in digestion. A number of species have probably not yet been identified.

IMPORTANT NON-SPORE-FORMING ANAEROBES: AN OVERVIEW

We have concentrated below on the more important groups and species.

Gram-Negative Rods

Many of the disease-producing, non-spore-forming, anaerobic, gram-negative bacteria causing disease in humans and animals are in the family Bacteroidaceae. This family contains many genera; the most significant from a veterinary standpoint is *Bacteroides*.

What is referred to as the *Bacteroides fragilis* group (10 species) is particularly important from a disease standpoint in horses, dogs, cats, farm animals, and humans.

Some species previously classified in the *Bacteroides* genus have been transferred to other families and genera.

Bacteroides corrodens has been renamed *Eikenella corrodens*. It causes infections in humans and animals.

The genera *Prevotella* and *Porphyromonas* are each in a different family. *Prevotella melaninogenica*, formerly *Bacteroides melaninogenica*, is frequently involved in infections in animals.

Prevotella heparinolyticus was formerly *Bacteroides heparinolyticus*. It has been associated with oral infections in horses and cats. *Porphyromonas levii* was formerly *Bacteroides levii*. This organism has been associated with summer mastitis in cattle.

The new genus *Dichelobacter* is in the family Cardiobacteriaceae. *Dichelobacter nodosus*, formerly *Bacteroides nodosus*, is the cause of the economically important disease, contagious foot rot of sheep.

The genus *Fusobacterium*, formerly in the family Bacteroidaceae, is now in the family Fusobacteriaceae. *Fusobacterium necrophorum* subsp. *necrophorum* and *F. necrophorum* subsp. *funduliforme* are involved in many infections in animals. *Fusobacterium nucleatum* infections in animals are infrequent.

Gram-Positive Anaerobic Cocci

The gram-positive anaerobic cocci belong in two genera: *Peptostreptococcus* and *Peptococcus*. The former has numerous species and the latter only one species, *Peptococcus niger*. They are normal flora on mucous membranes and participate with other species in mixed anaerobic infections. *Peptostreptococcus anaerobius* has been isolated from a variety of veterinary clinical specimens, and *Peptococcus indolicus* has been implicated as a cause of mastitis in cows. *Peptococcus niger*, has been associated with ovine foot rot and recovered infrequently from other animal infections.

Anaerobic Non-Spore-Forming Gram-Positive Rods

The anaerobic diphtheroid, *Actinobaculum (Eubacterium) suis*, is the causal agent of cystitis and pyelonephritis in swine. Boars carry *A. suis* in the preputial diverticulum and serve as the source of infection. Transmission takes place during breeding. The disease, which is ascending and limited to females, may result in the death of sows without clinical signs being observed. Penicillin may be effective if given early, but treatment of chronic cases is unsuccessful. *Actinobaculum suis* is also discussed in Chapter 27.

Members of the genus *Lactobacillus* are frequently isolated from animals, but they are not considered to be pathogenic. They are normal flora of the female genital tract.

Species of *Propionibacterium* are usually associated with dairy products and the skin and are not pathogenic in animals.

INFECTIONS INVOLVING NON-SPORE-FORMING ANAEROBES

These organisms frequently invade tissues that are damaged and in which some necrosis provides a favorable anaerobic milieu for their growth. They also are frequently secondary in primary infections.

They are often recovered from the following infectious processes and diseases in many animal species.

- Necrotic, gangrenous (often with clostridia), and suppurative processes. They may be foul smelling.
- Abscesses in the lung, liver, and brain; pyometritis; infrequently, cystitis and urinary tract infections, some postsurgical abscesses, diarrheal diseases, pneumonia, abortion, septicemias and bacteremias, foot rot of cattle and sheep, cellulitis, periodontal abscesses, guttural pouch infection (horses), chronic sinusitis, and suppurative mastitis and osteomyelitis.

METHODS FOR THE CULTIVATION OF ANAEROBES

1. Anaerobic jars: Brewer, Torbal, and GasPak systems. Plates and other media are placed in sealed jars. These use catalytic systems to eliminate oxygen.
2. An anaerobic plastic chamber or glove box is preferred. All procedures are conducted in the anaerobic chamber.
3. Prereduced media and media containing reducing agents, such as cooked meat media and thioglycolate broth, are used. Special oxygen-free differential media are used for biochemical tests.
4. Gas–liquid chromatographic analysis of volatile and nonvolatile fatty acids produced by anaerobes provides definitive identification of many anaerobes.

SPECIMENS: GENERAL

Affected tissue and pus from abscesses and suppurative processes should be used. Of utmost importance is the exclusion of oxygen from clinical specimens and cultures. Conventional swabs and other clinical specimens not protected from oxygen are not satisfactory. Special precautions must be taken in submitting specimens. Satisfactory anaerobic transport systems are available commercially. Fluid material can be submitted in a syringe, and some laboratories provide special tubes with oxygen excluded. Specimens should be cultured immediately, or precautions must be taken to prevent exposure to oxygen.

IMPORTANT NON-SPORE-FORMING ANAEROBES

Fusobacterium necrophorum

This species occurs worldwide. It is a commensal in the alimentary tract and on mucous membranes. Infections are endogenous.

Four biotypes or biovars of *F. necrophorum* have been described: A, B, AB, and C. Biotypes A and B are recovered from bovine liver abscesses and a variety of infections. Biotype B predominates in ruminal contents and lesions. Biotype A is more virulent than biotype B. Biotype AB is rarely isolated from animals, and its pathogenicity is intermediate between biotype A and biotype B. Biotype C strains were given the species name, *Fusobacterium pseudonecrophorum*, which has recently been changed to *Fusobacterium varium*. The latter species is an infrequent opportunist in humans.

Based on a number of characteristics and DNA analysis, biotypes A and B have been designated subspecies *necrophorum* and *funduliforme*, respectively, of *F. necrophorum*.

PATHOGENESIS. *Fusobacterium necrophorum* invades and multiplies in the anaerobic environment provided by damaged tissue. It is frequently a secondary invader. Infections are characterized by a necrotic process and are frequently mixed, such as in liver abscesses in cattle, where it is often found with *Archanobacterium pyogenes*.

The major factors in virulence are considered to be endotoxin and a potent leukotoxin. In addition, *F. necrophorum* produces a variety of extracellular products including hemolysin, hemagglutinin, adhesins (pili), platelet aggregation factor, proteases, and DNase. The significance of these products relative to virulence is not clear. Capsulated strains of *F. necrophorum* are more virulent for mice than noncapsulated strains.

PATHOGENICITY.   *Fusobacterium necrophorum* may be isolated from numerous infections initiated by a variety of wounds and injuries in all domestic animals. It is a common secondary invader in necrotic stomatitis, pharyngitis, and enteritis. Enteritis involving *F. necrophorum* is seen most commonly in swine. The general term used for *F. necrophorum* infections is necrobacillosis.

Some of the better-known diseases with which *F. necrophorum* is associated in various animals are as follows.

Horse.   It is usually involved in the infectious process called "thrush," involving the frog of the hoof. Infrequent cases of pneumonia and septicemia also have been reported.

Cattle.   It is associated with metritis, cellulitis, mastitis, and calf diphtheria and is found in necrotic foci in the mouth, larynx, and trachea. It is also seen in necrotic laryngitis in feeder cattle. *Fusobacterium necrophorum* is the primary cause of liver abscesses and foot rot.

Sheep.   It is a frequent secondary invader in lip and leg ulcerations (primary cause is the ulcerative dermatosis virus). In combination with *Archanobacterium pyogenes*, it causes foot abscess (ovine interdigital dermatitis) and abortion.

Swine.   It is considered the principal cause of "bull nose" resulting from the injury caused by "ringing" boars. It is a secondary invader in swine dysentery and necrotic enteritis.

Fowl.   It is involved in avian diphtheria, the primary cause of which is the fowl pox virus.

DIRECT EXAMINATION.   Gram-stained smears of affected tissues reveal gram-negative rods of variable length with characteristically beaded filaments.

Laboratory diagnosis and treatment of *F. necrophorum* are discussed at the end of the chapter.

Dichelobacter nodosus

This organism is a large gram-negative, nonmotile, anaerobic rod. It is the primary cause of contagious foot rot of sheep. *Fusobacterium necrophorum* and *Archanobacterium pyogenes* are common secondary invaders, and *Treponema penortha*, although present, is not pathogenic.

PATHOGENICITY AND PATHOGENESIS.   *Dichelobacter nodosus* can cause infections of the foot in goats, pigs, and cattle, where it is resident. It is not a commensal in the alimentary tract. Virulence appears to be associated with the production of proteolytic enzymes, resulting in the breakdown of keratin. Several acidic and basic extracellular serine proteases are produced by both virulent and avirulent strains. The disease is aggravated by moist environmental conditions.

Some evidence suggests the involvement of two chromosomally distinct regions associated with virulent phenotypes. Virulent strains of *D. nodosus* possess **pili (type IV)**,

which are thought to play a major role in the attachment and colonization of the epidermal matrix of the ovine hoof. In addition, these fimbrae are highly immunogenic.

Based on pilus antigens, at least 10 serologically distinctive groups of *D. nodosus* have been identified with an agglutination test and an ELISA.

LABORATORY DIAGNOSIS.   Contagious footrot of sheep can be diagnosed by the demonstration of the characteristic organism in gram-stained smears from typical lesions. Smears are made from material taken well down in the lesion after the horn has been pared away. The rods of *D. nodosus* may be straight or slightly curved and vary from 0.6 to 1.2 μm in length. They do not form spores and are gram-negative. When stained with Loffler's methylene blue, one, two, or more red-staining granules can be seen at either end or along the rod.

A nonpathogenic organism called *Treponema penortha* can be seen in large numbers in positive smears as slender filaments displaying loose, irregular curves. The organism is gram-negative and stains faintly compared with *D. nodosus*.

Cultural procedures are not usually carried out. The isolation and identification procedures recommended for other gram-negative anaerobes (discussed below) are applicable to *D. nodosus*.

TREATMENT AND CONTROL.   Foot trimming should be carried out before treatment. Formalin, copper, or zinc sulfate footbaths and 10% tincture of chloromycetin are used. The organism does not survive for longer than 2 weeks in pastures. Systemic use of penicillin, tetracyclines, tylosin, erythromysin, and streptomycin is of value when accompanied by other control measures such as culling, segregating affected sheep, only adding noninfected sheep, using dry pastures, and vaccination.

Alum-precipitated, oil-adjuvant, and other vaccines have been helpful in prevention.

Prevotella melaninogenica

This saccharolytic organism, which produces a dark colonial pigment, has been renamed *Prevotella melaninogenica* (formerly *Bacteroides melaninogenicus*). This species has been found in a considerable number of specimens from suppurative processes in farm and companion animals. It is frequently associated with *Fusobacterium necrophorum* in foot rot of cattle and sheep.

Bacteroides fragilis Group

The *B. fragilis* group comprises 10 species. All are recovered from clinical specimens. *Bacteroides fragilis* is the most common anaerobe causing infections in humans. It is encountered occasionally in various anaerobic infections in farm and companion animals.

Some strains of *B. fragilis* produce enterotoxin, which causes accumulation of fluid in ligated intestinal loops of lambs and calves. The enterotoxin, fragilysin, is an extracellular zinc **metalloprotease**. Enterotoxigenic strains have been implicated as the cause of diarrheal diseases in calves, lambs, foals, piglets, and humans.

LABORATORY DIAGNOSIS: GENERAL

Methods for the cultivation of anaerobes in general were described earlier.

Fusobacterium necrophorum

The organism is a strict anaerobe and grows best on enriched media. Two to 4 days of incubation are required. Many strains produce some L-forms on initial isolation. L-forms are cell-wall-deficient forms that resemble mycoplasmas in some respects.

Colonies are small, smooth, convex, and whitish-yellow in color, with a narrow zone of alpha- or beta-hemolysis. Initially, cultures may be pleomorphic; short rods, long filaments, and "moniliform" bodies may be seen. *Fusobacterium necrophorum* can be recovered frequently in pure culture from bovine liver abscesses. Pus or caseous material is taken aseptically by syringe or pipette and inoculated into previously heated thioglycolate broth.

Definitive identification is made on the basis of biochemical tests.

General Procedures for Laboratory Diagnosis

These will vary with laboratories and are only discussed briefly below.

1. A direct gram stain may give an indication of the kind of organism or organisms involved.
2. Various primary media are used: one with hemin and **menadione**, blood agar, laked blood agar (enhances pigment production), selective agar to suppress facultative anaerobes, and bile esculin agar for the *B. fragilis* group.
3. Incubate for at least a week.
4. Colony morphology, pigmentation, fluorescence, and antimicrobial susceptibility may indicate the genus involved.
5. Biochemical tests, gas–liquid chromatographic analysis, commercial systems, and DNA probes are used for final identification.

TREATMENT: GENERAL

Where applicable, establish and maintain drainage.

Antimicrobial susceptibility tests should be carried out; antibiotic resistance has been encountered, particularly in the *B. fragilis* group. Treatment will usually need to be started before the results of the susceptibility test are obtained. Amoxicillin, ampicillin, tetracyclines, chloramphenicol, metronidizole, clindamycin, clavulanic acid-amoxicillin, and cephalosporins are used. One must keep in mind that anaerobic infections are usually mixed; a facultative anaerobe is often involved. Tylosin has been the most effective drug as a food additive to prevent bovine liver abscesses.

Vaccination against *F. necrophorum* infections has thus far not been very successful.

GLOSSARY

Eh Symbol for oxidation-reduction potential.
menadione Compound having physiological effects similar to vitamin K.
metalloprotease One of several groups of enzymes that degrade proteins but that have a metal ion as a prosthetic group.
pili (type IV) Fimbrae that have a highly conserved amino terminal region, known as type IV.

34 Miscellaneous Potential Pathogens

Included in this chapter are some potential pathogens and opportunistic bacteria that were not, for taxonomic and other reasons, discussed in other chapters. Most are of minor pathogenic significance; however, some are encountered frequently in the veterinary diagnostic laboratory.

STREPTOBACILLUS MONILIFORMIS

Streptobacillus moniliformis is a facultatively anaerobic, gram-negative, highly pleomorphic rod that forms filaments with moniliform swellings and L-forms under certain conditions. Pioneering studies on L-forms were carried out with this species. Although its precise taxonomic position has not been determined, it is thought to be related to members of the order Mycoplasmatales. *Streptobacillus moniliformis* is a normal inhabitant of the oropharynx and nasopharynx of wild and laboratory rats and some other rodents.

The organism is a secondary invader in chronic murine pneumonia of rats and a primary cause of a disease of mice, characterized by septicemia, septic arthritis, hepatitis, and lymphadenitis. Serious systemic infections with polyarthritis and synovitis in turkeys have been attributed to rat bites.

Infections in humans initiated by rat bites (rat-bite fever) are characterized by septicemia and polyarthritis; abscesses and endocarditis have also been reported. Outbreaks of infection in humans caused by ingestion of contaminated food, including milk, are called Haverhill fever. Respiratory and gastrointestinal symptoms are more common in these infections.

The organism can be grown in blood or serum-enriched media incubated for at least 8 days. Isolation from humans is most readily accomplished with blood cultures. Identification is usually based on the characteristic cultural and morphologic features of the organism. Identification is confirmed by a number of biochemical tests.

Penicillin G is effective against the bacillary forms, and an aminoglycoside, tetracycline, or chloramphenicol must also be used to eliminate the L-forms.

NEISSERIA

In animals they occur as commensals, most commonly on the mucous membranes of the nasopharynx and conjunctiva. They are in the section β-Proteobacteria and,

thus, are related to *Bordetella* and *Burkholderia*. The taxonomic position of *Neisseria ovis*, *Neisseria caviae* (guinea pig), and *Neisseria cuniculi* (rabbits) is uncertain. Neisseriae have only infrequently been reported as causing disease in animals. *Neisseria ovis* is considered a potential cause of conjunctivitis in sheep.

Neisseria canis occurs in the nasopharynx of cats and dogs and has been recovered from cat- and dog-bite wounds in humans.

Neisseria weaveri (formerly CDC Group M-5), which occurs in the mouth and nasopharynx of dogs, has been recovered from dog-bite wounds in humans.

In clinical materials, they may appear as diplococci with adjacent sides flattened. They grow well on blood agar. In smears from cultures, these gram-negative cocci occur singly or in clumps. Identification requires a number of biochemical tests.

Neisseria meningococcus and *Neisseria gonorrhoeae* cause, respectively, the important human diseases meningococcal meningitis and gonorrhea.

CDC GROUP EF-4

These short, nonmotile, gram-negative rod or coccobacillus gives rise to small convex, mucoid, yellow-to-tan colonies. They are closely related to the *Neisseria*.

They are commensals in the mouth and nasopharynx of dogs and cats and are occasionally isolated from bite wounds in humans. They do not ordinarily cause infections in dogs or cats.

CHROMOBACTERIUM

Chromobacteria are short to medium-sized, gram-negative, motile rods that occur in soil and water. They are in the family Neisseriaceae and give rise to characteristic violet to purple colonies on media. Two species are recognized, *Chromobacterium violaceum* and *Chromobacterium fluviatile*. Only the former has been incriminated in disease.

Most infections, mainly suppurative pneumonia in swine and cattle, occur in tropical and subtropical countries, including the southern United States.

Chromobacterium violaceum is usually identified on the basis of microscopic and colonial morphology and the characteristic colonial pigmentation.

ACINETOBACTER

Acinetobacter spp. occur frequently in soil, water, and sewage and as part of the normal flora of animals and humans. They are isolated frequently from clinical specimens. On occasion, they cause opportunistic infections in animals.

Studies of *Acinetobacter* isolates have identified 21 hybridization groups (genospecies). Until species are clearly delineated, isolates are best identified as *Acinetobacter* spp. They are closely related to *Moraxella*.

They are strictly aerobic, nonmotile, gram-negative, coccobacillary rods. Some characteristics that aid in their identification are growth on MacConkey agar, oxidase negative, nitrate negative, and nonfermentative, and thus negative in the **O/F test**.

An *Acinetobacter*-like organism (CDC Control Group NO-l) has been recovered from dog- and cat-bite wounds in humans.

VIBRIO

Members of the genus *Vibrio* are closely related to enterobacteria. They are motile, facultatively anaerobic, gram-negative, straight or curved rods. *Vibrio* species are found in seawater and fresh water, where they can cause diseases in aquatic animals.

Vibrio metschnikovii causes an infrequent fatal disease of young chickens and other avian species. Sources of the organism are river water, birds, shellfish, sewage, and marine environments. The disease is characterized by the sudden onset of severe enteritis with diarrhea. Human infections have also been attributed to this species.

A number of *Vibrio* spp. cause a variety of infections, but most commonly, gastrointestinal disease in humans. Among these are particular strains of *Vibrio cholerae*, the cause of human cholera. *Vibrio parahaemolyticus* is a major cause of gastroenteritis in humans. The disease is associated with the consumption of inadequately cooked seafood. *Vibrio vulnificus*, which is occasionally found in raw oysters, produce the most serious disease.

Vibrio spp. grow well at 30°–35°C on commonly used laboratory media including MacConkey agar. They ferment glucose, are oxidase positive, and reduce nitrate (except *V. metschnikovii*). Nonfermentative colonies from MacConkey agar disclosing characteristic curved rods are used to initiate biochemical tests for final identification.

AEROMONAS

Aeromonads are closely related to enteric bacteria. Most are motile, oxidase positive, facultatively anaerobic, gram-negative rods. The taxonomy of aeromonads is unsettled, and *Aeromonas hydrophila* is not a homogeneous species. Aeromonads occur widely in freshwater, sewage, and soil and on fish. *Aeromonas hydrophila* is a pathogen of reptiles, fish, and amphibians. It has been recovered from a variety of animals and birds, including cattle, swine, dogs, horses,

several avian species, and wild, zoo, and laboratory animals; however, it is only rarely pathogenic in these animals. It causes furunculosis in salmonid fishes. *Aeromonas salmonicda* and *Aeromonas sobria* are pathogens of fish.

Aeromonas spp., of which there are many, have been implicated as the cause of cellulitis, diarrhea, septicemia, urinary tract infections, osteomyelitis, meningitis, peritonitis, otitis, endocarditis, and other infections in humans.

Known virulence factors of *A. hydrophila* are a heat-stable cytotoxin, a heat-labile cytotoxin, hemolysins (beta-hemolytic), and surface adhesins.

They produce catalase and oxidase and use glucose and other carbohydrates. They grow well on most laboratory media at room temperature (optimum 22°–28°C); however, most can be cultivated satisfactorily at 37°C. Some strains of *A. hydrophila* produce a brown pigment in 2–3 days on infusion agar. Most strains of *A. hydrophila* are beta-hemolytic.

LACTOBACILLUS

These long, slender, pleomorphic, gram-positive rods, which are part of the normal flora of the mouth, vagina, and intestinal tract of animals, are rarely pathogenic. There are more than 30 species, consisting of both facultative strains and those that are strict anaerobes. They are nonmotile and are oxidase, indole, and nitrate negative.

Various *Lactobacillus* spp. are isolated from animal clinical specimens. Cultures of *Lactobacillus acidophilus*, sometimes in milk (sweet acidophilus milk), have been administered orally to animals and humans to treat intestinal disorders. The idea is to replace the "undesirable" intestinal bacteria. The presence of large numbers of lactobacilli in vaginal secretions indicates a healthy vagina.

CAPNOCYTOPHAGA

Capnocytophaga canimorsus and *Capnocytophaga cynodegmi* are in the family Flavobacteriaceae. They are thin, spindle-shaped, gram-negative rods that resemble fusobacteria morhpologically. They are commensals in the mouth and nasopharynx of dogs. *Capnocytophaga cynodegmi* is mainly involved in dog-bite or scratch infections. *Capnocytophaga canimorsus* is more pathogenic and is responsible for a variety of infections including septicemia, meningitis, endocarditis, cellulitis, septic arthritis, diarrhea, lymphadenitis, and keratitis in humans. Many of the infections have been in those with impaired immune systems.

They are facultatively anaerobic and grow readily on blood agar, producing small, nonhemolytic colonies.

RIEMERELLA ANATIPESTIFER

Formerly *Pasteurella anatipestifer*, *R. anatipestifer* belongs in the family Flavobacteriaceae (12 genera) along with the genus *Flavobacterium*.

Riemerella anatipestifer causes infectious serositis, a widely occurring, highly acute disease of ducklings (up to 6 weeks), various waterfowl, chickens, turkey poults, and pheasants. Stress is thought to initiate outbreaks. A serofibrinous exudate is found in various locations in the acute form of the disease. Signs include nasal and ocular discharge, weakness, and lack of coordination. Mortality may reach 70%, and the effect on the commercial duck industry can be very severe.

The organism grows readily on blood or chocolate agar in a candle jar or with 5% CO_2. It is nonmotile, **asaccharolytic**, gram-negative, and nonhemolytic and does not grow on MacConkey agar. Definitive identification is based on biochemical tests. Three serotypes or immunotypes have been identified.

Both sulfaquinoxaline and a combination of penicillin and streptomycin have been effective treatments. A bacterin and a live avirulent vaccine are used. The appropriate immunotypes should be included.

WEEKSELLA

Bacteria that were related to flavobacteria and called CDC group IIj were subsequently named *Weeksella zoohelcum*. This species has recently been renamed *Bergeyella zoohelcum*. It is of interest because it is part of the normal flora of the mouth and paws of dogs and cats and possibly other animals. Wounds in humans caused by animal bites (particularly dog bites) are occasionally infected with *B. zoohelcum*. They do not appear to cause significant infections in dogs and cats.

They are gram-negative rods with rounded ends, and their colonies on blood agar are large, mucoid, sticky, tan to yellow, and difficult to remove from the agar surface. All strains hydrolyze urea rapidly (less than 5 min). They fail to grow on MacConkey agar and are nonfermentative, oxidase and indole positive, and penicillin sensitive.

PROTOTHECA

Members of this genus are microscopic, colorless achlorophyllic algae. They are ubiquitous in nature and are occasionally recovered from clinical specimens in which they are not usually significant. However, there have been a number of reports of animal and human infections. Two species are involved: *Prototheca zopfi*, which is usually associated with animals, and *Prototheca wickerharmii*, which causes most human infections.

These algae are infrequent opportunists that mainly produce disease if the host's resistance is impaired. Prothecae cause chronic bovine mastitis, cutaneous infections in cats, disseminated prothecosis in dogs, and infections involving the central nervous system. The disease has also been reported in other animals, including snakes and fish. Human infections most commonly involve the skin. The tissue reaction is mainly granulomatous.

The characteristic cells can be readily demonstrated in wet mounts from clinical materials. Small colonies, white to cream colored, that resemble those of *Cryptococcus* spp. appear on Sabouraud agar (25°C) and blood agar (37°C) in 24 hours; however, they grow best at 30°C. The cells (sporangia) are larger than bacteria and are globose or round in form and without a capsule. Eight or more characteristic sporangiospores are produced by internal segmentation. They are nonfermentative, and carbohydrate assimilation tests are used to identify species.

Treatment with amphotericin B or ketoconazole has shown promise in human infections; however, treatment of animal infections, which are often more severe than most human infections, has been disappointing.

GLOSSARY

asaccharolytic Does not break down sugars metabolically.
O/F test This test is used to determine whether a bacterium uses carbohydrates by oxidation or fermentation.

PART III

Fungi

Introduction to the Fungi and Fungal Infections

This chapter is a brief introduction to basic and practical aspects of fungi and the diseases they cause. At present, it is estimated that there are over 1 million different species of fungi. Of these, about 70,000 have been described. These numbers should suggest to the reader that there are a vast number of these organisms that have yet to be identified.

We begin this chapter with a discussion of the general characteristics of the fungi, specifics of fungal classification, some general aspects of fungal infections, antifungal chemotherapy, and laboratory diagnosis.

GENERAL CHARACTERISTICS OF FUNGI

For the most part, the fungi are heterotrophic, perform extracellular digestion and absorb their nutrients, are nonmotile, are spore-bearing, and possess cell walls that somewhat resemble those of plants in chemical composition and structure. Fungi are unicellular—the yeasts—or multicellular filamentous colonies—the molds and mushrooms. The fungi are not photosynthetic, and consequently, they are restricted to a saprophytic or parasitic existence.

They are abundant and widespread in the soil, on vegetation, and in water, where they subsist on decaying vegetation and wood. Digestion of these materials is accomplished by the production of specific proteolytic, lipolytic, and glycolytic enzymes. Most fungi grow best at an acidic pH of about 5.0 and a temperature of about 25°C. They store glycogen for energy and use maltose and glucose for energy metabolism. Most fungi are aerobic; yeasts are fermentative and grow both aerobically and anaerobically. The cell wall prevents osmotic lysis and protects against mechanical injury and entrance by harmful macromolecules.

MOLDS

The two principal kinds of fungi are the molds and the yeasts. The main element of the vegetative or growing form of the mold is the hypha, a branching tubular structure 2–10 μm in diameter. As growth begins, hyphae become intertwined to form a mycelium. The vegetative mycelium consists of the surface hyphae, whereas the hyphae that arise above the surface are referred to as the aerial mycelium. Under certain conditions, the hyphae of the aerial mycelium produce reproductive cells or spores. These are collectively referred to as fruiting bodies. The hyphae of many fungi are divided by cross-walls called septa. Some hyphae grow into the culture medium, whereas others grow upward as "aerial hyphae." Some of the latter produce stalklike structures referred to as conidiophores or sporangiophores, which give rise to asexual spores called conidia. They are referred to by a variety of names (see Glossary). The asexual spores or conidia are more resistant to physical and chemical agents than hyphae. Free conidia promote the aerial dissemination of fungi.

YEASTS

The yeasts are oval or spherical cells ranging in diameter from 3 to 5 μm. Some varieties of yeasts or yeastlike fungi produce chains of irregular yeast cells that are referred to as pseudohyphae. Some fungi that exist in the mycelial form at room temperature will convert to a yeast form at 37°C or when in the tissues of animals. These fungi are called dimorphic.

CLASSIFICATION SYSTEMS AND REPRODUCTION

There are two independent classification systems for the fungi. One is based on anamorphs (asexual structures) and the other on teleomorphs (sexual structures). Sexual reproduction takes place by fusion of two haploid nuclei (karyogamy) followed by meiotic division of the diploid nucleus. Two hyphal **protoplasts** may unite (plasmogamy) and be followed immediately by karyogamy. The sexual state of many of the medically important fungi has not been demonstrated. Asexual reproduction, which involves the division of nuclei by mitosis, would appear to be so efficient that sexual elements rarely occur with these fungi.

With regard to asexual reproduction, the three mechanisms are sporulation followed by germination of the spores (examples *Aspergillus* and *Penicillium*), fragmentation of hyphae (as with *Coccidioides immitis* and *Geotrichum candidum*), and budding of yeast cells (as demonstrated by *Candida* and *Cryptococcus*).

The various reproductive structures are defined below and are referred to later under the specific disease-producing fungi. The sexual stage of a number of the dermatophytic (ringworm) fungi has been observed. For example, the sexual or perfect stage of *Microsporum nanum* is called

Nannizzia obtusa (ascomycetes). Only the asexual stage is found in infected skin. The sexual stage of *Cryptococcus neoformans* is called *Filobasidiella neoformans*.

SUBCELLULAR STRUCTURES OF FUNGI

In general, fungal cells are larger than most bacteria and are eukaryotic. They possess all the cytoplasmic organelles indicated in Table 1.1 and Fig. 35.1, with the exception of chloroplasts, and consequently are not photosynthetic. The medically important structures of a fungus are capsule, cell wall, and cytoplasmic membrane.

Capsule

Some fungi produce an external coating of slime or a more compact capsule. The capsule, or slime layer, is composed of amorphous polysaccharides that may cause the cells to adhere and clump together. The fungal capsule may be antigenic and antiphagocytic, as in *Filobasidiella* (formerly *Cryptococcus*) *neoformans*.

Cell Wall

The cell wall is the major structure of a fungus, and it determines its shape and the process of fungal morphogenesis (such as sporulation or yeast–mold dimorphism). It lies immediately external to the cytoplasmic membrane. Unlike that found in bacteria, most of the fungal cell wall is a thatch work of polysaccharide (chitin, glucan, mannan, cellulose) chains called microfibrils. The rest is protein and glycoprotein, which cross-link the polysaccharide chains. Because a wide variety of species of fungi share the same polysaccharides, many have common surface antigens. However, many unique antigenic determinants, resulting from the different branching patterns of the polysaccharides, are also found within certain groups. These antigens are useful for classification. Detection of species-specific surface antigens in solution provides a sensitive means of identification of slow-growing or poorly sporulating pathogenic fungi or both.

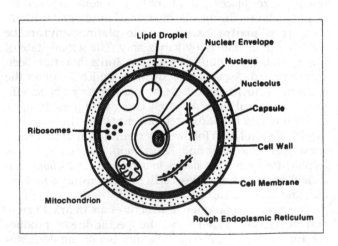

FIGURE 35.1   Schematic drawing of a yeast cell.

Cytoplasmic Membrane

Fungi possess a bilayered membrane similar in structure and composition to the cell membranes of higher eukaryotes. Unlike the bacterial membrane (except for the mycoplasmas), but similar to that of other eukaryotes, the fungal membrane contains sterols. The principal fungal sterols are ergosterol and zymosterol (mammalian cell membrane possesses cholesterol). This difference has been exploited in the successful use of the polyene antibiotics (such as amphotericin B), which have greater affinity for fungal sterol than for cholesterol.

CLASSIFICATION OF FUNGI

The taxonomy of fungi is in a state of flux; it undergoes continual refinement and revision. The products of sexual reproduction such as ascospores, basidiospores, and zygospores have been used to define large, major groups of fungi. The sexual cycle, if present, can be used to confirm species identity. However, the sexual cycle of many fungi is not known, and consequently, classification is based on asexual and vegetative morphology. The criteria for establishing genera and families are frequently unreliable. However, comparisons of guanine and cytosine content, and DNA homology, have helped establish some relationships. Some of the salient features of the principal fungus groups are given below.

Some organisms that are referred to as "fungi" are no longer in the Kingdom Fungi, but have been moved to the Kingdom Protista. Some of the reasons underlying this taxonomic movement are based on features of the mitochondria, presence of motile cells, cell wall carbohydrates, and lysine biosynthesis pathways. These organisms are considered the "fungal-like" protistans.

Kingdom Protista

There are five phyla representing this kingdom. These include Oomycota, Hyphochytriomycota, Labyrithulomycota, Myxomycota, and Acrasiomycota. In this discussion, however, we will only consider the Oomycota.

Largely aquatic protistans that are either unicellular or filamentous, Phylum Oomycota contain the sterol fucosterol, and store carbohydrates as beta 1–3 glucans called mycolaminarins. They are pathogens of plants and fish.

Order Saproleginales: The water molds. The majority are saprophytic; however, some are parasitic, such as *Saprolegnia parasitica*, a parasite of salmon.

Order Leptomitales: This order contains organisms that are primarily saprophytic and that are very similar to the Saproleginales.

Order Peronosporales: Considered evolutionarily the most advanced group of Oomycota. They are largely parasitic and have a range of environments: aquatic, amphibious, and terrestrial. The order comprises three families: Pythiaceae (*Phytophthora infestans*, the cause of the 1847 Irish potato famine); Peronosporaceae (*Peronospora tabacina*, the cause of the blue mold of tobacco); and Albuginaceae (*Albugo candida*, the cause of the white rust of **crucifers**).

Kingdom Fungi

PHYLUM CHYTRIDIOMYCOTA (CHYTRIDS).   Formerly known as Phycomycetes. They are thought to be the evolutionarily oldest group of fungi. This group is predominantly aquatic (both freshwater and marine forms) fungi, which range from unicellular to **coencytic** to those producing mycelium. They have chitin in their cell walls and are the only group that produces flagellated gametes. Many species are saprophytic; others are parasites of protists, invertebrates, fungi, and plants; a few anaerobic species are found in the rumen of herbivores. Each of the orders is distinguished largely based on morphology of the flagellated gametes.

Order Chytridiales: Lack a true mycelium. The majority of species are found in freshwater. However, some species are found in soil or in marine environments. A few are parasitic on algae, other fungi, and higher plants. Examples include *Chytriomyces* and *Rhizophidium*.

Order Spizellomycetales: Primarily found in soil. The order comprises saprophytic and parasitic forms. Examples include *Olpidium*, *Rozella*, and *Spizellomyces*.

Order Blastocladiales: Thought to be the most advanced group of Chytridiomycota. Several members are facultatively anaerobic. The order contains saprophytic and parasitic forms, including *Physoderma* (parasitic on higher plants) and *Coelomomyces* (parasitic on animals).

Order Monoblepharidales: Members are primarily aquatic and possess nonmotile eggs. Includes *Oedogoniomyces* and *Monoblepharis* spp.

Order Neocallimastigales: Obligate anaerobes in rumen, caecum, or hindgut of mammalian herbivores. There they break down cellulose and reduce the size of lignin deposits. Representatives include *Caecomyces*, *Orpinomyces*, *Pyromyces*, and *Neocallimastix*.

PHYLUM ZYGOMYCOTA (BREAD MOLDS).   Characterized by nonseptate mycelium and asexual and sexual reproduction by zygosporangia and zygospores. Several of these fungi cause infrequent diseases in animals. They have chitin in their cell walls, have no flagellated cells, and do not have **centrioles**. Zygomycota species can be saprophytic, parasitic, or **mutualistic**.

Order Mucorales. Largest order of Zygomycota. Many representatives of this order are used in industry and food production. This order is composed of three families: Mucoraceae (*Rhizopus*, used in the production of a variety of acids, such as lactic and succinic), Pilobolaceae (*Pilobolus*, common name "hat thrower fungus"), and

Entomorphthorales (*Entomorphthora*, parasites of insects).

Orders Endogonales and Glomales. Comprises organisms that are saprophytic or that live in symbioses with plants comprising structures known as mycorrhiza.

PHYLUM BASIDIOMYCOTA (CLUB FUNGI).   Septate mycelium, sexual reproduction by basidiospores on a basidium. Some are associated with a variety of plant diseases. Examples include puffballs, mushrooms, rusts, smuts, and *Filobasidiella neoformans*.

Order Agaricales: Contains the mushrooms.
Order Ustilaginomycetes. Primarily plant pathogens; includes smuts.
Orders Uredinales, Septobasidiales, and Sporidiales: Includes rusts, plant pathogens, marine yeasts, and insect symbionts.

PHYLUM ASCOMYCOTA (SAC FUNGI).   Septate mycelium, sexual reproduction by a saclike structure (ascus) that contain ascospores. *Neurospora*, morels, truffles, yeasts (*Saccharomyces cerevisiae*), *Emmonsiella capsulata*. Contains teleomorphic states of dermatophytes, *Aspergillus*, *Penicillium*, and some other fungi. Cause plant diseases, including Dutch elm disease, and some species are parasites of or mutualists with insects.

Order Taphrinales: *Taphrina deformans*.
Order Saccharomycetales: Includes *Saccharomyces cerevisiae*.
Class Euascomycetes: Includes *Peziza*, *Neurospora*, *Talaromyces*, and *Dothidea*.

DEUTEROMYCOTA (FUNGI IMPERFECTI).   Deuteromycota is not a recognized taxonomic group of fungi. However, those fungi that do not fit neatly above are often placed here until such time that more accurate phylogenic relationships are established. These organisms possess septate mycelium, and a sexual stage is either not present or not identified. However, this group includes most fungi of medical and veterinary significance, including *Candida*, *Microsporum*, and *Trichophyton*.

FUNGAL INFECTIONS: GENERAL CONSIDERATIONS

Fungi, excepting the dermatophytes, rarely cause disease in healthy, immunocompetent animals. Disease usually results when there are debilitating conditions that favor the growth of fungi or when fungi accidentally penetrate host barriers. The fungi causing disease in animals and humans are broadly classified as follows:

- Pathogenic fungi: Those that cause ringworm and the more common mycoses, such as blastomycosis and histoplasmosis.
- Opportunistic fungi: Those that seldom cause disease. Typically, disease is associated with immunocompromised individuals. These fungi are

numerous and widespread in nature, constituting species of a number of genera, including *Penicillium*, *Aspergillus*, *Mucor*, *Absidia*, and *Rhizopus*. Many fungi have the capacity to cause disease when introduced to tissues as a result of abrasions or other trauma.

A number of circumstances may give rise to systemic fungal infections:

1. Prolonged administration of antibiotics. Mode of action:
   - Lowered host resistance; mechanisms not understood; effect may be on phagocytosis or antibody production.
   - Interfere with synthesis of vitamins by effect on normal microflora, such as vitamin K and vitamin B complex components.
   - Upsets the microfloral balance, suppressing bacteria growth and favoring fungal growth, as in intestinal candidiasis.
2. Radiation, steroid therapy, urethane, mustard gas, and folic acid antagonists may activate latent fungal and bacterial infections. Steroids inhibit inflammatory as well as antibody response.
3. Cancer: Fungal infections occur in patients with leukemia or lymphoma, particularly if they are being treated with antibiotics or anticancer drugs. Some of the latter are strongly immunosuppressive. Fungal infections are not uncommon in debilitated patients with terminal malignancies.
4. Immunosuppressive therapy, as with azathioprine; patients are more susceptible to aspergillosis, cryptococcosis, and various opportunistic fungi.
5. Cytotoxic drugs: ablation of the bone marrow in the treatment of leukemia.
6. Immune deficiencies: acquired immune deficiency syndrome, T-cell deficiency, thymic hypoplasia, and anergy.
7. Humans and probably some animals with endocrine disorders are prone to opportunistic fungal infections.

SOME GENERAL FEATURES OF FUNGAL INFECTIONS

1. Most fungi capable of causing disease in animals and humans are classified among the Fungi Imperfecti.
2. Diseases caused by fungi do not usually assume epidemic proportions. Some exceptions are the dermatophytoses and infrequently, aspergillosis, histoplasmosis, and cryptococcosis. Only the dermatophytoses are communicable.
3. Conclusive proof that pathogenic fungi produce classic exotoxins or endotoxins is as yet lacking.
4. Some features of most fungous diseases are low invasiveness and low virulence of the organism. Certain predisposing factors contributing to the establishment of infection are:

- Tissue damage or necrosis resulting from trauma, infection, or ischemia.
- Lowered general resistance and immunosuppression, particularly of cell-mediated immunity.
- Moist environment, as with *Candida* infections in humans and animals.
- Exposure to a large number of organisms, as, in brooder pneumonia (aspergillosis).

Chronicity of some infections leads to a granulomatous process that resembles the reaction to a foreign body. Immunity is considered to be more cell-mediated than antibody-mediated.

5. Infected and exposed animals may develop a sensitivity to the fungus in question. This hypersensitivity is responsible in part for the pathologic effects produced. Hypersensitivity may contribute to dissemination of the infection within the host.
6. Many pathogenic fungi exhibit a significant tissue tropism. For example, *Histoplasma capsulatum* lives within macrophages, and dermatophytes thrive on keratin.
7. The causal fungi are identified principally by the study of cultural characteristics and the microscopic morphology of the so-called "fruiting bodies" or reproductive elements.

IMMUNITY TO FUNGAL INFECTIONS

Most of the fungi produce diseases that are characterized by granulomatous lesions resembling those produced by mycobacteria and other bacterial facultative intracellular parasites. Most fungal infections are asymptomatic, limited, and readily eliminated by the animal. Such exposed animals will usually manifest a positive delayed-type hypersensitivity skin reaction.

Antibodies to the various fungi are found in all the mycotic diseases except the dermatophytoses. In these superficial infections, the antibody-producing cells are not stimulated. Antibody titers may be negative or low in asymptomatic or mild infections. Immunity to fungal infections is more cell-mediated than humoral. Serum antibodies from infected animals do not protect normal animals from experimental infections.

Most animals exposed to or infected by fungi develop a hypersensitivity of the delayed type that is detectable by inoculation of fungi or their products into the skin. Hypersensitivity to products of fungi spread hematogenously is responsible for the skin eruptions accompanying the dermatophytoses ("id" eruptions), candidiasis, and coccidioidomycosis. Hypersensitivity and resistance are closely related in the animal's response to infection. There is a correlation between recovery and the development and persistence of delayed hypersensitivity. When a state of anergy (absence of delayed hypersensitivity reaction) develops in a serious systemic infection, the prognosis is usually poor.

Skin tests analogous to the tuberculin test are used in blastomycosis, histoplasmosis, coccidioidomycosis, and sporotrichosis. Various elements of the fungus are inoculated intradermally. A reaction of the delayed hypersensitivity type constitutes a positive test. A positive test indicates either past or current infection, and the result is considered along with other information in arriving at a diagnosis. The test result may be negative if the animal is anergic.

SEROLOGY OF MYCOTIC INFECTIONS

The serologic diagnosis of mycotic infections of animals has received little attention. Some of the serologic procedures that are employed in important mycoses of humans are mentioned under specific diseases. Not all veterinary diagnostic microbiology laboratories are prepared to carry out these procedures. Assistance is sometimes available through the courtesy of some hospital and public health laboratories.

It should be kept in mind that many of the skin tests and serologic procedures referred to under specific diseases were developed for use in human beings and that animals may respond somewhat differently.

ANTIFUNGAL CHEMOTHERAPY

Treatment of particular fungal diseases is discussed with the disease in subsequent chapters.

The polyene antibiotics produced by various *Streptomyces* spp. have revolutionized the treatment of mycotic diseases. The principal drugs in the polyene group are amphotericin B, nystatin, and pimaricin (natamycin). They combine with sterols in the cytoplasmic membrane of fungi and adversely affect its permeability. However, they may also bind to sterols in mammalian cell membranes, resulting in toxicity. Sterols are not present in bacteria, with the exception of mycoplasmas. They are present in red blood cells, however, and hemolytic anemia can be a side effect. Renal toxicity is the most serious side effect seen with amphotericin B. Because of its potential toxicity, this drug is reserved for serious infections. Nystatin is used topically or orally for candida infections. Pimaricin is used to treat mycotic keratitis.

The drug 5-fluorocytosine (flucytosine) is useful in the treatment of candidiasis and cryptococcosis. Flucytosine is transported into fungal cells and hydrolyzed to 5-fluorouracil. The latter is incorporated into fungal RNA, resulting in errors in the production of RNA. It is relatively nontoxic when given orally. Resistance of *Candida albicans* has been encountered.

The synthetic benzimidazole derivatives, called imidazoles, (two nitrogen molecules) and triazoles (three nitrogen molecules) have considerable antifungal activity. They affect the fungal cell wall and cell membrane, resulting in interference with nutrient use. Among the imidizoles, miconazole, clotrimazole, econazole, and ketoconazole appear to be the most useful. Two important triazoles are fluconazole and itraconazole. Although side effects are seen, they are not as serious as those that can accompany amphotericin B therapy. These drugs are be-

ing used to treat blastomycosis, histoplasmosis, dermatophytosis, and candidiasis.

Griseofulvin is produced by *Penicillium griseofulvum*. It is a selectively toxic antibiotic that is specific for fungi whose walls contain chitin. It accumulates in the keratin layer where it inhibits the nucleic acid synthesis of dermatophytes.

The aromatic diamidine 2-hydroxy-stilbamidine was the first effective treatment for blastomycosis. It is still used in humans who tolerate it better than amphotericin B.

Iodides, usually given orally, are effective in the treatment of sporotrichosis. These compounds do not affect in vitro growth of *Sporothrix schenckii*. Their mechanism of action is not clear.

GROUPING OF FUNGOUS DISEASES

The fungus diseases are discussed in the following chapters: Chapter 36, Dermatophytosis; Chapter 37, Mycoses Caused by Yeasts and Yeastlike Fungi; Chapter 38, Subcutaneous and Inoculation Mycoses; and Chapter 39, Respiratory and Systemic Mycoses.

This is an arbitrary grouping, and occasionally, the subcutaneous mycoses may produce systemic disease; conversely, some of the agents causing systemic disease may cause nonsystemic infections.

LABORATORY PROCEDURES

Laboratory procedures commonly used in the diagnosis of fungous infections are summarized in Table 35.1.

Most fungi grow well on simple media at room temperature (22°–25°C). The most commonly used media are variations of Sabouraud dextrose agar. Sabouraud's contains peptone, dextrose, and agar and has a pH of 5.6. The low pH inhibits the growth of bacteria. All fungi grow aerobically. A number of fungi will grow in the yeast phase at 37°C. The media most commonly used at this temperature are blood agar and brain heart infusion agar.

Inocula should be large, and incubation periods exceeding a month may be required. Cycloheximide (actidione) may be added to Sabouraud agar to inhibit the growth of many saprophytic fungi. It should be remembered that it also inhibits some important fungi, such as *Pseudoallescheria boydii*, *Aspergillus fumigatus*, and *Cryptococcus neoformans*. Chloramphenicol is added to Sabouraud agar to inhibit bacterial growth.

Indication for culture may come from the detection of fungi in tissue sections particularly after special fungal stains are used.

A variety of media are used in mycology laboratories for special purposes, such as demonstration of chlamydospores, growth of some dermatophytes, and the presumptive identification of certain yeasts. Slide cultures are particularly helpful in identifying many fungi.

General diagnostic procedures typically involve direct microscopic examination with specimens that have been stained with lactophenol cotton blue (fungal hyphae),

Table 35.1   Common Laboratory Procedures Used in the Diagnosis of Fungal Infections

Procedure	Purpose
Wet mount of tissue or mucus-containing specimens in 10% KOH	Strong alkali degrades tissue and mucus, permitting visualization of fungi
Wet mount portions teased from fungal colonies and mounted in lactophenol cotton blue	Permits observation of fungal morphology and presence of spores; kills fungi and provides good contrast for visualization
Tissue sections and clinical material stained with periodic acid–Schiff (PAS) or methenamine silver stains	Both PAS and silver stain fungal cell walls to give good contrast with background in tissue sections and clinical materials
Sabouraud glucose agar for culture; incubation at room temperature (RT) for up to 6 weeks	Low pH of the medium and RT incubation favor growth of fungi over bacteria; antibiotics (chloramphenical, cyclohexamide) may also be added to discourage bacterial and fungal growth
Blood agar or brain heart infusion agar at 37°C for 1 week or more	Various fungi grow at 37°C; the yeast phase of dimorphic fungi grow on these media at 37°C
Slide cultures, with incubated blocks of Sabouraud's glucose agar (about 1 cm square and 2 or 3 mm deep) on a glass slide covered with a coverslip and incubated in a moist chamber at room temperature; when spores form, the coverslip is carefully removed and examined in a lactophenol cotton blue wet mount	Permits observation of relatively undisturbed fungal growth; particularly useful for identification of fruiting bodies

Source: Adapted from G. N. Myrvik and R. S. Weiser. Introduction to Medical Mycology. In *Fundamentals of Medical Bacteriology and Mycology, 2nd ed.* Philadelphia, Lea & Febiger, 1988.

10% potassium hydroxide (arthrospores or fungus in hair, skin scrapings, and tissue), India ink (capsules), Gram stain (presence of yeasts), Kinyoun acid-fast stain (*Nocardia*), or Giemsa stain (dermatophytes).

A variety of commercially available identification systems are available. These include Dermatophyte Test Medium, for the isolation of identification of dermatophyte infections, and the Yeast Identification Systems, which are tests designed for the rapid identification of yeasts. Various probe-based methods, including the polymerase chain reaction, are being developed to aid in the identification of pathogenic fungi in cultures and clinical materials. They are not yet widely used in veterinary diagnostic laboratories.

COMMONLY USED MYCOLOGICAL TERMS

Arthrospore: An asexual spore formed by the disarticulation of the mycelium, as can be seen in *Geotrichum candidum*.

Ascospore: A sexual spore characteristic of the true yeasts or ascomycetes. It is produced in a saclike structure called an ascus. This ascospore results from the fusion of two nuclei and is seen in *Saccharomyces* spp.

Ascus: The specialized saclike structure characteristic of the true yeasts in which ascospores are produced. This is found in *Saccharomyces* spp.

Blastospore: A spore produced as a result of a budding process along the mycelium or from a single spore, as in *Saccharomyces* spp.

Chlamydospores: Thick-walled, resistant spores formed by the direct differentiation of hyphae, as seen in *Candida albicans* and *Histoplasma capsulatum*.

Clavate: Club-shaped, as the microconidia of *Microsporum nanum*.

Columella: The persisting dome-shaped upper portion of the sporangiophore, which can be seen in *Mucor* spp.

Conidium: An asexual spore formed from hyphae by abstriction, budding, or septal division, as in *Penicillium* spp.

Conidiophore: A stalklike branch of the mycelium on which conidia develop either singly or in numbers as found in *Penicillium* spp.

Dematiaceous: A term used to denote the dark brown or black fungi such as *Phialophora* spp. and *Hormodendrum* spp.

Dimorphic: Having two forms or phases, referred to as the yeast form and mycelial form. *Blastomyces dermatitidis* is dimorphic.

Echinulate: Spiny; for example, the macroconidia of *Microsporum*.

Ectothrix: Occurring outside the hair shaft, as *Microsporum* spp.

Endogenous: Originating or produced from within. *Candida albicans* infections are usually considered endogenous.

Endothrix: Occurring inside the hair shaft, as *Trichophyton* spp. on occasion.

Exogenous: Originating from without, as *Histoplasma capsulatum* infection.

Geophilic: Denotes fungi whose natural habitat is the soil, such as *Coccidioides immitis*.

Germ Tube: Tubelike structures produced by germinating spores. They develop into hyphae, as in *Candida albicans*.

Glabrous: The smooth form; for example, the glabrous form of *Geotrichum candidum*.

Hyaline: Fungi whose hyphae are colorless (transparent), as observed with many dermatophytes.

Hyphae: The filaments that compose the body or thallus of a fungus.

Macroconidia: Large, multinucleate conidia; they may be fusiform (spindle-shaped) or clavate (club-shaped). If divided by transverse and longitudinal septations, they are termed "muriform" (having walls). *Microsporum canis* produces them.

Microconidia: Small, single-celled conidia borne laterally on hyphae. They may be spherical, elliptical, oval, pyriform (pear-shaped), or clavate. *Trichophyton mentagrophytes* produces them.

Mycelium: A mat made up of intertwining, thread-like hyphae.

Nodes: The points on the stolons from which the rhizoids arise, as in *Rhizopus* spp.

Obovoid: Egg-shaped and having the larger portion at the distal end.

Pseudohyphae: Filaments composed of elongated budding cells that have failed to detach, as seen in *Candida albicans*.

Rhizoid: Rootlike, branched hyphae extending into the medium, as in *Rhizopus* spp.

Ringworm: A term used to refer to dermatophyte infections. Throughout history, peoples have thought these infections to be caused by worms that arrange themselves in ring formation.

Septate: Has cross-walls or septa in the hyphae, as found in the hyphae of *Aspergillus*.

Sessile: Denotes attachment directly to a hypha without a stalk.

Sporangiophore: A specialized hypha bearing a sporangium; for example, in *Rhizopus* spp.

Sporangium: A closed, often spherical structure in which asexual spores are produced by cleavage, as seen in *Mucor* spp.

Sterigmata: Specialized structures, short or elongated, borne on a vesicle and producing conidia, as seen in *Aspergillus*.

Stolon: A horizontal hypha or runner that sprouts where it touches the substrate. It forms rhizoids in the substrate, as observed in *Absidia* spp.

Vesicle: The terminal swollen portion of a conidiophore, which is seen in *Aspergillus*.

Yeasts: An ill-defined group of unicellular fungi lacking mycelium and reproducing asexually by blastospores and occasionally by sexually produced ascospores. The latter are the true yeasts (such as *Saccharomyces* spp.).

Zygospore: A thick-walled, sexual spore of the true fungi that results from the fusion of two similar gametangia, as in *Phycomycetes*.

GLOSSARY

centriole Structure in the nucleus composed of microtubules that is involved in the formation of the spindle apparatus that aids in the parceling out of duplicated chromosomes to daughter cells during cell division.

coencytic Multinucleate cells, as observed in the mycelium of the Zyogmycota.

crucifers Refers to the crucifer family of plants, including broccoli, Brussels sprouts, cabbage, cauliflower, Chinese cabbage, kale, mustard, radish, rutabaga, and turnip.

mutualistic Relationship between different cells (organisms) that is mutually beneficial.

protoplast Cell from which the cell wall has been removed.

36   Dermatophytosis

The dermatophytes that cause infections in animals and humans, and whose sexual stages have been characterized, belong to the group Deuteromycota. (Deuteromycota is not a recognized taxonomic group of fungi. However, those fungi that do not fit neatly are often placed here until such time that more accurate phylogenic relationships are established.) At one time, this group was referred to as the Fungi Imperfecti, as no sexual spores had been identified to classify them among the various phyla described in Chapter 35. All dermatophytes of veterinary importance are in the genera of *Trichophyton* and *Microsporum*. Several species of dermatophytes in the subdivision Deuteromycotina are known to have sexual life cycles (perfect state or teleomorphs) and to produce ascospores. These species are now classified in the family Gymnoascaceae of the subdivision Ascomycotina. The species that have perfect states in the genera *Trichophyton* and *Microsporum* are placed in the genera *Arthroderma* and *Nannizzia*, respectively. The perfect state is useful in the identification of certain species; its demonstration requires special technique. For purposes of identification, diagnostic microbiologists are primarily concerned with the conidial state of isolates.

The term "ringworm" denotes a clinical entity rather than an infection caused by a specific dermatophyte. Dermatophytes are able to penetrate all layers of the skin but are generally restricted to the cornified, nonliving keratin layer of the skin and its appendages (hairs, nails, horns, and feathers). These fungi do not penetrate beyond the stratum corneum because of antifungal activity of serum and body fluids and possibly because of a lack of tolerance for temperature above 35°C.

Most dermatophytes are not fastidious in their nutritional needs. They are aerobic and require a moist milieu for growth. The formation of arthrospores, which are responsible for infectivity, is stimulated by carbon dioxide.

EVOLUTION AND DISTRIBUTION

The dermatophytes occur in all parts of the world. All ringworm fungi may have originated from soil forms, but a significant number of them appear to have abandoned their saprophytic existence to become parasites. This adaptive process appears to entail loss of their perfect state (sexual life cycle). Increasing adaptability to the human and animal host is thought to result in the gradual loss of both the perfect state and the ability to produce asexual spores.

Dermatophytes are highly host-adapted parasites, although several, such as *Microsporum gypseum* and *Microsporum nanum*, can survive for long periods in soil. Ringworm fungi are categorized as geophilic, zoophilic, or anthropophilic depending on their habitat and host preference. Geophilic fungi inhabit the soil, whereas zoophilic and anthropophilic fungi are primarily found as parasites of animals and humans, respectively. Some have a broad host range, whereas others infect only a few animal species (Table 36.1).

TRANSMISSION

Dermatophytes may be transmitted from animal to animal, from animals to humans, from one human to another, and from soil to either animals or humans by direct or indirect contact.

PATHOGENESIS AND PATHOGENICITY

Very little is known about the extracellular products of the dermatophytes that may be important in pathogenesis. They produce keratinases, some elaborate elastase, and collagenase. These enzymes help provide nutrients by digesting host tissues. The extracellular products of certain dermatophytes may induce severe inflammation at the site of infection.

Infections caused by dermatophytes or keratinophilic fungi are referred to as dermatophytoses. The term formerly used, dermatomycosis, includes all fungal infections involving the skin. Many species of *Microsporum* and *Trichophyton* cause ringworm in animals. The principal differential characteristics of important veterinary dermatophytes are listed in Table 36.1.

Infection by a dermatophyte may result in a state of hypersensitivity to the dermatophyte. The nature of the lesion depends to some extent on the immunologic response. The inflammation is most severe if there is a hypersensitivity reaction; however, this response may contribute to the resolution of the infection. The local inflammatory response and the delayed-type hypersensitivity are attributed to galactomannan glycopeptides. It has been suggested that chronic dermatophytosis may be related to a modification of cell-mediated immunity. Vesicular lesions may appear on various parts of the body as part of a general allergic reaction. They result from the

Table 36.1 Summary of Principal Characteristics of Important Veterinary Dermatophytes

Characteristic	M. canis	Microsporum gypseum	Microsporum nanum	Trichophyton mentagrophytes*	Trichophyton verrucosum	Trichophyton gallinae	Trichophyton equinum
Principal hosts	Dog and cat (most cases), humans, monkey, horse	Dog, horse, cat	Swine	Many animal species, including all domestic animals	Cattle, sheep	Fowl	Horse
Fluorescence	+	–	–	–	–	–	–
Arthrospores	Ectothrix, small, mosaic	Ectothrix, large, chains	Ectothrix, large, chains	Ectothrix, large, chains	Ectothrix, large, chains	Ectothrix, large, chains	Ectothrix, long chains
Cultural features	White to buff; reverse: yellow to orange; rapid grower	Buff; reverse: orange brown to yellow; moderately rapid	White to buff; reverse: red; moderately rapid	Granular, light buff to tan; reverse: variable red, yellow, etc.; fairly rapid	Deeply folded, white to brilliant yellow; slow	Radial folds, white to pale rose; reverse: red; moderately rapid	White, cottony, yellow edge; old colony velvety to cream-tan; reverse: yellow to red-brown
Macroconidia	Spindle-shaped, frequent	Ellipsoidal, septa 2–6, frequent	Obovoid to ellipsoidal ovate; frequent	Occurrence variable; spindle or clavate; 5–6 septa	Requires thiamine; long and thin walled; rare	Infrequent; club-shaped and clavate	Rare; clavate; requires nicotinic acid
Microconidia	Few, sessile	Sessile or on short sterigmata; clavate	Clavate	Abundant, pyriform or clavate, sessile	Abundant with thiamine; singly ovoid; pyriform or clavate	Singly on hyphae, pyriform to clavate	Many, spherical to pyriform
Other	Accessory structures similar to those of T. gallinae	Persists in soil; accessory structures similar to those of T. gallinae	Persists in soil	T. equinum resembles T. mentagrophytes (see below)	Chlamydospores; grows better at 37° than 25°C	Chalmydospores, nodular bodies, racquet hyphae	

Note: Other deramatophytes are encountered less frequently in domestic animals. Among these are *Trichophyton rubrum*, reported in the dog; *Microsporum audouinii*, reported in dog and monkey; and *Trichophyton schoenleinii*, reported in horses and cats in Europe.

*Consists of three varieties, *erinacei*, *mentagrophytes*, and *quinckaenum*.

hematogenous spread of the fungi or its products. These lesions, which do not contain the organism, are called dermatophytids, or "id" lesions or reactions. They are well known in humans and occasionally occur in animals. In addition, infections with *Microsporium canis* frequently possess **kerions**, the result of vesicles in and around the lesions.

Secondary bacterial invaders such as *Staphylococcus aureus* and *Staphylococcus intermedius* are common, and they may cause pustules in hair follicles. Dermatophytes can hydrolyze keratin, and the infection is localized in the keratinized epidermis. This is thought to be caused by the lack of sufficient concentration of available iron elsewhere. The epidermis and hair are the principal structures attacked in lower animals. Dermatophytosis is almost always superficial, and most infections are self-limiting and rarely lead to death. However, long-lasting infection can cause severe lesions, with concomitant discomfort for the animals and economic loss.

Characteristically, dermatophytosis is more frequently observed in stabled farm animals than in pastured animals. The incidence is usually higher during winter months in temperate regions, and the disease may resolve itself spontaneously in the spring and summer.

In domestic animals there are no apparent differences in the clinical appearances of infections produced by the different dermatophytes. The lesions in domestic animals are usually characterized by circular, scaly areas of alopecia with or without crust formation. In dogs and cats, lesions occur most frequently on the head and extremities. The head and tail are the most frequent locations in horses and cattle. Remissions are seen frequently in animals that have been treated for clinical dermatophytosis.

LABORATORY DIAGNOSIS

First, if feasible, examine patient in the dark with a Wood's lamp (filtered ultraviolet light, 3650 Å) to determine whether fluorescence is present. If present, remove some fluorescing hairs with forceps for microscopic examination. Also remove hairs at edge of lesions for examination.

Second, hairs, nails, and skin scrapings are examined in 10% or 20% KOH under a coverslip for the presence of arthrospores or hyphae. The preparation should be gently warmed for about 10 minutes or allowed to stand for about 30 minutes at room temperature to digest proteinaceous debris. The penetration and clarity can be enhanced by the addition of DMSO (36%; dimethylsulfoxide) to the KOH (20%; potassium hydroxide). Special staining procedures such as lactophenol cotton blue are used for better visualization before examining.

Third, regardless of whether arthrospores are found, material is inoculated onto Sabouraud agar containing cycloheximide and chloramphenicol. The former inhibits contaminating fungi, and the latter inhibits contaminating bacteria. Do not discard plates until they have been incubated at room temperature (25°–30°C) for at least a month. If *Trichophyton verrucosum* is suspected, the culture

plate should also be incubated at 37°C, as this temperature enhances growth of this fungus. For production of macroconidia, *T. verrucosum* (cattle) requires a medium supplemented with inositol and thiamine; *Trichophyton equinum* requires nicotinic acid. Yeast extract is a satisfactory source of these growth supplements.

Fourth, if fungi grow, examine colonies grossly for morphology, texture, and pigment as seen under the colonies. Then examine the mycelium or other material microscopically in a lactophenol cotton blue wet mount. A **tape mount** is a convenient procedure. The principal morphologic and cultural characteristics of the important dermatophytes of animals are summarized in Table 36.1. The morphology of the macroconidia of the major animal dermatophytes is shown in Fig. 36.1. Their demonstration in cultures is significant in identification.

IDENTIFICATION

Knowledge of colony characteristics, microscopic morphology, and nutritional requirements are essential for identification of dermatophytes (Table 36.1). The size and shape of macro- and microconidia and the thickness of their cell walls are important microscopic characteristics for speciation. Detection of arthrospores outside (ectothrix) or inside (endothrix) the hair shaft may make possible the rapid diagnosis of ringworm. Additional characteristics used for the identification of some species are urease production, geographic occurrence, **auxotrophy**, requirement for vitamins and amino acids, hair perforation tests, and temperature stimulation of growth. Speciation of dermatophytes may require the expertise of a reference laboratory. Commercially available *Trichophyton* agars, Nos. 1 to 7 containing various growth factors (vitamins and amino acids), are available to aid in the identification of species by determining the nutritional responses of species.

Dermatophyte Test Medium (DTM) and Rapid Sporulation Medium (RSM) are available commercially under a number of trade names. When dermatophytes grow on DTM, a modified Sabouraud agar (that contains phenol red), they change the yellow medium to red (alkaline), usually within 2 weeks. This is a useful screening medium. It is advisable to submit positive cultures to a microbiology laboratory for confirmatory examination, as false-positive reactions occur.

TREATMENT

The affected animal or animals, if part of a group, should preferably be isolated. All affected animals should be treated topically with an antifungal solution. Systemic treatment is usually economically prohibitive for cattle and horses. Clipping is indicated in animals with medium-to-long hair. Among the solutions used are lime–sulfur, sodium hypochlorite (1:10 household bleach), chlorhexidine, captan, and povidone–iodine. If topical treatment

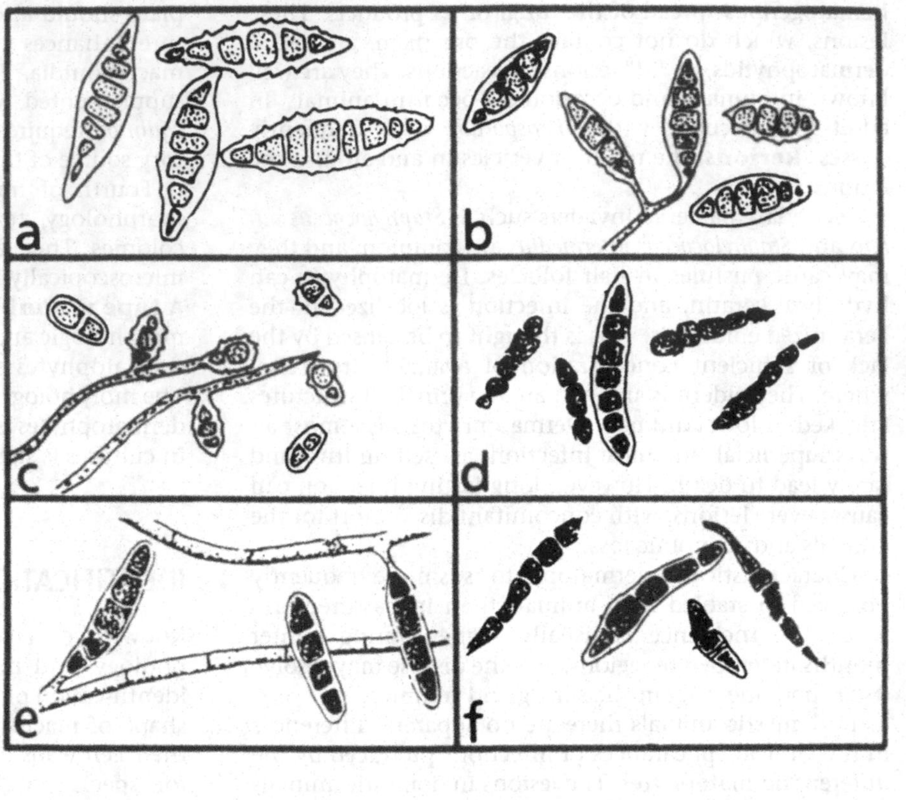

FIGURE 36.1   Macroconidia of important dermatophytes: (a) *Microsporum canis*, (b) *Microsporum gypseum*, (c) *Microsporum nanum*, (d) *Trichophyton mentagrophytes*, (e) *Trichophyton equinum*, and (f) *Trichophyton verrucosum*.

alone is not effective, systemic therapy is indicated, particularly in dogs and cats. Griseofulvin, ketoconazole, and itraconazole are used for systemic treatment. Griseofulvin and itraconazole are less toxic for cats. They should be given for at least 2 weeks past clinical cure. The spot treatment of lesions is not recommended, as unapparent areas of infection may be missed.

Dogs and cats in particular can be reinfected from an asymptomatic carrier. To determine whether an animal is a carrier, the entire body should be combed thoroughly with a new toothbrush. Collected hairs should be cultured. Topical treatment is carried out if the culture is positive. Systemic treatment may be necessary.

Cattle ringworm is often a problem in stabled animals in temperate regions. It usually clears up when the cattle leave the stable. The topical antifungal solutions referred to above, applied as sprays, are effective.

A live attenuated *T. verrucosum* vaccine, widely used in Europe, reduces the severity of infections.

An inactivated fungal cell wall vaccine for cats reduces the severity of the clinical disease.

Cages, pens, rubbing posts, saddles, grooming tools, tack, and so forth should be thoroughly disinfected. Although dermatophytes can survive for years off the animal, they are susceptible to commonly used disinfectants.

Precautions should be taken to prevent human infections.

PUBLIC HEALTH SIGNIFICANCE

Human dermatophytosis is occasionally acquired from infected animals. The species involved are: *M. canis*, most commonly from dogs and cats; *Trichophyton mentagrophytes* from horses and other animals; and *T. verrucosum* from cattle.

GLOSSARY

auxotrophy Organisms that are unable to synthesize certain nutrients (growth factors) that need to be provided to obtain growth. These include amino acids, nicotinamide adenine dinucleotide, biotin, and so forth.

kerions Pus-filled inflammatory swellings that may resemble bacterial abscesses.

tape mount In this procedure, a small length of clear Scotch-brand tape is applied, adhesive side down, to the fungal colony. Elements of the fungus adhere to the tape, which is applied to a microscope slide, then examined under the microscope.

37

Infections Caused by Yeasts and Yeastlike Fungi

CANDIDIASIS

A number of species of *Candida* can be differentiated by biochemical tests. All *Candida* spp., of which there are more than 200, occur saprophytically. The important species from the standpoint of disease is *Candida albicans*. It is a normal inhabitant of the digestive tract, oral cavity, and vagina. Infections are usually endogenous.

The following *Candida* species have been implicated as causes of bovine mastitis: *C. albicans, C. parapsilosis, C. guilliermondii, C. krusei, C. pseudotropicalis, C. rugosa,* and *C. tropicalis. C. parapsilosis* has caused bovine abortion, and *Candida rugosa* has been implicated in pyometra in a mare.

Pathogenesis

Candida albicans possess adhesins consisting of fibrillar, peptide-mannans that have an affinity for the fibronectin on the surface of host cells. The yeast forms are responsible for tissue damage. Secreted aspartic proteinases (Saps), which are encoded by 10 genes, are thought to contribute to tissue damage and are currently considered to be important virulence factors. Inhibition of yeast cell division results in hyphal elements that invade tissues. These hyphal elements are also thought to be important virulence factors. They are associated with the ability to penetrate host tissues and localize *C. albicans* infections. Other possible virulence factors include cell wall glycoprotein, proteases, neuraminidase, chitin, mannoprotein, and lipids. The cell wall glycoproteins appear to have endotoxin-like activity. Both polymorphonuclear leukocytes and macrophages have candidacidal activity, and the latter are involved when there is a granulomatous response. The investigation into the specific mechanisms of *C. albicans* pathogenesis is ongoing.

Pathogenicity

Infections by *C. albicans* occur most frequently on mucous membranes of the digestive and genital tracts. The young are especially susceptible. Candidiasis involving the gastrointestinal tract may result from prolonged antibiotic therapy. Disseminated candidiasis has been reported occasionally in immunocompromised animals and in those undergoing prolonged antibiotic treatment and chemotherapy. Natural infections in animals appear to be uncommon.

PUPPIES, KITTENS, CALVES, AND FOALS. Infection of the oral and intestinal mucous membrane is uncommon. Mycotic stomatitis and enteritis occur, and white-to-gray patches representing pseudomembranous inflammation of the mucous membrane are seen. Pyothorax and cystitis in adult cats have been attributed to *C. albicans*.

SWINE. Infections of the lower esophagus and esophageal region of the stomach occur. *Candida albicans* may be found in stomach ulcers. Diarrhea and cutaneous candidiasis have been reported in swine.

CHICKENS, TURKEYS, AND OTHER BIRDS. Infections of the mouth, esophagus, and crop occur, with pseudomembranous whitish areas, usually in the young. Crop mycosis (thrush) may affect a considerable number of young chickens and turkeys.

COWS. Mastitis caused by various *Candida* spp. is common. Genital infections are rare.

MARES. *Candida albicans* causes metritis and vaginitis.

STALLIONS AND BULLS. Genital candidiasis is seen in stallions and bulls.

HUMANS. The mucous membranes of the mouth, tongue, and genital tract are more commonly involved than the nails and skin. Recurring candidal vulvovaginitis occurs frequently in women. The oral form (thrush), characterized by white patches, occurs commonly in infants. Several defects in cell-mediated immunity predispose humans to chronic mucocutaneous candidiasis. *Candida* infections are frequently seen in acquired immune deficiency syndrome patients, and disseminated candidiasis occurs in advanced malignancies.

Immune Response

Both cell-mediated and humoral immunity are important in defense. Although more information is currently being obtained, little is known about the immune response to *C. albicans*. It has long been recognized that protection is dependent on cell-mediated immunity, and studies have indicated an essential role of type 1 cytokines in protection against *Candida* spp. However, antibodies also play a role in that antibodies directed against mannan constituents and secretory aspartyl proteinases of *C. albicans* also are protective, as indicated by passive transfer experiments. In addition, *C. albicans* can stimulate the release of histamine by mast cells and induce the production of IgE antibodies associated with the induction of *C. albicans* allergies.

Laboratory Diagnosis

Organisms can frequently be seen in wet mounts (20% KOH, india ink, or lactophenol cotton blue) and in smears stained with Gram's stain (gram-positive), where they appear as oval, thin-walled, budding cells and hyphal fragments (pseudohyphae); see Fig. 37.1.

1. They are readily cultivated on blood agar and Sabouraud agar at 25° and 37°C. Soft, creamy colonies resembling those of staphylococci are seen in 24–48 hours.
2. Identification is accomplished by the demonstration of the large chlamydospores (see Fig. 37.1) or germ tubes characteristic of *C. albicans*. Plates of corn meal or Chlamydospore agar are inoculated by cutting into the agar at an angle to the bottom of the plate. If present, the chlamydospores can be seen below the surface in 24–48 hours by focusing directly on the line of inoculation.
3. To demonstrate germ tubes, a small amount of fetal bovine serum is inoculated with a light inoculum of growth. After incubation for 2–4 hours at 37°C, a drop from the serum sediment is examined microscopically. A germ tube is a filamentous outgrowth from the yeast cell. Unlike pseudohyphae, there is no restriction at the point of origin.
4. Species of *Candida* other than *C. albicans* are identified by carbohydrate fermentation and **assimilation tests**. These reactions are used to identify species in several commercial systems.

Treatment

Nystatin (mycostatin) is used in ointments for skin infections and locally for oral and genital infections. It is administered in the feed to treat candidiasis in chickens and turkeys and intestinal and oral candidiasis in swine, dogs, and cats. Very little of the drug is absorbed orally. It has been administered into the mammary gland to treat mastitis caused by *Candida* spp. Clotrimazole and ketoconazole are also used in topical preparations.

Amphotericin B is the most effective drug for the treatment of systemic candidiasis. Ketoconazole and clotrimazole have been effective in the treatment of mucocutaneous candidiasis in human beings. Clotrimazole infusions have been used to treat mycotic endometritis in mares and cows. Clotrimazole is an effective treatment for bovine mastitis caused by *Candida* spp.

CRYPTOCOCCOSIS

There are many species in the genus *Cryptococcus*, but only *Cryptococcus neoformans* is considered potentially pathogenic. There are two varieties, *C. neoformans* var. *neoformans* (serotypes A and D) and *C. neoformans* var. *gattii* (serotypes B and C). *Filobasidiella neoformans* is the telemorphic state of serotypes A and D and the telemorphic state of serotypes B and C. These serotypes are based on differences in capsular antigens.

Most strains from clinical disease in animals and humans are var. *neoformans*, and the reservoir of this variety is the feces of birds, particularly pigeons, and soil contaminated by avian excreta. This variety occurs in nature and reaches high concentrations in pigeon droppings and nests. The pigeon is not infected; the organisms colonize feces after they have been passed.

Var. *gattii* occurs in tropical and subtropical regions and is not associated with avian habitats. It has been associated with meningitis in humans, specifically serotype C. It has also caused infrequent disease in dolphins (serotype B), cats, dogs and koalas.

Infections are exogenous and are usually acquired by inhalation. Primary foci are most often in the respiratory system, including the paranasal sinuses, with possible subsequent spread. Animal-to-animal transmission is not known to occur.

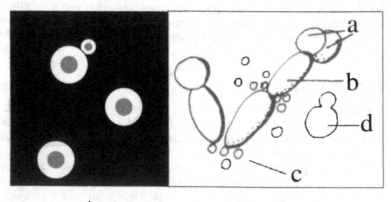

FIGURE 37.1   Elements of *Cryptococcus neoformans* and *Candida albicans*. **(A)** India ink stain of *C. neoformans* showing the large capsule. **(B)** *C. albicans* showing the **(a)** chlamydospores, **(b)** pseudohyphae, **(c)** blastospores, and **(d)** yeast cells of *C. albicans*.

A   B

Pathogenesis

The thick capsule of *C. neoformans*, which is composed mainly of polysaccharide with mannose units, is antiphagocytic and immunosuppressive. Secretion of capsular antigen into body fluids binds antibody before it reaches *C. neoformans* cells and also induces **suppressor cells**. Both humoral and cell-mediated immunity (CMI) are important defense mechanisms, although CMI is more effective in eliminating the fungus.

The majority of animals are protected from cryptococcal infection by macrophages, **natural killer cells**, and polymorphonuclear leukocytes. There may be a granulomatous response with infiltration of macrophages and neutrophils.

Pathogenicity

Only sporadic cases of cryptococcal mastitis have been reported in cattle. The disease is uncommon in sheep and goats.

In the dog and cat, infections of the pharynx and paranasal sinuses are seen, occasionally with dissemination to the central nervous system and other tissues including lungs, kidney, and joints. A mycetoma form with subcutaneous granulomas is also seen.

In horses, it is most frequently seen as a paranasal infection, which may or may not spread to other tissues, including the brain. Abortion in mares has also been reported.

Cryptococcosis has been reported in a number of animals including fox, dolphin, monkey, ferret, guinea pig, cheetah, and some avian species.

In humans, infections involving the lungs and central nervous system (cryptococcal meningitis) are most common.

Direct Examination

Yeastlike cells can be seen in wet mounts of cerebrospinal fluid and pus. The large capsule can be seen if clinical material is mixed with india ink or nigrosin (see Fig. 37.1). The yeastlike cells are gram-positive and can be seen in stained smears.

Laboratory Diagnosis

The organism grows at 37° and 25°C on blood agar and Sabouraud agar, respectively; it is inhibited by cycloheximide. Wrinkled, whitish granular colonies usually appear within a week. They become slimy, mucoid, and cream to brownish in color on further incubation. Budding yeastlike cells with large capsules can be seen in wet mounts.

1. Most saprophytic strains of *Cryptococcus* species do not grow at 37°C.
2. Identification is based in part on cultural and morphologic characteristics, especially the presence of the large capsule (see Fig. 37.1). Members of the genus *Cryptococcus* produce urease on Christensen's urea agar, whereas *Candida* spp. do not.
3. Several species of *Cryptococcus* possess capsules, but only *C. neoformans* produces brown colonies on birdseed agar. The latter medium, which contains *Guzotia abysinica* seeds, can also be used as a selective medium for *C. neoformans*. In this medium, *C. neoformans* produces melanin, and the enzyme responsible for its initial production is phenoloxidase. The seeds of birdseed agar are rich in compounds that are substrates for the cryptococcal phenoloxidase.
4. The various species can be identified by carbohydrate assimilation tests. Commercial kits are available for the identification of most *Cryptococcus* spp. A deoxyribonucleic acid probe is available for the identification of the cultured organism.
5. A highly presumptive diagnosis of cryptococcosis can be made on basis of the demonstration of yeastlike cells with large capsules from lesions and characteristic colonial growth on blood and Sabouraud agar.
6. Strains of the true yeast *Saccharomyces* can be distinguished from cryptococci by the presence of ascospores in the former. The ascospores stain well with methylene blue.
7. *Geotrichum* and *Trichosporon* both produce true mycelia.

A latex agglutination procedure is available as a test for antigen in body fluids; it is not ordinarily used in animals. Tube agglutination, complement fixation, enzyme-linked immunosorbent assay, and immunofluorescence assay are used for detection of specific antibody in humans but infrequently in animals.

Treatment

Amphotericin B is effective and is sometimes combined with flucytosine; the toxicity may be substantial. The imidazole derivatives such as ketoconazole, fluconazole, and itraconazole have shown some promise.

Public Health Significance

Although cryptococcosis is not considered to be acquired from animals, one should avoid contact with infectious materials.

GEOTRICHOSIS

This disease is caused by the yeastlike fungus *Geotrichum candidum*. It is an uncommon disease rarely diagnosed clinically. This fungus is found widely in nature, and its isolation from clinical materials is not necessarily significant. Two cultural forms occur: the glabrous or yeastlike form and the fluffy form. The latter strains are sometimes given the name *Oospora*. The glabrous form of *G. candidum* is the one usually associated with disease.

Pathogenicity

Infections have been reported from cattle, pigs, horses, dogs, fowl, penguins, ocelot, nonhuman primates, and humans. They are usually identified on postmortem examination. The bronchi, lungs, udder (mastitis), and mucous membranes of the alimentary tract are most frequently affected. The disease is usually mild and is characterized by the formation of granulomas that may suppurate. *Geotrichum candidum* is occasionally recovered from otitis externa in the dog. It has caused rare systemic disease in dogs, abortion and mastitis in cattle, and cutaneous lesions in flamingoes and snakes.

Laboratory Diagnosis

Purulent material or scrapings from lesions are examined in wet mounts. The organism appears as rectangular or spherical arthrospores. They are thick-walled, nonbudding, and in gram-stained smears, they are strongly gram-positive.

The organisms grow fairly rapidly at room temperature (25°C) on Sabouraud agar. The colonies are membranous with radial furrows and soft, with a dry, granular surface. The mycelium is made up of septate hyphae that fragment, producing chains of characteristic rectangular-to-round arthrospores. The organism does not grow well on blood agar at 37°C.

Differentiation from other fungi is based on cultural and morphologic characteristics. *Geotrichum candidum* can be distinguished from *Coccidioides immitis* and *Blastomyces dermatitidis* by the fact that the latter two species produce cottony, filamentous colonies at room temperature. *Geotrichum candidum* produces a soft, yeastlike colony at room temperature and does not form blastospores; this differentiates it from *Trichosporon* spp.

Indications of geotrichosis may come from histopathological examination of tissues.

Treatment

Specific treatment is rarely administered. In vitro tests indicate susceptibility to amphotericin-B and flucytosine. There appear to be few to no reports of the use of antifungal drugs in animal geotrichosis.

MALASSEZIA

Malessezia pachydermatis, a lipophilic yeast, occurs as a commensal on the oily areas of the skin and ears of dogs and cats. In some cases of otitis externa, they are present in larger numbers than normal and it is generally concluded that in such cases they have pathogenic significance. This species is now recognized as an important cause of chronic dermatitis in dogs.

Malessezia furfur causes blepharitis, folliculitis, seborrhea, dandruff, and **tinea versicolor** in human beings.

Malassezia are bottle-shaped, small budding cells that reproduce by a process known as bud fission in which the bud detaches from the parent cell by the production of a septum (see Fig. 37.2). They can be demonstrated in wet

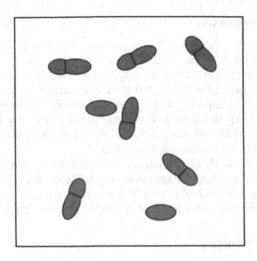

FIGURE 37.2   Characteristic morphology of *Malassezia*. Note the characteristic small, bottle-shaped, budding cells.

mounts (10% KOH) of clinical material, such as from dogs' ears. No telemorphic state has been described for this fungus.

They can be readily recovered on Sabouraud glucose agar to which sterile olive oil and Tween 80 have been applied to the surface. They are obligate lipophiles. Incubation is 2–4 days at 37°C; growth is slower at 25°C. Identification is based on microscopic morphology and growth characteristics. *Malassezia* spp. are nonfermentative and urease positive.

Treatment

Treatement will depend on the location and nature of the infection. Topical preparations containing clotrimazole, ketoconazole, or other antifungal agents are used.

TRICHOSPORONOSIS

Trichosporonosis is caused by the soilborne yeast *Trichosporon beigelii*. However, it is now known based on nucleic acid and ultrastructure studies that *T. beigelii* includes a number of potentially pathogenic species. We will continue to refer to these yeasts as *T. beigelii*. It is an imperfect fungus within the family Tremellomycetidae. It produces blastoconidia, well-developed hyphae, pseudohyphae, and arthroconidia.

Trichosporon beigelii is an opportunist yeast that causes superficial and deep-seated mycoses in humans and, less frequently, in animals. Infection of hair in humans is called white piedra. The severe infections are usually seen in individuals that are immunocompromised. Disseminated trichosporonosis has been reported in cats infected with feline leukemia virus. *Trichosporon beigelii* has been recovered infrequently from various infections in animals including a nasal granuloma in a cat, skin infections in the horse and monkey, and mastitis in cattle and sheep. This saprophytic yeast is occasionally a contaminant in clinical specimens.

Trichosporon can be recovered on Sabouraud glucose agar after 7 days' incubation. Initially, colonies are cream colored, shiny, and smooth and later become dry and membranous. Definitive identification is based on assimilation tests and growth characteristics. All species are urease positive.

Treatment

There is little information on the treatment of trichosporonosis in animals. Clotrimazole or miconazole, used topically, and fluconazole have been effective in human trichosporonosis, and presumably, other azole drugs would be effective.

OTHER YEASTS

Torulopsis glabrata occurs as a commensal in animals and is found in soil. It has been implicated as the cause of pyelonephritis, pneumonia, septicemia, and meningitis in immunocompromised human patients; mastitis and abortion in cattle; and systemic infections in dogs and monkeys.

The fungi *Rhodotorula minuta* and *Rhodotorula rubra* have been recovered from the canine ear and equine uterus and are associated infrequently with infections in animals.

GLOSSARY

assimilation tests These tests use broth media to detect carbohydrate use in the presence of oxygen.

natural killer cell Lymphocyte that recognizes and destroys, in a nonspecific manner, infected host cells and foreign cells.

suppressor cells Type of T cell thought to "turn off" an immune response.

tinea versicolor Human infection of the skin (neck, torso, or limbs) caused by lipophilic yeasts of the *Malassezia furfur* complex.

38

Subcutaneous and Inoculation Mycoses

SPOROTRICHOSIS

Sporotrichosis is caused by *Sporothrix schenckii*, a dimorphic fungus that occurs in nature in association with soil, wood, and vegetation. Infections are exogenous and worldwide in occurrence. The portal of entry is usually a wound. The presence of the organism on thorny plants and traumatic introduction of the organism may account for some infections.

Pathogenesis and Pathogenicity

Proteases are possible virulence factors of *S. schenckii*. It has been noted that the cell wall sugar composition is also reflective of virulence. The more virulent forms have a rhamnose:mannose molar ratio of 1.7:1.0, whereas the avirulent forms have a ratio of 1.0:1.7. The relationship of this observation to virulence has yet to be determined.

Infections in humans and some animals are characterized by the formation of subcutaneous nodules or pyogranulomas. The organisms usually enter through wounds in the skin and spread via the lymphatics. The parasitic form of growth is the blastoconidia. The nodules eventually ulcerate and discharge pus. Involvement of bones, joints, and visceral organs with fatal termination is rare but has been reported in the dog, cat, and horse. Infections have been described in humans and in the dog, cat, horse, donkey, mule, camel, cattle, fowl, and wild rodents. In veterinary practice, the disease occurs most commonly in the horse, in which it is seen most frequently as an ascending lymphocutaneous infection of the leg.

Direct Examination

In pus and tissue, the organism appears as a single-celled cigar-shaped body, usually within neutrophils. These structures (yeast phase) are very difficult to demonstrate in stained smears and wet mounts of pus and tissue scrapings except in feline specimens, which contain numerous yeast cells. Fluorescent antibody, **periodic acid-Schiff**, and **calcofluor white** staining of clinical materials frequently yield positive results. Characteristic "asteroid bodies" consisting of clusters of yeast cells with peripheral eosinophilic rays are seen in tissue sections.

Laboratory Diagnosis

Sporothrix schenckii is readily grown on brain heart infusion agar, blood agar (37°C), and Sabouraud agar with cycloheximide and chloramphenicol (25°–27°C) in 1–3 weeks.

TISSUE PHASE. At 37°C, colonies appear in 3–5 days. They are yeastlike, smooth, soft, and cream to tan in color. There is no mycelium. Colonies are composed of the same elements that occur in pus and tissue, specifically, cigar-shaped cells and spherical or oval budding cells. Some large pyriform cells may also be seen (Fig. 38.1).

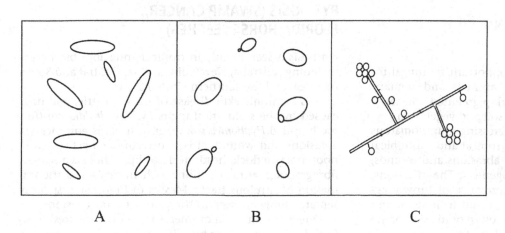

A   B   C

FIGURE 38.1 Morphologic elements of *Sporothrix schenckii*. **(A)** Cigar-shaped bodies (yeast form) of the organism in tissues. **(B)** Mature and budding yeast cells from growth on blood agar at 37°C. **(C)** Growth at 25°C on Sabouraud's agar: hyphae with microconidia, sometimes in a characteristic "flowerette" arrangement.

MYCELIAL PHASE. At 25°–27°C, colonies appear early, but the characteristic structures are not evident until the aerial mycelium is produced. Colonies are white and soft at first and then become tan to brown to black. The texture is leathery, wrinkled, and coarsely tufted.

The mycelium consists of fine, branching septate hyphae that bear pyriform or ovoid microconidia, which are borne in clusters from the ends of conidiophores or as sessile forms directly on the sides of hyphae (Fig. 38.1). Thick-walled, large chlamydospores may be seen in old cultures.

The mold phase of *S. schenckii* can be converted to the yeast phase by subculturing from Sabouraud agar to brain heart infusion agar with 10% blood. The latter is incubated for 3–5 days at 37°C in 5% CO_2.

A latex agglutination test and a tube agglutination test are used to detect antibodies in humans. The presence of the latter are not always diagnostic. The immunodiffusion test is reliable and easy to perform.

Factors involved in the immune response have thus far received little attention.

Animal Inoculation

Mice are susceptible. Suspected material or cultures are inoculated intraperitoneally. The mice are sacrificed in 3 weeks, and if infected, cigar-shaped bodies can be seen in smears from the peritoneal exudate and granulomata.

Treatment

Potassium iodide is administered orally to the point of producing iodinism. It is continued for several weeks after apparent recovery to prevent recrudescence. Other drugs that have been effective are amphotericin B, itraconazole, fluconazole, and other imidazoles.

Public Health Sigificance

Great care must be exercised in handling animal infections, both on the part of the veterinarian and those in contact with the patient. Infection is readily acquired from infectious material.

CHROMOBLASTOMYCOSIS AND PHAEOHYPHOMYCOSIS

These names denote infrequent opportunistic fungal infections of domestic and other animals and humans caused by a wide variety of dark-pigmented (dematiaceous) fungi that occur widely in soil and vegetation.

These are chronic, slowly progressing granulomatous diseases occurring principally in tropical and subtropical regions. Fungi are introduced via abrasions and wounds, but little is known of their pathogenesis. The infections, which are characterized by the presence of brown-pigmented fungal elements in tissue, result in nodular and frequently ulcerating lesions, most often of the skin of the feet and legs, with regional granulomatous lymphadeni-

tis; systemic infection is infrequent. Both normal and compromised animals can be infected. Ocular infections, central nervous system infections and systemic disease have been reported in turkeys and other avian species.

Chromoblastomycosis is caused by several species, mainly of the genera *Cladosporium*, *Phialofora*, *Fonsecaea*, and *Rhinocladiella*. Phaeohyphomycosis can be caused by more than 100 species of dematiaceous fungi of various genera, including *Alternaria*, *Bipolaris*, *Dactylaria*, *Curvularia*, *Exophiala*, *Scolecobasidium*, and *Exophilia*. These two diseases also differ in the morphology of the forms seen in tissues.

Direct Examination

Material from granulomatous or ulcerous lesions is examined in 10% sodium hydroxide. The organisms causing chromoblastomycosis are single-celled or clustered, spherical, thick-walled muriform or sclerotic bodies with a black or dark brown pigment. The same fungal elements are seen in sections of biopsies. They multiply by cross-wall formation or splitting rather than budding. In phaeohyphomycosis, the fungal forms are yeastlike, pseudohyphal, or hyphal and without muriform cells.

Laboratory Diagnosis

Material from lesions or biopsies is cultured. The organisms grow on Sabouraud agar at room temperature; growth is slow, requiring up to a month. The colonies are compact and deep brown to black, and their surface is velvety and often wrinkled. Their identification is based on their method of conidiation. Identification of the genus is usually not difficult, but a specialist may be required to identify the species.

Treatment

Surgical excision with large margins is appropriate for some lesions; recurrence is common. Amphotericin B (locally or systemically), flucytosine, and itraconazole have been effective in humans but have not been adequately tested in animals.

PYTHIOSIS (SWAMP CANCER, FLORIDA HORSE LEECHES)

Pythiosis is seen mainly in tropical and subtropical areas including Australia, New Guinea, Asia, Central and South America, and the southern United States.

It is a chronic skin disease of horses, cattle, and dogs caused by the soilborne fungus *Pythium insidiosum* (formerly called *Hyphomyces destruens*). It gains entrance via abrasions and wounds, frequently involving the limbs, hoof, hock, fetlock, head, neck, or lips. There is a pyo- or fibrogranulomatous reaction, with necrosis and the formation of fistulous tracts. Masses of branching, sparsely septated fungi are seen in the yellow necrotic lesions.

Direct examination of smears from exudate, freshly affected tissue including biopsies, and histopathologic examination of tissue sections with a finding of septate hyphae suggests a mycosis that may be pithiosis. However, definitive diagnosis requires the isolation and identification of the causal fungus. The presence of characteristic zoospores in cultures will suggest *P. insidosum*. Final identification may require the aid of a mycologist.

An immunodiffusion test is available in some reference laboratories.

The disease is progressive but not usually systemic, and there have been no remissions reported in the absence of treatment, which involves surgery and administration of amphotericin B or imidazole drugs.

MYCETOMA

A mycetoma is a pyogranulomatous, subcutaneous abscess of animals and humans resulting from traumatic inoculation of a saprophytic fungus or an actinomycete. We will refer here only to mycotic mycetomas.

A number of fungi, both pigmented and unpigmented, have been recovered including *Pseudoallescheria boydii*, *Curvularia* spp., *Cochliobolus spicifer*, *Madurella* spp., and *Helminthosporium* spp. These fungi occur in soil and are implanted via abrasions or wounds. Mycetomas have been characterized by the triad, tumefaction (swelling), draining sinuses, and grains.

Microcolonies (grains or granules), which frequently are pigmented, can sometimes be seen grossly in lesions and exudates. These infrequent infections have been reported in horses, cattle, dogs, and cats. The lesions occur most commonly on the extremities but may also be found involving the nasal mucosa (e.g., bovine nasal granuloma), the peritoneum, and the skin in various locations.

Incision of the lesions in the case of the dematiaceous fungi reveals discrete brown or black fungal microcolonies embedded in a large mass of granulation tissue.

Laboratory Diagnosis

Scrapings or biopsy tissue are examined grossly for the characteristic microcolonies, which are small (0.5–3.0 μm), irregularly shaped, and variously colored. These colonies or "grains" are placed in 10% sodium hydroxide and then pressed out by means of a coverslip and observed microscopically. They reveal mycelia that are usually 2–4 μm in width, in contrast to the narrower filaments found in the actinomycotic granule. Also of significance is the presence of chlamydospores.

The species involved grow readily and usually slowly (2–3 weeks) on Sabouraud agar at room temperature. Identification is based on cultural characteristics and microscopic morphology. Speciation may require the aid of a mycologist.

Treatment

Surgical debridement or excision of the lesion is usually indicated. Amphotericin B, iodides, itraconazole, and ketoconazole given for long periods have been effective in some cases.

EPIZOOTIC LYMPHANGITIS

This disease caused by *Histoplasma farciminosum* (also referred to as *Histoplasma capsuatum* var. *farciminosum*) occurs in equidae in Asia and Mediterranean regions. The organism occurs in nature, and the mode of infection is via wounds and abrasions and possibly blood-sucking arthropods.

It is a chronic disease involving the lymph nodes, superficial lymph vessels, and skin mainly of the limbs, back, and neck. It is characterized by the formation of suppurative, nodular, ulcerating lesions along the lymphatics of the legs. More than 90% of cases occur in horses. A pulmonary form has also been described as well as disseminated disease. The mortality rate can reach 15% in fully susceptible animals. Although the organism occurs in nature, most cases are considered to derive from other infected animals. Although rare, respiratory, conjunctival, and gastrointestinal infections have been reported.

Laboratory Diagnosis

The oval or pear-shaped cells can be seen in pus from fresh lesions. A diagnosis is usually made by demonstration of the characteristic double-contoured yeast cells in wet mounts from typical lesions.

The organism is dimorphic, growing in the mycelial phase at room temperature and in the yeast phase at 37°C. Growth of the two phases is often slow, taking up to 8 weeks. Yeastlike cells with some hyphae are seen at 37°C. At room temperature, hyphae yield characteristic thick-walled chlamydospores.

An enzyme-linked immunosorbent assay and an immunofluorescence assay have been used to detect specific antibodies, which support a diagnosis.

Treatment

Iodides orally, and local application of iodine and silver nitrate, are reported to be effective. Modern antifungal drugs have not been adequately tested.

RHINOSPORIDIOSIS

The cause of this disease is *Rhinosporidium seeberi*, a fungus presumed to occur in nature (water) and that has not been cultivated as yet on artificial media but has been propagated in cell cultures.

Recently, *R. seeberi* has been determined to be a single-celled protist that has the characteristics of both pathogenic fungi and protozoans. Analysis of 18S rRNA sequences has confirmed this taxonomic move.

Rhinosporidium seeberi causes a chronic, generally benign disease of cattle, horses, mules, dogs, aquatic birds, and humans characterized by the formation of polyps on the nasal and ocular mucous membranes. More than 90% of the nasal cases involve male animals. The disease occurs mostly in tropical and subtropical countries. Infrequent cases have been reported in dogs in the United States.

Direct Examination

Wet mounts from nasal discharge and sections from polyps disclose large sporangia (200 to 300 μm) that contain thousands of endospores (Fig. 38.2). The latter are released when the sporangia rupture. Sporangia develop in tissue from small, globose spores. Typical sporangia are seen in stained sections of biopsy specimens.

The disease is treated by surgical excision of polyps. Recurrence is not uncommon.

GLOSSARY

calcofluor white Nonspecific fluorochrome that binds to the cellulose of fungal cell walls. Depending on the ultraviolet filters used, the fungi fluoresce blue-white or green.

periodic acid-Schiff stain Stain used to detect fungi, particularly yeasts and hyphae, in clinical specimens. After the several steps required, the cell wall carbohydrates appear a bright pink-magenta.

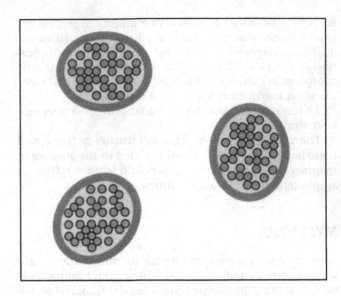

FIGURE 38.2   Sporangia of *Rhinosporidium seeberi*. These are large, ovoid, thick-walled sporangia containing thousands of endospores.

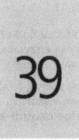

39 Respiratory and Systemic Mycoses

ZYGOMYCOSIS

Zygomycosis is a disease of animals and humans caused by fungi of the order Mucorales, class Zygomycetes. Included are the genera *Mucor*, *Rhizomucor*, *Absidia*, *Rhizopus*, *Mortierella*, *Cunninghamella*, and *Saksenaea*, which occur widely as thermotolerant saprophytes in soil and decaying vegetation.

Pathogenicity

The mode of infection is mainly by inhalation or ingestion. These fungi are opportunistic and are frequently secondary to concurrent infections, metabolic acidosis, or immunosuppression.

They have various disease manifestations caused by a number of species. They may infect lymph nodes of the respiratory and alimentary tracts. Lesions are granulomatous and occasionally ulcerative and caseocalcareous. They are usually localized but, on occasion, may become generalized, with lesions in several organs. Ulceration of stomach and intestines has been attributed to zygomycosis. Focal lesions are seen occasionally on body surfaces.

Lesions in swine are mainly found in mediastinal and submandibular lymph nodes, embolic "tumors" are seen in the liver and lungs, and fungi of this group may be found in gastric ulcers.

Lesions in cattle are found in the bronchial, mesenteric, and mediastinal lymph nodes; there may be nasal and abomasal ulcers. Abortions are attributed to these fungi, and *Mortierella wolfii* in particular is an important cause of bovine abortion (mycotic placentitis), which is sometimes followed by acute pneumonia and death. However, it should be kept in mind that placentas are frequently contaminated by fungi of these genera.

Zygomycosis has also been reported in horses, dogs, cats, sheep, mink, avian species, guinea pigs, wild animals, nonhuman primates, rodents, and humans.

Direct Examination

Fragments and pieces of coarse, nonseptate (pauciseptate), branching hyphae are seen in smears from lesions and biopsies. The coarseness and considerable thickness of fungal elements is especially significant. These infections are frequently detected in stained tissue sections.

Laboratory Diagnosis

Fungi of this group grow rapidly at room temperature on Sabouraud agar. Because they are common contaminants, isolation alone is not necessarily considered significant. Repeated isolation, characteristic lesions, and the presence of fungal elements in sections indicate significance.

All have round sporangia borne on sporangiophores; sporangia contain numerous sporangiospores.

Identification of species may require the aid of a mycologist.

Rhizomucor **species.** These fungi produce a thick, gray mycelium with few if any rhizoids. Sporangiophores are short, with black, spherical sporangia.

Mucor **species.** They have a thick, colorless mycelium without rhizoids. Sporangiophores are simple or branched, and globose sporangia contain small spores (see Fig. 39.1).

Absidia **species.** The sporangiophores do not arise from the stolons opposite the rhizoids as in *Rhizopus*. However, *Absidia* resemble *Rhizopus* species grossly (Fig. 39.1).

Rhizopus **species.** They have dense, cottony, aerial mycelium that are first white and then turn grey. Sporangiophores arise from the stolons where the stolons contact the medium through rhizoids (see Fig. 39.1).

Mortierella **species.** *Mortierella wolfii* grows on blood agar and Sabouraud agar at 25°–27°C and 37°C. The colonies on Sabouraud and blood agars are white, velvety, dense, and characteristically lobulated. The hyphae are hyaline, and sporangia are produced on special media. Definitive identification is based on the morphology of the sporangia and spores.

Treatment

Amphotericin B is the preferred drug. Surgical measures may be indicated.

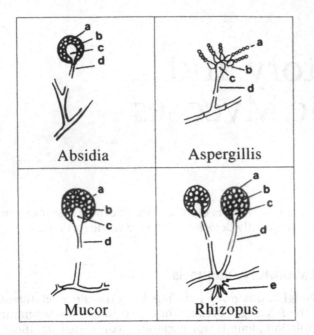

FIGURE 39.1   *Absidia*: (a) sporangium, (b) sporangiospores, (c) columnella, (d) sporangiophore. *Aspergillis*: (a) conidia, (b) sterigmata, (c) vesicle, (d) conidiospore. *Mucor*: same basic structure as *Absidia*. *Rhizopus*: (a) sporangium, (b) sporangiospores, (c) columnella, (d) sporangiophore, (e) rhizoids.

ENTOMOPHTHOROMYCOSIS

This disease, mainly of horses, caused by ubiquitous saprophytic fungi in the genera *Basidiobolus* and *Conidiobolus*. *Conidiobolus coronatus* cause ulcerative granulomas of the lips and oral and nasal mucous membranes, involving subcutaneous tissues. Lesions caused by *Basidiobolus ranarum* may be large and involve the skin of the head, neck, and chest. They are circular, usually single, ulcerative, and nodular. There may be fistulous tracts with extension to lymph nodes.

Unlike the Mucorales, these fungi produce colonies that are flat and waxy, which later become fuzzy and white. The hyphae are septate, and the characteristic conidia and sporangia are used in identification. Species identification is usually made by a mycologist.

Surgical excision and treatment with amphotericin B (locally or systemically) or ketoconazole have been effective.

ASPERGILLOSIS

Aspergillosis is mainly caused by *Aspergillus fumigatus*, which occurs widely in nature and is a common laboratory contaminant. Other species are infrequent causes of the disease.

Pathogenicity

At present, the mechanisms of pathogenicity are not known. However, it is thought that toxic components may be, in part, associated with formation of hemorrhagic lesions. In addition, the activity of enzymes, such as elastase, may be associated with tissue damage.

CATTLE.   Infections involve the uterus, fetal membranes, and fetal skin and, on occasion, result in abortion. Aspergilli occasionally cause bovine mastitis and ocular infections and diarrhea in calves.

HORSES.   Infection causes abortion, keratomycosis, occasionally pulmonary aspergillosis, and guttural pouch aspergillosis, an important mycosis seen mainly in stabled horses. It involves fungus invasion of the roof of the medial compartment of the guttural pouch. The two most important clinical signs, in addition to the nasal discharge, are epistaxis, caused by fungal erosion of the wall of the internal carotid artery, and dysphagia, caused by neuritis of the laryngeal and pharyngeal nerves.

DOGS.   Nasal aspergillosis is an important chronic disease of dogs (rarely in cats and horses) and is usually caused by the colonization of *A. fumigatus* in the nasal cavity and paranasal sinuses. The disease is characterized clinically by a persistent unilateral or bilateral nasal discharge, sometimes bloody or purulent (secondary bacteria), sneezing, open-mouth breathing, and such less commonly seen signs as facial and palatal swelling, loss of appetite, and depression. Ordinarily, the disease does not become systemic, although if untreated it results in an intractable process with extensive local tissue damage. Disseminated aspergillosis with multiple granulomas and infarcts has been reported in dogs.

OTHER ANIMALS.   Infrequent infections occur, most often involving the lungs. Pulmonary and intestinal aspergillosis occurs infrequently in cats.

AVIAN SPECIES.   Several manifestations of aspergillosis are seen in chickens, turkeys, and other wild and domestic avian species including penguins in captivity: (1) a diffuse infection of the air sacs, (2) a diffuse pneumonic form, and (3) a nodular form involving the lungs.

The disease is called "brooder pneumonia" in chicks and poults; many birds may be affected. The spores are acquired by inhalation from the fungi growing on feed or litter. The principal gross lesion consists of yellow nodules found in the lungs and air sacs.

HUMANS.   Primary and secondary infections occur in a wide variety of tissues and locations: lungs, skin, nasal sinuses, external ear, bronchi, bones, and meninges. Infections occur most frequently in immunocompromised patients.

Laboratory Diagnosis

Specimens will depend on the character and location of the lesion. Material scraped or curetted is examined for fungal elements in 10% NaOH and is also cultured. Short pieces of thick, septate hyphae are characteristic of aspergillosis. The typical conidial heads are seen only in the lungs and air sacs, where there is access to oxygen. Biopsies and tissues are cultured and saved for histopathological examination. Aspergilli grow rapidly on blood and Sabouraud agar at room and incubator temperatures. Colonies are white at first but later turn green to dark-green, flat, and velvety. Colony color varies with different species.

The genus is identified by the presence of the conidiophores, with large terminal vesicles bearing sterigmata from which chains of spores or conidia are produced (see Fig. 39.1). The vesicle of *A. fumigatus* is flask-shaped. Identification of species is based on colony and microscopic morphology.

Because *Aspergillus* spp. occur widely as contaminants, repeated isolation or histological evidence may be required for diagnosis.

An agar gel immunodiffusion test has been of value in the diagnosis of nasal aspergillosis in dogs.

Treatment

Surgery and local and systemic drug treatment are used in nasal aspergillosis and guttural pouch mycosis. The regimens used are often complex, and the results have been variable. Ketonazole, other imidazole drugs, thiabendazole, and oral potassium iodide (guttural pouch mycosis) have been used with varying success.

Avian aspergillosis is not usually treated.

PAECILOMYCOSIS

This is an infrequent, systemic mycosis, caused by *Paecilomyces lilacinus* and *Paecilomyces variotii*, which usually begins as a pulmonary infection. The fungi are widely distributed in soil and decaying organic material.

Although generally considered nonpathogenic, these fungi have the capacity to produce infections in animals, including the horse, dog, and cat, that are immunocompromised, debilitated, or subject to prolonged administration of antibiotics. Occurrence in captive amphibians and reptiles has been reported. Lesions consisting of multiple gray-white nodules occur in the lungs and other tissues and organs.

Laboratory Diagnosis

A strongly presumptive diagnosis is made on the basis of demonstrating the characteristic elements in wet mounts and sections from lesions. These elements consist of septate pseudohyphae, oval conidia, and thin-walled spores.

Definitive diagnosis is based on the demonstration of the characteristic fungal elements and the isolation and identification of the fungi. *Paecilomyces* spp. grow better at 25°C than at 37°C.

Treatment

There is little information on treatment. Ketaconazole and other azole antifungal drugs may be effective, although the economics of extended treatment in the horse may be a limiting consideration.

PNEUMOCYSTIS PNEUMONIA

Pneumocystis carinii is the causative agent of diffuse pneumonia, typically observed in immunocompromised individuals. This form of pneumonia is rarely observed in healthy individuals. The organism has been observed in the lungs of a variety of animals, including rats, rabbits, mice, ferrets, guinea pigs, dogs, sheep, goats, horses, chimpanzees, and monkeys.

The habitat is exclusively the pulmonary alveoli. Organisms develop and multiply extracellularly. Experimental studies have shown that the organism can be transmitted by inhalation.

Pneumocystis carinii, a fungus (although its current taxonomic location is highly debated), has been observed in three forms associated with the organism's life cycle. These forms include a thick-walled cyst, a sporozoite, and a thin-walled trophozoite.

A great deal about the mode of replication of this organism and its transition to the various stages is not currently known. However, the cyst is a spherical to ovoid structure (4–6 μm in diameter) that contains up to eight pleomorphic sporozoites. Sporozoites are eventually released from the cyst via breaks in the cyst wall and are then termed trophozoites. Trophozoites do not enter the host cell directly but, rather, attach to the surface of the cell during a phase in the life cycle. The mechanism by which the trophozoites transition back into cysts is not known.

Strains differ antigenically and are host specific. Animal strains are therefore an unlikely source of human infections.

Pathogenicity

The mode of infection is mainly by inhalation of aerosol organisms.

Normal, healthy animals carry the organism in their lungs with impunity. Disease is associated with immunosuppression resulting from treatment, concurrent infections (e.g., HIV infection), and various defects of the immune system. Although the incubation period is not known in humans and animals, the disease usually begins 1–2 months after the onset of immunosuppression.

Organisms attach to **type 1 pneumocytes**, and as infection progresses, there is interstitial edema with infiltration of neutrophils and lymphocytes. As lungs become infiltrated in the severe disease, there is respiratory distress and often a fatal outcome in the absence of effective treatment.

Necropsy reveals heavy, airless, infiltrated lungs, thickened alveolar septa, and foamy material containing *P. carinii* in the alveoli.

There is a dearth of information on the disease in animals. Most cases have been in foals with immune deficiency, dogs, and pigs. It has been reported in mice and rats receiving immunosuppressive agents.

Immune Response

Pneumocystis carinii pneumonitis is often observed in hosts with compromised cell-mediated immunity. Both

IgM and IgG antibodies are observed in response to infection, but the presence of antibody does not protect against the disease. However, the presence of specific antibody stimulates alveolar macrophages to actively engulf and digest the parasite.

Although it is a major infection in acquired immune deficiency syndrome patients, other conditions, such as severe protein–calorie malnutrition, may exacerbate the disease. Furthermore, treatment with immunosuppressive drugs can cause an individual to become susceptible.

Laboratory Diagnosis

Diagnosis is based on demonstration of cysts of the organism in material from lungs, including sputum (humans), bronchial brushings, lung aspirates, tracheobronchial mucus, and transtracheal needle biopsies. Giemsa, methenamine silver, and indirect immunoflorescent antibody stains are used to demonstrate the characteristic morphological forms of the organism.

The organism has only been cultivated in cell cultures.

Treatment

There is little information on the treatment of the disease in animals. The following agents have been of value in the human disease: trimethoprim-sulfonamide, a combination of the antimalarial drug primaquine and clindamycin, and the antiprotozoal drug atovaquone.

BLASTOMYCOSIS

The causative agent, *Blastomyces dermatitidis*, occurs in moist soil, particularly in wooded areas. In the United States, the disease is most common in the north-central and southeastern states; although referred to as North American blastomycosis, the disease is worldwide in distribution.

Pathogenicity

The mode of infection is usually via the respiratory tract, and the initial lesions are found in the lung. Infection via wounds is rare. The disease is characterized by the formation of granulomatous nodules and occurs principally in dogs and humans. It has also been reported in the horse, cat, dolphin, ferret, and sealion, but it is uncommon in these animals. In dogs, the lesions are usually found in the lungs and on the skin. Skin lesions and generalized blastomycosis result from hematogenous dissemination from the original pulmonary lesions. The fungus can usually be demonstrated and recovered from all lesions including those involving bone, eyes, brain, and genitalia. Unless treated, the disseminated disease terminates fatally. The skin lesions, which are circumscribed and granulomatous, may ulcerate.

Laboratory Diagnosis

The large, spherical, thick-walled cells (5–20 μm in diameter) are readily demonstrable in wet mounts. A single bud connected to the larger mother cell by a wide base is frequently seen. Some cells give a double contoured effect.

The organism grows slowly at 25° and 37°C on Sabouraud agar and blood agar, respectively. On Sabouraud agar at 25°C, a moist, greyish, yeastlike colony is seen that develops a white cottony mycelium. As it ages, it becomes tan to dark brown to black. The septate hyphae bear small, oval, or pyriform conidia laterally, close to the point of septation. Older cultures form chlamydospores with thickened walls (see Fig. 39.2).

On blood agar at 37°C, creamy, waxy, wrinkled colonies, cream to tan in color, are observed. Thick-walled budding yeast cells similar to those in tissue sections and exudate are seen (see Fig. 39.2).

The sexual or teleomorphic form has been described and is named *Ajellomyces dermatitidis*. The complement fixation test can be of value; rising titers are significant. A positive immunodiffusion test indicates recent or current infection. Falling antibody titers during the course of the disease indicates a poor prognosis. An enzyme-linked immunosorbent assay and counterimmunoelectrophoresis using a commercially available antigen have been effective in diagnosis.

Treatment

Primary focal cutaneous lesions, which are infrequent, should be removed surgically. Amphotericin B is preferred for severe cases. The disseminated disease usually responds poorly to treatment. Ketaconazole has been used effectively in human beings and dogs.

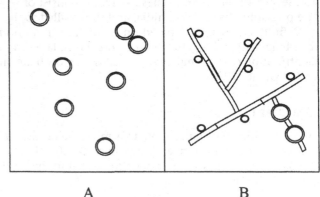

FIGURE 39.2   Dimorphism of *Blastomyces dermatitidis*. **(A)** Yeast cells (thick walled); growth in tissues at 37°C. **(B)** Hyphae, microconidia and chlamydospores; growth on Sabouraud agar at 25°C.

A   B

Public Health Significance

Although one should avoid contact with infectious material, transmission from infected animals to humans is extremely rare.

HISTOPLASMOSIS

Histoplasmosis is caused by *Histoplasma capsulatum*, a dimorphic fungus that is found in soil and decaying vegetation. A heavy concentration has been encountered in soils containing the feces of bats and birds, such as starlings and pigeons. Infection is exogenous, usually by inhalation, less frequently by ingestion. Apparently, soils with avian and bat feces—those with a high nitrogen content—provide a favorable milieu for multiplication. It only occurs passively in the intestines of live birds.

There are many subclinical, transient infections.

Pathogenicity

Clinical histoplasmosis is a generalized disease involving the reticuloendothelial system. The mode of infection is usually via inhalation, with primary infection of the respiratory tract. Infection via wounds or ingestion is rare. Infections have been reported from dogs, cattle, nonhuman primates, cats, horses, sheep, swine, humans, and various wild animals.

Some of the lesions seen in dogs and cats are ulcerations of the intestinal tract. There may be enlargement and swelling of the liver, spleen, and lymph nodes caused by tubercle-like lesions. Acute and chronic forms are seen. Although the clinical disease is generalized, it usually assumes either a predominantly pulmonary or an intestinal form in animals. Osteomyelitis in cats, caused by *H. capsulatum*, has been reported.

Direct Examination

Because *H. capsulatum* is small and rarely found extracellularly, it is extremely difficult to demonstrate in clinical materials. Smears are made from scrapings of ulcers, from cut surfaces of lymph nodes, from biopsies, and from material from sternal puncture and buffy coat. They are stained by the Giemsa or Wright method and examined under oil immersion objective. The organisms occur intracellularly (mononuclear cells) as small, round or oval, yeastlike, single, or budding cells. A clear halo is seen around the darker-staining central material. The characteristic small yeast cells can be seen in the cytoplasm of macrophages in stained sections of affected tissues. Fluorescent antibody staining has been used to identify the organism in cultures and clinical specimens.

Laboratory Diagnosis

On Sabouraud agar at 25°C, colonies are cottony-white to cream at first, later becoming tan to brown. Two kinds of spores are borne on the septate hyphae: small, smooth, round to pyriform microconidia, either on short lateral branches or attached directly by the base; and small and large macroconidia or chlamydospores (7–18 μm in diameter) that are round and thick-walled and may be covered with knoblike projections (tuberculate chlamydospores; see Fig. 39.3).

On blood agar at 37°C, colonies are small, white, and yeastlike and yield yeastlike cells (see Fig. 39.3).

The organism can be recovered from contaminated specimens by mouse inoculation.

The complement fixation test is useful; rising titers are significant; titers disappear after about 9 months. The immunodiffusion test and counterimmunoelectrophoresis are useful. The skin test is of little value in diagnosis, as it may only indicate exposure.

Treatment

Amphotericin B is the preferred drug. The azoles, miconazole, ketoconazole, and itraconazole are also of value. The prognosis in acute and disseminated histoplasmosis is poor.

COCCIDIOIDOMYCOSIS

The cause of coccidioidomycosis is *Coccidioides immitis*, a fungus that occurs widely in the soil of certain arid areas of

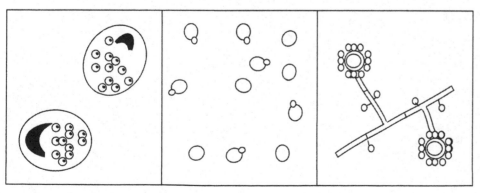

FIGURE 39.3 Dimorphic growth of *Histoplasma capsulatum*. **(A)** Small, intracellular yeast cells with dark central areas; growth in tissues at 37°C. **(B)** Yeast cells; growth on blood agar at 37°C. **(C)** Tuberculate chlamydospores; growth on Sabouraud agar at 25°C.

A   B   C

the southwestern United States and South America. Its occurrence is infrequent outside the Americas. There are many subclinical, transient infections in animals and humans.

Pathogenicity

The mode of infection is by inhalation.

The disease is characterized by the formation of nodules or granulomas that are usually minimal and localized. It has been encountered in cattle, sheep, dogs, cats, horses, swine, nonhuman primates, various wild animals, and humans. The gross lesions in cattle resemble tuberculosis and are usually seen in the bronchial and mediastinal lymph nodes and, less frequently, in the lungs. Lesions have been found in the lungs, brain, liver, spleen, bones, and kidneys of dogs. Disseminated, progressive disease occurs most frequently in immunocompromised dogs and humans. Abortion and infrequent disseminated infections have been reported in horses.

Direct Examination

In unstained wet mounts, the organisms are seen as nonbudding, thick-walled sporangia having diameters varying from 10 to 80 μm. These large sporangia or spherules contain numerous endospores 2–5 μm in diameter. The large sporangia burst, releasing the endospores and leaving "ghost" spherules.

Laboratory Diagnosis

Caution: *Coccidioides immitis* is highly infectious. It grows readily in 1–2 weeks at 25° and 37°C on Sabouraud and blood agars, respectively. Colonies are flat, moist, and membranous at both temperatures, later developing a coarse, cottony, aerial mycelium, the color of which varies from white to brown. The tissue phase is not seen on artificial media unless a special spherule medium is used with incubation at 40°C. The yeast form can be obtained by inoculating cultures into mice (see Fig. 39.4).

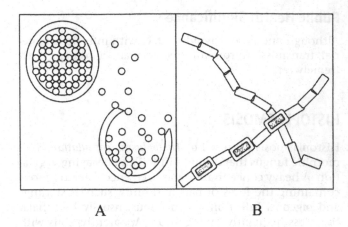

FIGURE 39.4 Dimorphism of *Coccidioides immitis*. **(A)** Intra- and extracellular spherules containing round endospores; growth in tissues at 37°C. **(B)** Hyphae, arthrospores with collarettes; growth on blood agar at 37°C and Sabouraud agar at 25°C.

When stained by lactose phenol cotton blue, the culture shows branching septate mycelia that form chains of thick-walled, barrel-shaped arthrospores (2–3 μm long) separated by clear spaces, the remnants of empty cells.

The complement fixation test is useful; rising titers are significant. Other serologic procedures that have been useful are immunodiffusion, the tube precipitin test, and the latex agglutination test. A positive skin test indicates exposure.

Treatment

Amphotericin B is the preferred drug. The imidazole compounds including ketoconazole and fluconazole have been effective.

GLOSSARY

type 1 pneumocytes Those cells lining the alveolar sacs associated with gas exchange.

Cumulative Glossary

acidosis A condition of decreased alkalinity of tissue and blood that is accompanied by various signs including vomiting and general malaise.

adjuvant A substance that increases the potency (immunogenicity) of an antigen or immunogen.

ADP ribosylation Addition of ribose to the ADP molecule.

anergy Failure to react immunologically to the injection of an allergen or antigen.

anoxygenic Does not form oxygen as a product of photosynthesis.

antigen Molecule or substance that is recognized by an animal as foreign (nonself) and that elicits an immune or specific antibody response.

apoptosis Programmed cell death; that is, a regulated set of events that result in cell death.

asaccharolytic Does not break down sugars metabolically.

assimilation tests These tests use broth media to detect carbohydrate use in the presence of oxygen.

atelectasis Collapse of the lung.

autogenous bacterin Bacterin prepared from bacteria isolated from an infected animal or animals in a herd, flock, and so forth.

auxotrophy Refers to those organisms that are unable to synthesize certain nutrients (growth factors) that need to be provided to obtain growth. These include amino acids, nicotinamide adenine dinucleotide, biotin, and so forth.

bacillary angiomatosis Disorder characterized by proliferation of neovascular tissues (angiomas). The lesions may be single or many and involve many organs. They are red (cranberry-like) initially, then enlarge to several centimeters in diameter and may ulcerate.

bacteremia Presence of viable bacteria in the blood.

bacterial sepsis Presence of bacteria and their toxins in the blood or tissues.

bacterin Killed suspension of bacteria.

bacteriocins Agents produced by some bacteria that kill or inhibit the growth of closely related bacteria.

bacteriophage Virus capable of infecting bacterial cells.

Biosafety Level The Centers for Disease Control and Prevention has classified etiological agents on the basis of their human hazard. The levels of hazard are 1 through 4. Level 1 agents are the least infectious, and Level 4 (some viruses) are the most infectious. The safety measures to be employed for each level have been described.

blepharospasm Involuntary spasmodic winking caused by contraction of the orbital muscle of the eyelids.

bradykinin Composed of a chain of nine amino acid residues that is formed in injured tissues and acts in the inflammatory process by dilating small vessels.

brucellosis ring test Test for agglutinins in the milk. A stained *B. abortus* antigen is added to several milliliters of milk. If agglutinins are present, they combine with the antigen and rise to the top of the milk sample, producing a discernable ring.

calcofluor white Nonspecific fluorochrome that binds to the cellulose of fungal cell walls. Depending on the ultraviolet filters used, the fungi fluoresce blue-white or green.

capsid The protein coat that surrounds the nucleic acid core of a virus particle.

carboxyphilic Growth requires CO_2.

carbuncle Local purulent, necrotic, inflammatory process involving the skin and deeper tissues with multiple openings from which pus is discharged.

catecholamines Substances that act as hormones or neurotransmitters or both.

centriole Structure in the nucleus composed of microtubules and involved in the formation of the spindle apparatus that aids in the parceling out of duplicated chromosomes to daughter cells during cell division.

chiggers Six-legged larvae of harvest mites that suck blood from vertebrates and, thus, cause intense itching.

citrulline ureidase This enzyme, which is also known as citrullinase, converts citrulline + H_2O to ornithine + CO_2 + NH_3 in amino acid metabolism.

coencytic Multinucleate cells, as observed in the mycelium of the Zyogmycota.

commensalism State in which one organism (e.g., a bacterium) lives on another organism (e.g., an animal), obtaining food and other benefits but imposing no damage on the latter.

competent Refers to a cell able to take up DNA from its environment.

Coombs test This is a test that employs an antibody directed against immunoglobulins to agglutinate particles (e.g., erythrocytes) carrying nonagglutinating ("incomplete") antibody on their surface.

Crohn's disease Disease mainly affecting the small intestine (regional ileitis) and characterized by cramps, diarrhea, local abscesses, weight loss, and inappetance. The cause is not known.

crucifers This refers to the crucifer family of plants, including broccoli, Brussels sprouts, cabbage, cauliflower, Chinese cabbage, kale, mustard, radish, rutabaga, and turnip.

cytoskeletal elements Refers to the cytoskeleton or scaffold of eukaryotic cells; for example, microtubules, microfilaments, and intermediate filaments.

cytosol Refers to the fluid portion of the cytoplasm.

dalton Unit of mass used to express masses of atoms, molecules, and nuclear particles. It is equal to one-twelfth of the weight of the carbon 12 atom; it is also called atomic mass unit.

defensins Small, cationic, bactericidal peptides generated by phagocytes, such as neutrophils and macrophages.

Dermatobia hominis This tropical warble fly is an important parasite of cattle in South America. Its larval stages are found in many animals including cattle, sheep, goats, swine, rabbits, dogs, cats, and humans.

desmosome   One of the types of cell junctions by which cells join or communicate with each other. The desmosome of one cell adheres to the desmosome of another. This system of joining cells is designed to resist mechanical separation. Desmosomes are important in the structure of the epithelium, for example.

diphtheroid   Synonym of coryneform (*Corynebacterium*-like). Usually refers to nonpathogenic corynebacteria.

diskospondylitis   Inflammation of the vertebrae and vertebral disk.

diterpene   Terpene containing twice as many atoms in a molecule as a monoterpene. Terpenes are present in essential oils and used as organic solvents.

DNA-gyrase   Enzyme that catalyzes the conversion of double-helical DNA to the superhelix form.

Eh   Symbol for oxidation-reduction potential.

electroporation   Technique for introducing DNA or RNA into a cell, using a pulsed electric field, which creates temporary pores in the cell membrane that allow the DNA or RNA to enter the cell.

endospore   Structure formed within certain gram-positive bacteria, such as *Bacillus anthracis*, that is extremely resistant to heat, drying, and other harmful influences.

endosymbiosis   State whereby an organism that lives in a symbiotic relationship within another organism or cell.

enzootic   Present in a district or region at all times.

epitope   Local chemical configuration on the antigen molecule (antigenic determinant) that elicits specific antibody.

exotoxin   Toxic substance of a microorganism released into the surrounding medium during its growth.

Forssman's antibodies   Antibodies to glycolipid antigens that are found on the tissues cells of many species including the dog, cat, horse, and sheep but not humans, rabbit, rat, pig, or cow.

furuncle   Localized inflammatory process of the skin and subcutis that discharges pus and is caused by an infection.

fusion protein   Protein that is the result of two genes that have been put together via recombinant techniques, transcribed into mRNA and then translated.

"gated porins"   Specific proteins that can act as gates (channels or pores) into the cell for specific substances.

Gb4 receptor   Refers to the globotetraosyl ceramide receptor located on the surface of some eukaryotic cells. The gene encoding this receptor in humans is located on chromosome 4.

gene gun   Technique that involves the coating of small metallic beads with a genetically engineered plasmid. Once coated, the beads are "shot" into living target cells. The apparatus looks very similar to a gun.

habronemiasis   Cutaneous habronemiasis is a granulomatous skin disease of horses caused in part by the larvae of spirurid stomach worms.

halophilic   Halophilic organisms require salt (NaCl) for growth.

hemorrhagic septicemia   Specifically, this is an acute disease of mainly cattle and water buffalo, caused by a variety of the bacterial species *Pasteurella multocida*.

histamine   This compound is a vasodilator and smooth muscle constrictor widely distributed in tissues and in high concentrations in mast cells. It is released when cell-bound IgE (an antibody) reacts with antigen.

horizontal gene transfer   Movement of genetic information from one cell to another (not an offspring).

hypoplasia   A condition in which an organ or tissue does not fully develop or mature.

impetigo   An acute, contagious staphylococcal or streptococcal skin disease characterized by vesicles, pustules, and crusts.

indirect hemagglutination   In this type of hemagglutination, the antigen is adsorbed to the red cells. There is hemagglutination when specific antibody is added.

inspissated   Thickening in consistency of, frequently, pus.

interleukin-1   One of a number of interleukins that mainly function in the regulation of the immune system. They are produced by lymphocytes and monocytes.

intrapalpebral   Within an area near the eyelid.

introns   Portion of a gene that does not encode any part of the final gene and that is removed by the process of splicing.

iridocyclitis   Inflammation of the iris and ciliary body.

IS6110   Insertion sequences, typically associated with transposons.

ischemia   Deficiency of blood in tissue caused by obstruction or functional constriction of a blood vessel.

kerions   Pus-filled inflammatory swellings that may resemble bacterial abscesses.

kilobase (kb)   Measure of the length of a nucleic-acid strand equal to 1000 nucleotides.

LD$_{50}$ Least number of microorganisms or toxic substance required to kill 50% of the test animals.

leukotrienes   Group of metabolites of arachidonic acid that have a number of pharmacological effects. They may be released from mast cells, leukocytes, and platelets.

lipoglycans   Long-chain heteropolysaccharides linked to membrane lipids and embedded in the cytoplasmic membranes of many mycoplasmas.

lysate   Contents that are the result of lysis of a cell.

lysozyme   Enzyme, also known as muramidase, present in many body fluids that breaks down murein, a component of the cell walls of gram-positive bacteria.

lytic (virulent) phage   Bacteriophage that, on entering a target cell, is replicated and results in the lysis and ultimate death of the host cell.

mannose-resistant adhesins   Adhesins capable of binding in the presence of large quantities of mannose, in contrast with those that are unable to bind as mannose blocks their ability to do so.

megabase (Mb)   One million nucleotide bases.

M cells   Also known as microfold cells. M cells are specific cells of the intestinal epithelium near lymphoid follicles that endocytose a variety of protein and peptide antigens. The endocytosed antigens are then directly transported into the underlying tissue, where they are taken up by macrophages. Note that the antigens are not degraded by the M cells, merely transported to the regional macrophages.

Medusa-head   From Greek mythology: One of the Gorgons with snakes for hair.

menadione   Compound having physiological effects similar to vitamin K.

menaquinones   Family of compounds that are structurally similar to vitamin K2.

mesosome   Bacterial structure associated with an invagination of the plasma membrane. It is the site of respiratory enzymes.

metalloprotease   One of several groups of enzymes that degrade proteins but that have a metal ion as a prosthetic group.

MHC   Acronym for major histocompatability complex. These are a group of cell-surface proteins that are involved in the immune discretion of "self" versus "nonself" and that are important in the generation of specific immune responses.

mitogen Any agent that causes a cell to divide.

mordant Chemical (in the gram-stain iodine) that fixes a dye (crystal violet in the gram-stain) by combining with it to form an insoluble compound.

multiplex PCR Polymerase chain reaction designed for the amplification of more than one DNA fragment per reaction.

mutualistic Relationship between different cells (organisms) that is mutually beneficial.

NADH Acronym for nicotinamide adenine dinucleotide, reduced form. NAD is a coenzyme that carries or releases protons and electrons to and from metabolic reactions. The NADH form is NAD with protons and electrons (thus, reduced).

natural killer cell Lymphocyte that recognizes and destroys, in a nonspecific manner, infected host cells and foreign cells.

negative stain Demonstration of the form of bacteria by surrounding them with a substance, for example, india ink, that they do not take up. They appear as unstained bright bodies against a dark or colored background.

nephrosis Noninflammatory disease of the kidneys that mainly affects function of the nephrons.

nucleic acid fingerprinting Refers to PCR-RFLP (polymerase chain reaction–restriction fragment length polymorphism) used by De Voss et al. (1993) for the detection of *P. aeruginosa* species. The method amplifies the *OprI* lipoprotein gene by PCR, which is then digested with different restriction enzymes and separated by gel electrophoresis. This fingerprint is used in the molecular taxonomy of this genus. DNA fingerprinting is discussed at further length in Chapter 23 under *Bacillus anthracis* Genetics. The form of electrophoresis called pulsed field-gel electrophoresis (PFGE) is used in DNA fingerprinting for strain identification in clinical microbiology. PFGE allows the separation of extremely large (several thousand kilobases in length) DNA fragments.

O/F test Test used to determine whether a bacterium uses carbohydrates by oxidation or fermentation.

opportunistic This refers to microorganisms that do not normally cause disease, for example, many bacteria of the normal flora of animals, but that can be pathogenic under certain circumstances such as trauma and impairment of the immune system.

optochin Ethylhydrocuprein that strongly inhibits the growth of *S. pneumoniae* but not certain streptococci whose colonies resemble the pneumococcus.

palisade Arrangement resembling a picket fence.

pasteurization Involves the heating of milk or other liquids to the point that potential pathogens are killed. It has been particularly effective in the prevention of tuberculosis and brucellosis in humans (see Chapter 9 for details).

pathogenic Having the capacity to cause disease in a susceptible host.

peliosis hepatitis Liver disorder characterized by the presence of small, blood-filled cystic lesions containing the bacteria. It is accompanied by weight loss, fever, and abdominal pain.

periodic acid–Schiff stain Stain used to detect fungi, particularly yeasts and hyphae, in clinical specimens. After the several steps required, the cell wall carbohydrates appear a bright pink–magenta.

permease Enzyme that allows the movement of a substance into cells.

phage Synonym of bacteriophage.

pheromone Chemical signal, for example, odor, that is omitted by one animal and that affects the behavior of animals of the same species. Pheromones are used by animals to attract mates.

pili (type IV) These pili or fimbrae are generally classified as glycolipid binding proteins. Many gram-negative bacteria posses type IV pili. As a result, they are grouped based on amino acid similarities of the major pili component. In pseudomonads, type IV pili mediate adhesion to host cells.

pinnipeds Group of aquatic animals including walruses, seals, and similar animals that have finlike flippers for locomotion.

pleomorphic Assuming various forms.

polyserositis Inflammation of the serous membranes; namely, the pleura, peritoneum, and pericardium.

p-pili Refers to periplasmic pili.

primer Short, single-stranded oligonucleotide that anneals to a specific region on a RNA or DNA strand and that is employed by a polymerase as the location to begin synthesis of a complementary nucleotide strand.

prophage DNA of a lysogenic virus that has integrated into the host chromosome.

prostaglandins Number of hormone-like compounds that have a variety of functions as inflammatory mediators.

protoplast Cell from which the cell wall has been removed.

prozone The absence of serological reaction, for example, agglutination, at low dilutions of potent antisera.

pseudomembrane False membrane, sometimes called a diphtheritic membrane, composed mainly of fibrin and necrotic cells on the surface of an inflamed mucous membrane.

psychrophilic A pychrophilic organism is able to grow at low temperatures. Its optimum temperature for growth is less than 15°C.

pulmonary sequestration Loss of connection of lung tissue with the pulmonary veins and the bronchial tree.

purpura hemorrhagica This condition in horses, as a sequella of strangles, is mediated by immune complexes of antibody and streptococcal antigen in vascular basement membranes.

redox potential Oxidation-reduction potential.

restriction endonucleases (restriction enzyme) Bacterial enzymes that cleave DNA at locations defined by a specific sequence of nucleotide bases.

restriction enzymes Bacterial enzymes that recognize and cleave specific DNA sequences.

reverse transcriptase Enzyme made by retroviruses and used to synthesize DNA from a RNA template. The enzyme is used widely in molecular biology to make DNA clones from messenger RNA.

salpingitis Inflammation of a fallopian or eustachian tube.

septicemia Bacteria increasing in numbers in the blood, but also used as a synonym for bacteremia.

serotonin This compound found in platelets and mast cells is a neurotransmitter and causes smooth muscle contraction, increased vascular permeability, and vasoconstriction of larger vessels.

shock In general, a state of circulatory failure associated with reduced total blood volume and low blood pressure. It has various causes including endotoxin.

Shwartzman reaction This reaction follows the second of two doses of lipopolysaccharide. It is characterized by local skin necrosis or generalized disease of kidneys, liver, heart, and lungs.

species incertae sedis Species of uncertain affiliation.

spheroplasts Refers to a gram-negative bacterium that has had the cell wall removed but in which the cell itself is not ruptured.

sporadic (infection or disease) Scattered in occurrence; usually individual cases.

superantigen Antigens (mostly from bacterial toxins) that interact with a particular subset of T cells resulting in activation of large numbers of T cells directly.

suppressor cells Type of T cell thought to "turn off" an immune response.

tape mount In this procedure, a small length of clear Scotch brand tape is applied, adhesive side down, to the fungal colony. Elements of the fungus adhere to the tape, which is applied to a microscope slide, then examined under the microscope.

taxon Refers to any taxonomic group; for example, genus, family, order, and so forth.

temperate phage Lysogenic virus, the DNA of which is integrated into the host chromosome constituting a prophage. As part of the host chromosome, it is replicated with the chromosome and transferred to each daughter cell.

thylakoid membrane Flattened membrane discs in which chlorophyll and other components for photosynthesis are located.

thromboembolic Associated with thromboembolism, which is the blocking of a blood vessel by a fragment or particle that has broken away from a blood-clot at a particular location.

tinea versicolor Human infection of the skin (neck, torso, or limbs) caused by lipophilic yeasts of the *Malassezia furfur* complex.

TSI agar medium Bacteriological medium, triple sugar iron agar, used mainly for preliminary screening of enterobacteria.

transferrin Beta globulin in blood plasma, which can combine with ferric ions and thus transport iron throughout the body.

type 1 pneumocytes Cells lining the alveolar sacs associated with gas exchange.

tyrosine kinase One of a group of enzymes that preferentially phosphorylate the tyrosine residues of particular proteins. Typically observed in cell signaling mechanisms.

ungulate Hoofed mammals, many of which are herbivorous and horned.

uveitis Inflammation of the iris, ciliary body and choroid.

virulence Degree of pathogenicity of a microorganism.

Western blot Performed in three stages: first, the antigen mixture is electrophoresed on a gel; second, it is blotted onto nitrocellulose paper; and third, the blot is exposed to the antibody of interest. The dark band, if present, represents the antigen recognized by the antibody.

wet mounts Suspension of clinical material in saline or other solutions to facilitate microscopic examination.

Index